Genetic Patterns in Neuroimaging

Editor

L. CELSO HYGINO DA CRUZ Jr

NEUROIMAGING CLINICS OF NORTH AMERICA

www.neuroimaging.theclinics.com

Consulting Editor
SURESH K. MUKHERJI

February 2015 • Volume 25 • Number 1

ELSEVIER

1600 John F. Kennedy Boulevard • Suite 1800 • Philadelphia, Pennsylvania, 19103-2899

http://www.neuroimaging.theclinics.com

NEUROIMAGING CLINICS OF NORTH AMERICA Volume 25, Number 1
February 2015 ISSN 1052-5149, ISBN 13: 978-0-323-35445-5

Editor: John Vassallo (j.vassallo@elsevier.com)
Developmental Editor: Donald Mumford

Neuroimaging Clinics of North America (ISSN 1052-5149) is published quarterly by Elsevier Inc., 360 Park Avenue South, New York, NY 10010-1710. Months of issue are February, May, August, and November. Business and editorial offices: 1600 John F. Kennedy Blvd., Suite 1800, Philadelphia, PA 19103-2899. Business and editorial offices: 6277 Sea Harbor Drive, Orlando, FL 32887-4800. Periodicals postage paid at New York, NY, and additional mailing offices. Subscription prices are USD 360 per year for US individuals, USD 514 per year for US institutions, USD 180 per year for US students and residents, USD 415 per year for Canadian individuals, USD 655 per year for Canadian institutions, USD 525 per year for international individuals, USD 655 per year for international institutions and USD 260 per year for Canadian and foreign students and residents. To receive student/resident rate, orders must be accompanied by name of affiliated institution, date of term, and the *signature* of program/residency coordinator on institution letterhead. Orders will be billed at individual rate until proof of status is received. Foreign air speed delivery is included in all *Clinics* subscription prices. All prices are subject to change without notice. POSTMASTER: Send address changes to *Neuroimaging Clinics of North America*, Elsevier Health Sciences Division, Subscription Customer Service, 3251 Riverport Lane, Maryland Heights, MO 63043. Telephone: 1-800-654-2452 (U.S. and Canada); 314-447-8871 (outside U.S. and Canada). Fax: 314-447-8029. E-mail: journalscustomerservice-usa@elsevier.com (for print support); journalsonlinesupport-usa@elsevier.com (for online support).

Reprints. For copies of 100 or more of articles in this publication, please contact the Commercial Reprints Department, Elsevier Inc., 360 Park Avenue South, New York, NY 10010-1710. Tel.: 212-633-3874; Fax: 212-633-3820; E-mail: reprints@elsevier.com.

Neuroimaging Clinics of North America is covered by *Excerpta Medical/EMBASE,* the RSNA Index of Imaging Literature, *MEDLINE/PubMed (Index Medicus),* MEDLINE/MEDLARS, SciSearch, Research Alert, and Neuroscience Citation Index.

PROGRAM OBJECTIVE

The goal of *Neuroimaging Clinics of North America* is to keep practicing radiologists and radiology residents up to date with current clinical practice in radiology by providing timely articles reviewing the state of the art in patient care.

TARGET AUDIENCE

Practicing radiologists, radiology residents, and other healthcare professionals who utilize neuroimaging findings to provide patient care.

LEARNING OBJECTIVES

Upon completion of this activity, participants will be able to:
1. Review genetics in neuropathology and neuroimaging
2. Recognize applications for neuroimaging in brain tumors, multiple sclerosis, cerebrovascular malformations.
3. Discuss brain imaging and genetic risk in the pediatric population.

ACCREDITATION

The Elsevier Office of Continuing Medical Education (EOCME) is accredited by the Accreditation Council for Continuing Medical Education (ACCME) to provide continuing medical education for physicians.

The EOCME designates this enduring material for a maximum of 15 *AMA PRA Category 1 Credit*(s)™. Physicians should claim only the credit commensurate with the extent of their participation in the activity.

All other health care professionals requesting continuing education credit for this enduring material will be issued a certificate of participation.

DISCLOSURE OF CONFLICTS OF INTEREST

The EOCME assesses conflict of interest with its instructors, faculty, planners, and other individuals who are in a position to control the content of CME activities. All relevant conflicts of interest that are identified are thoroughly vetted by EOCME for fair balance, scientific objectivity, and patient care recommendations. EOCME is committed to providing its learners with CME activities that promote improvements or quality in healthcare and not a specific proprietary business or a commercial interest.

The planning committee, staff, authors and editors listed below have identified no financial relationships or relationships to products or devices they or their spouse/life partner have with commercial interest related to the content of this CME activity:

Hortensia Alvarez, MD; Ahmed M. Amer, MD; Patricia Ashton-Prolla, MD, PhD; Carlos Alberto Buchpiguel, MD, PhD; Mauricio Castillo, MD, FACR; Rivka R. Colen, MD; L. Celso Hygino da Cruz, Jr, MD; Mohamed G. ElBanan, MD; Themis Maria Félix, MD, PhD; Roberto Giugliani, MD, PhD; Denise Golgher, PhD; Kristen Helm; Roberta Hespanhol, MD; Brynne Hunter; Margareth Kimura, MD; Sandy Lavery; José Leite, MD, MBA, MSc; Maria Gabriela Longo, MD; Jill McNair; Suresh K. Mukherji, MD, MBA, FACR; Whitney B. Pope, MD, PhD; Ilana Zalcberg Renault, MD, PhD; Stefan D. Roosendaal, MD, PhD; Carolina Fischinger Souza, MD; Karthikeyan Subramaniam; Filippo Vairo, MD, MSc; Marina Lipkin Vasquez, MSc, PhD; John Vassallo; Leonardo Modesti Vedolin, MD, PhD; Pascal O. Zinn, MD, PhD.

The planning committee, staff, authors and editors listed below have identified financial relationships or relationships to products or devices they or their spouse/life partner have with commercial interest related to the content of this CME activity:

Frederik Barkhof, MD, PhD, is a consultant/advisor for Bayer Schering Pharma AG, Biogen Idec, Inc., Genzyme Corporation, Janssen Research & Development, Merck Serono, Novartis Pharmaceuticals Corporation and Roche; has a research grant from Dutch MS Society, EU-FP7; and is on speakers bureau for MedScape.

UNAPPROVED/OFF-LABEL USE DISCLOSURE

The EOCME requires CME faculty to disclose to the participants:
1. When products or procedures being discussed are off-label, unlabelled, experimental, and/or investigational (not US Food and Drug Administration [FDA] approved); and
2. Any limitations on the information presented, such as data that are preliminary or that represent ongoing research, interim analyses, and/or unsupported opinions. Faculty may discuss information about pharmaceutical agents that is outside of FDA-approved labelling. This information is intended solely for CME and is not intended to promote off-label use of these medications. If you have any questions, contact the medical affairs department of the manufacturer for the most recent prescribing information.

TO ENROLL

To enroll in the *Neuroimaging Clinics of North America* Continuing Medical Education program, call customer service at 1-800-654-2452 or sign up online at http://www.theclinics.com/home/cme. The CME program is available to subscribers for an additional annual fee of USD 235.

METHOD OF PARTICIPATION

In order to claim credit, participants must complete the following:

1. Complete enrolment as indicated above.
2. Read the activity.
3. Complete the CME Test and Evaluation. Participants must achieve a score of 70% on the test. All CME Tests and Evaluations must be completed online.

CME INQUIRIES/SPECIAL NEEDS

For all CME inquiries or special needs, please contact elsevierCME@elsevier.com.

NEUROIMAGING CLINICS OF NORTH AMERICA

FORTHCOMING ISSUES

May 2015
Spinal Infections
E. Turgut Tali, *Editor*

August 2015
Orbit and Neuro-ophthalmic Imaging
Juan E. Gutierrez and Bundhit Tantiwongkosi,
Editors

November 2015
Imaging of Paranasal Sinuses
Varsha Joshi, *Editor*

RECENT ISSUES

November 2014
Clinical Applications of Functional MRI
Jay J. Pillai, *Editor*

August 2014
Craniofacial Trauma
Deborah R. Shatzkes, *Editor*

May 2014
Imaging of the Postoperative Spine
A. Orlando Ortiz, *Editor*

Contributors

CONSULTING EDITOR

SURESH K. MUKHERJI, MD, MBA, FACR
Professor and Chairman, W.F. Patenge
Endowed Chair, Department of Radiology,
Michigan State University, East Lansing,
Michigan

EDITOR

L. CELSO HYGINO DA CRUZ Jr, MD
Radiologist, Clínica de Diagnóstico Por
Imagem (CDPI) and IRM, Department of
Radiology, Federal University of Rio de
Janeiro, Rio de Janeiro, Brazil

AUTHORS

HORTENSIA ALVAREZ, MD
Professor of Radiology, Interventional
Neuroradiology, University of North Carolina at
Chapel Hill, Chapel Hill, North Carolina

AHMED M. AMER, MD
Research Fellow, Department of Diagnostic
Radiology, MD Anderson Cancer Center,
University of Texas, Houston, Texas

PATRICIA ASHTON-PROLLA, MD, PhD
Medical Genetics Service, Hospital de
Clínicas de Porto Alegre; Post Graduation
Program on Genetics and Molecular Biology,
Department of Genetics, Universidade
Federal do Rio Grande do Sul, Porto Alegre,
Rio Grande do Sul, Brazil

FREDERIK BARKHOF, MD, PhD
Department of Radiology & Nuclear Medicine,
Neuroscience Campus Amsterdam,
VU University Medical Center, Amsterdam,
The Netherlands

CARLOS ALBERTO BUCHPIGUEL, MD, PhD
Professor and Director, Department of Nuclear
Medicine and Molecular Imaging, São Paulo
University (USP), São Paulo, Brazil

MAURICIO CASTILLO, MD, FACR
Professor of Radiology; Chief of
Neuroradiology, University of North Carolina
at Chapel Hill, Chapel Hill, North Carolina

RIVKA R. COLEN, MD
Assistant Professor, Department of Diagnostic
Radiology, MD Anderson Cancer Center,
University of Texas, Houston, Texas

MOHAMED G. ELBANAN, MD
Research Fellow, Department of Diagnostic
Radiology, MD Anderson Cancer Center,
University of Texas, Houston, Texas

THEMIS MARIA FÉLIX, MD, PhD
Medical Genetics Service, Hospital de
Clínicas de Porto Alegre, Porto Alegre,
Rio Grande do Sul, Brazil

ROBERTO GIUGLIANI, MD, PhD
Medical Genetics Service, Hospital de
Clínicas de Porto Alegre; Department of
Genetics, Universidade Federal do Rio
Grande do Sul, Porto Alegre, Rio Grande do
Sul, Brazil

DENISE GOLGHER, PhD
Symbiosis-Biotechnology Consultancy,
Rio de Janeiro, Brazil

ROBERTA HESPANHOL, MD
Consultant, PET/CT, Clínica de Diagnóstico
Por Imagem (CDPI), Rio de Janeiro, Brazil

L. CELSO HYGINO DA CRUZ Jr, MD
Radiologist, Clínica de Diagnóstico Por
Imagem (CDPI) and IRM, Department of
Radiology, Federal University of Rio de
Janeiro, Rio de Janeiro, Brazil

MARGARETH KIMURA, MD
Radiologist, MRI Department of Clínica de
Diagnóstico Por Imagem (CDPI), Rio de
Janeiro, Brazil

JOSÉ LEITE, MD, MBA, MSc
Chief, PET/CT, Clínica de Diagnóstico Por
Imagem (CDPI), Rio de Janeiro, Brazil

MARIA GABRIELA LONGO, MD
Radiology Service, Hospital de Clínicas de Porto
Alegre; Post Graduation Program on Medical
Sciences, Medicine, Department of Internal
Medicine, Universidade Federal do Rio
Grande do Sul, Porto Alegre, Rio Grande do
Sul, Brazil

WHITNEY B. POPE, MD, PhD
Department of Radiological Sciences, David
Geffen School of Medicine at UCLA,
Los Angeles, California

ILANA ZALCBERG RENAULT, MD, PhD
Researcher at INCA; Consultant in
Molecular Genetics at DASA, Rio de
Janeiro, Brazil

STEFAN DIRK ROOSENDAAL, MD, PhD
Department of Radiology & Nuclear
Medicine, Neuroscience Campus
Amsterdam, VU University Medical Center,
Amsterdam, The Netherlands

CAROLINA FISCHINGER SOUZA, MD
Medical Genetics Service, Hospital de
Clínicas de Porto Alegre, Porto Alegre,
Rio Grande do Sul, Brazil

FILIPPO VAIRO, MD, MSc
Medical Genetics Service, Hospital de
Clínicas de Porto Alegre; Post Graduation
Program on Genetics and Molecular
Biology, Universidade Federal do Rio
Grande do Sul, Porto Alegre, Rio Grande do
Sul, Brazil

MARINA LIPKIN VASQUEZ, MSc, PhD
Researcher Staff, Molecular Biology
Laboratory; Manager of Tumor Bank,
Instituto Estadual do Cérebro Paulo
Niemeyer (IECPN), Rio de Janeiro, Brazil

LEONARDO MODESTI VEDOLIN, MD, PhD
Radiology Service, Hospital de Clínicas de
Porto Alegre and Hospital Moinhos de Vento;
Post Graduation Program on Medical
Sciences, Medicine, Department of Internal
Medicine, Universidade Federal do
Rio Grande do Sul, Porto Alegre,
Rio Grande do Sul, Brazil

PASCAL O. ZINN, MD, PhD
Neurosurgery Resident, Department of
Neurosurgery, Baylor College of Medicine,
Houston, Texas

Contents

Foreword   xiii

Suresh K. Mukherji

Preface: Genetic Patterns in Neuroimaging   xv

L. Celso Hygino da Cruz Jr

Understanding Genetics in Neuroimaging   1

Marina Lipkin Vasquez and Ilana Zalcberg Renault

Gene expression is a process of DNA sequence reading into protein synthesis. In cases of problems in DNA repair/apoptosis mechanisms, cells accumulate genomic abnormalities and pass them through generations of cells. The accumulation of mutations causes diseases and even tumors. In addition to cancer, many other neurologic conditions have been associated with genetic mutations. Some trials are testing patients with epigenetic treatments. Epigenetic therapy must be used with caution because epigenetic processes and changes happen constantly in normal cells, giving rise to drug off-target effects. Scientists are making progress in specifically targeting abnormal cells with minimal damage to normal ones.

Molecular Imaging in Genetics   17

José Leite, Roberta Hespanhol, and Carlos Alberto Buchpiguel

Neuroimaging is a potentially valuable tool to link individual differences in the human genome to structure and functional variations, narrowing the gaps in the casual chain from a given genetic variation to a brain disorder. Because genes are not usually expressed at the level of mental behavior, but are mediated by their molecular and cellular effects, molecular imaging could play a key role. This article reviews the literature using molecular imaging as an intermediate phenotype and/or biomarker for illness related to certain genetic alterations, focusing on the most common neuro-degenerative disorders, Alzheimer's disease (AD) and Parkinson disease.

Brain Imaging and Genetic Risk in the Pediatric Population, Part 1: Inherited Metabolic Diseases   31

Maria Gabriela Longo, Filippo Vairo, Carolina Fischinger Souza, Roberto Giugliani, and Leonardo Modesti Vedolin

In this article, the genotype-MR phenotype correlation of the most common or clinically important inherited metabolic diseases (IMD) in the pediatric population is reviewed. A nonsystematic search of the PubMed/Medline database of relevant studies about "genotype-phenotype correlation" in IMD was performed. Some MR phenotypes related to specific gene mutations were found, such as bilateral hyper-trophy of inferior olives in patients harboring POLG and SURF1 mutations, and central lesions in the cervical spinal cord in patients with nonketotic hyperglycinemia harboring GLRX5 gene mutation.

Brain Imaging and Genetic Risk in the Pediatric Population, Part 2: Congenital Malformations of the Central Nervous System   53

Maria Gabriela Longo, Themis Maria Félix, Patricia Ashton-Prolla, and Leonardo Modesti Vedolin

In this article, an update is presented of the correlation of imaging and genetic findings in congenital malformations of the central nervous system (CMCNS).

A nonsystematic search of the PubMed/Medline database was performed. The congenital disorders were classified in 3 groups of malformation: ventral induction disorders, cortical malformations, and congenital malformations of the posterior fossa. The highlights of genotype-imaging phenotype correlation of some congenital malformations are provided. It is hoped that developments in genotype-MR phenotype in CMCNS will foster further prognostic and pathogenic breakthroughs for the frequently associated neurologic dysfunction in children affected by these common diseases.

Genetic Markers and Their Influence on Cerebrovascular Malformations   69

Hortensia Alvarez and Mauricio Castillo

Cerebrospinal vascular malformations are a group of anomalies affecting the arterial wall, the capillary arteriovenous interface, or the venous and lymphatic structures. Heritability and family studies allow identification of mutations in single genes associated with rare familial conditions causing cerebral or spinal vascular malformations, as is the case in hemorrhagic hereditary telangiectasia diseases. This article reviews the genetic and epigenetic influences increasingly reported in recent years as causal factors or triggers involved in the formation and growth of cerebromedullary vascular malformations.

Imaging Phenotypes in Multiple Sclerosis   83

Stefan Dirk Roosendaal and Frederik Barkhof

Multiple sclerosis (MS) is a common disease of the central nervous system, with various clinical symptoms and a heterogeneous disease course. MRI can depict focal and diffuse manifestations of the disease, and accurately measure progression over time. The precise pathogenesis of MS is unknown. Nevertheless, genetic influences have been found for susceptibility to MS in linkage and association studies. More recent genome-wide association studies have revealed other genes to be related to disease susceptibility and severity, explaining part of the variability in symptoms, radiological manifestations and disease course. Studies relating genetics and imaging in MS are discussed in this paper.

Molecular Genetics of Glioblastomas: Defining Subtypes and Understanding the Biology   97

Ilana Zalcberg Renault and Denise Golgher

Despite comprehensive therapy, which includes surgery, radiotherapy, and chemotherapy, the prognosis of glioblastoma multiforme is very poor. Diagnosed individuals present an average of 12 to 18 months of life. This article provides an overview of the molecular genetics of these tumors. Despite the overwhelming amount of data available, so far little has been translated into real benefits for the patient. Because this is such a complex topic, the goal is to point out the main alterations in the biological pathways that lead to tumor formation, and how this can contribute to the development of better therapies and clinical care.

Genomics of Brain Tumor Imaging   105

Whitney B. Pope

Imaging genomics combines imaging-defined phenotypes with molecular determinants of disease. Recent studies have examined the relationship between MRI-derived feature sets and gene expression in gliomas, including glioblastoma

(GBM). Several groups have identified correlations between the expression of particular molecularly defined oncogenic pathways in GBM and malignant phenotypes on MRI. The combination of clinical, genetic, and imaging data has improved prognostic modeling and has identified potential therapeutic targets. Many challenges remain in fully leveraging the associations between such large datasets, but even current methodology shows promise in helping to craft individually tailored treatments to patients with brain tumors and other diseases.

Neuroimaging and Genetic Influence in Treating Brain Neoplasms 121

L. Celso Hygino da Cruz Jr and Margareth Kimura

The current treatment of glioblastoma patients based on surgery, radiation, and chemotherapy has achieved modest improvement in progression-free survival. In this direction, personalized treatment is the next achievement for better patient management and increased overall survival. Genetic characterization of high-grade gliomas by MR imaging is the goal in neuroimaging. The main genetic alterations described in these neoplasms, implications in patient treatment, and prognosis are reviewed. MR imaging features and novel techniques are correlated with the main genetic aspects of such tumors. Posttreatment phenomena, such as pseudoprogression and pseudoresponse, are analyzed in association with the genetic expression of these tumors.

Imaging Genomics of Glioblastoma: State of the Art Bridge Between Genomics and Neuroradiology 141

Mohamed G. ElBanan, Ahmed M. Amer, Pascal O. Zinn, and Rivka R. Colen

Glioblastoma (GBM) is the most common and most aggressive primary malignant tumor of the central nervous system. Recently, researchers concluded that the "one-size-fits-all" approach for treatment of GBM is no longer valid and research should be directed toward more personalized and patient-tailored treatment protocols. Identification of the molecular and genomic pathways underlying GBM is essential for achieving this personalized and targeted therapeutic approach. Imaging genomics represents a new era as a noninvasive surrogate for genomic and molecular profile identification. This article discusses the basics of imaging genomics of GBM, its role in treatment decision-making, and its future potential in noninvasive genomic identification.

Index 155

Foreword

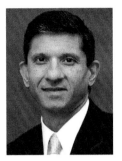

Suresh K. Mukherji, MD, MBA, FACR
Consulting Editor

Imaging genomics and proteomics is an emerging field aimed at identifying and characterizing genetic variants related to brain-related illnesses. This new imaging approach combines genetic information and neuroimaging data in the same subjects to discover neural mechanisms linked to numerous disorders. Numerous studies have shown the overall strength of imaging genetics and its impact on facilitating an understanding of the genetic underpinnings of various neurologic disorders and an improvement in early diagnosis and treatment.

This issue focuses on neurologic conditions in which imaging genetics may play an important role in daily practice and, more specifically, in clinical approaches. In essence, one can argue that this is the epitome of the role of imaging in personalized medicine: the ability to noninvasively predict and correlate genomics and proteomics with various neurologic disorders.

I feel this issue is both "overdue" yet "ahead of its time." The authors have done a wonderful job of introducing and also explaining the tangible clinical potential of this approach, and I sincerely thank this world-class group for their superb contributions. I also want to thank Dr Luiz Celso Hygino da Cruz Jr for accepting to undertake this monumental task. I am sure this singularly unique translational issue will be equally beneficial to imagers and scientists studying the molecular and genetic basis of neurologic disorders.

Suresh K. Mukherji, MD, MBA, FACR
Department of Radiology
Michigan State University
846 Service Road
East Lansing, MI 48824, USA

E-mail address:
mukherji@rad.msu.edu

Neuroimaging Clin N Am 25 (2015) xiii
http://dx.doi.org/10.1016/j.nic.2014.10.003
1052-5149/15/ – see front matter © 2015 Elsevier Inc. All rights reserved.

Preface
Genetic Patterns in Neuroimaging

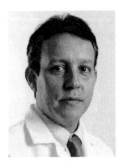

L. Celso Hygino da Cruz Jr, MD

Editor

The past decade has witnessed a tremendous growth in brain imaging as well as an enormous explosion of interest and success in genomics. Recent advances in neuroimaging technology and molecular genetics have provided the unique opportunity for investigation of genetic influence on the variation of brain attributes. As the initial publications on brain imaging and genetics are being released, imaging genetics has become a rapidly growing research approach with an increasing number of publications every year.

Imaging genetics has rapidly developed into a promising, high-impact research field and extended into a body of studies on cerebral disorders, including both neurologic and psychiatric studies. In this context, brain imaging measures sit in the pathway that connects genetic factors to brain illnesses.

Imaging genetics is an emerging field aimed at identifying and characterizing genetic variants that influence measures derived from anatomical or functional brain images, which are in turn related to brain-related illnesses. This new imaging approach combines genetic information and neuroimaging data in the same subjects to discover neural mechanisms linked to numerous disorders.

An increasing number of studies have shown the overall strength of imaging genetics and its impact on facilitating an understanding of the genetic underpinnings of various neurologic disorders and an improvement in early diagnosis and treatment. Noninvasive brain imaging techniques provide much more objective and reproducible phenotypes and can accommodate highly heterogeneous symptoms expressed by patients classified into the same diagnostic group.

Although standard imaging or genetic methods are well established and have many successful applications, merging the two fields is not straightforward. The overwhelming growth of this new imaging concept provides abundant promising results but also reveals challenges embedded within study designs. Another big challenge faced by both radiologists and geneticists is how to properly analyze the large amount of collected data. Although methods reviewed here attempt to tackle this complex problem, limitations are clear. The success of individual studies and the continuing growth of imaging genetics depend on the availability of imaging genetic analytic tools and their proper implementation. Further developing current methods and integrating more information relevant to imaging genetics will continue to be an important research frontier. It is very promising to see that some studies have taken steps in this direction.

Given that the future focus of imaging genetics is expected to ultimately help in understanding various neurologic disorders and turning basic science into clinical strategies, we believe that more effort should be focused on the development of methods that can confront these challenges.

In this issue, we focus on some neurologic conditions in which imaging genetics may play an important role in daily practice and, more specifically, in clinical approaches. The issue starts with an overview of analysis of genetics and brain

Neuroimag Clin N Am 25 (2015) xv–xvi
http://dx.doi.org/10.1016/j.nic.2014.10.001

imaging, trying to build a bridge between the two. The next article surveys the methods and organizes them according to their multivariate nature on specific clinic conditions, such as demyelinating diseases, vascular diseases, neoplasm, psychiatric and pediatric disorders, as well as dementia. Given detailed reviews of imaging data available, we provide a brief summary that includes a recently proposed method of analysis.

I hope the readers find these articles informative, entertaining, provocative, and helpful in their practice. I wish to express my sincere gratitude to all the contributors, who range from established experts to rising stars in the field, allowing this project to become a reality. I really appreciate all their efforts immensely.

I do not have words to express my thankfulness to Suresh Mukherji, MD, Consulting Editor, for the privilege of being chosen and for placing his trust in me to lead this important project. Thanks also must be given to the series editors, Donald Mumford and John Vassallo, for guidance, patience, and encouraging support through the process of preparation of this issue.

Last, and by no means least, I want to dedicate this conquest to my son, Bruno, and to my wife, Simone, for their support, love, and understanding during the process of preparing this work. And to my parents, Leonice and Luiz Celso, for their encouragement and enormous contribution to my career.

L. Celso Hygino da Cruz Jr, MD
Radiologist CDPI and IRM
Department of Radiology
Federal University of Rio de Janeiro
Avenida Pasteur 162/401
Rio de Janeiro, Brazil
CEP 22290-240

E-mail address:
celsohygino@hotmail.com

Understanding Genetics in Neuroimaging

Marina Lipkin Vasquez, MSc, PhD[a],*, Ilana Zalcberg Renault, MD, PhD[b]

KEYWORDS

- DNA • Genome • Mutations • Genetic diseases

KEY POINTS

- The history of genetics and the Human Genome Project.
- Understanding genetics: from DNA to Protein.
- Identification of different molecular abnormalities.
- Most used technologies to identify genetic injuries.
- Genetics and epigenetics mechanisms identified in neurological disorders.

INTRODUCTION

Genome is the term used to describe the group of genes and regulatory sequences from an individual. Genes carry all the information that distinguishes one organism from others. Genes were discovered in 1865 by Gregor Mendel. His observations led to the creation of laws regarding the transmission of hereditary characteristics from generation to generation, which have constituted the basis of genetics until now.[1] The nature of the genes was understood only in 1952, when the scientist Roselin Franklin showed a distinctive pattern that indicated the helical shape of DNA. One year later, James Watson and Francis Crick revealed the mechanisms of DNA structure: the double helix. In 1977, Frederick Sanger developed a rapid DNA sequencing technique.[2]

In 1983, Kary Mullis improved the technique of PCR for amplifying DNA and the first genetic disease, Huntington disease, was mapped.[3]

Since then, the development of techniques to analyze the genome has grown and different pathologies are associated with genetic abnormalities.

Recently, the DNA sequence of the entire human genome was sequenced by the international, collaborative research program called the Human Genome Project (HGP). The project was idealized in 1984 but launched in 1990. The full sequence of the human genome obtained by the HGP was completed in 2003 and provided the first complete view of human genetic code.

The complete human genome contains approximately 3 billion bases and approximately 20,500 protein-coding genes on 46 chromosomes (22 pairs of autosomal chromosomes and 2 sex chromosomes). The coding regions constitute less than 5% of the genome (the function of the remaining noncoding DNA is not yet well established) and some chromosomes have a higher density of genes than others. James Watson was one of the HGP heads and his own genome was sequenced and published on the Internet.[4]

Scientists are studying how the DNA sequences of human genes can vary among individuals and populations and how genetic changes can generate diseases.

A genetic disease is any illness caused by an abnormality in an individual's genome. The abnormality can range from a discrete mutation in 1 base in the DNA of a single gene to a chromosome aberration involving the gain or loss of the genes in

The author has nothing to disclose.
[a] Molecular Biology Laboratory, Instituto Estadual do Cérebro Paulo Niemeyer (IECPN), Rua do Resende 156, 2nd Floor, Centro, Rio de Janeiro CEP 20231-092, Brazil; [b] DASA, Rua João Borges 120/502, Gavea, Rio de Janeiro CEP 22451-100, Brazil
* Corresponding author.
E-mail address: Marina.lipkin@iecpnprosaude.org.br

neuroimaging.theclinics.com

an entire chromosome or set of chromosomes. Some genetic disorders are hereditary (inherited from the parents) whereas others are caused by acquired mutations in a somatic gene or group of genes. Mutations can happen either randomly or due to some environmental exposure.[5]

Most genetic diseases are the direct result of mutations in 1 or many genes. One of the most difficult questions to be further elucidated, however, is how genes contribute to diseases that have a complex pattern of inheritance, such as diabetes, asthma, cancer, and mental illness.[6]

In the nervous system, from depression to Alzheimer disease, familial genetic heritage has been observed. Other conditions, such as Parkinson disease and tumors in the central nervous system, have been associated with a variety of gene deregulations.[4]

In these cases, more than 1 mutation is responsible for the disease arising, and several genes may contribute to a person's susceptibility to a disease.[7] Moreover, genes may affect how someone reacts to environmental factors. To understand how genetics are involved in the genesis of a disease, it is important to understand the mechanisms of gene expression, cell cycle, and proliferation/death control.

FROM DNA TO PROTEIN

DNA is the molecule that carries hereditary information in almost all organisms. DNA consists of 2 polynucleotide strands. Each nucleotide comprises a sugar, a phosphate molecule, and a nitrogenous base (adenine, guanine, thymine, or cytosine). DNA is arranged in spiral forming a structure, called the double helix.[1]

During DNA replication each strand acts as a template for the synthesis of its complementary strand. The disposition of nucleotides along the DNA strand constitutes the genetic code. Every three nucleotide sequence, called codon, encodes one specific amino acid. A gene is a sequence of nucleotides along the DNA strand that determines the sequence of amino acids in a protein.[1]

Gene expression is a process of DNA sequence reading into protein synthesis. This process has 2 major steps: transcription and translation. During transcription, the information is shifted from the DNA to a messenger RNA (mRNA). The DNA serves as template for complementary base pairing catalyzed by an enzyme called RNA polymerase, forming a precursor RNA molecule (pre-mRNA). Then the pre-mRNA is processed to form a mature mRNA. During this phase, called splicing, noncoding regions named introns are excluded from the molecule and only the coding region, the exons,

remain in the mRNA structure. Alternative splicing occurs and different sequences are processed, giving rise to a huge variety of mature mRNAs. The mature mRNA receives some structural markers that signal for cytoplasmic exportation. In the cytoplasm, the step of protein synthesis called translation starts. The mature mRNA, a single-stranded copy of the gene, is then recruited by a protein complex in the ribosome and is translated into a protein molecule.

DNA Transcription—Control of Gene Expression

The process of transcription was first observed in 1970 by electron microscopy. During transcription, 1 DNA strand serves as template for RNA synthesis, whereas the other strand is considered noncoding.

The process of transcription starts when RNA polymerase attaches to the template DNA strand and begins to catalyze the production of RNA by matching complementary bases to the original DNA strand.[8]

Transcription factors bind to specific DNA sequences called enhancer and promoter/silence sequences to recruit RNA polymerase to an appropriate transcription site and signal which part of the gene will be transcribed.

The promoters and enhancers or silencers are located within regulatory regions of the gene as well as within introns. Enhancer sequences regulate gene activation by binding proteins and changing the conformational structure of the DNA, helping to attract RNA polymerase. Because DNA is tightly packed into chromatin, transcription also requires several specialized proteins that facilitate the access to the coding strand.

The Role of Chromatin Structure

In human cells, DNA is packaged around histones, which are proteins in chromatin that also perform a function in gene regulation. In general, they control whether transcription factors may access the DNA.

For transcription to occur, the transcription area needs to be unrolled. This process requires the coordination of histone modifications, transcription factors binding, and other chromatin remodeling activities.

Modifications of histones can open up a gene, whereas DNA modifications can shut it down. In general, methylation of DNA makes chromatin more tightly closed and results in down-regulation or inhibition of gene transcription. On the other hand, acetylation of histones unbends bindings and helps transcription. Methylation of histones can increase or decrease their acetylation, regulating gene expression. The mechanism of regulation of DNA 3-D structure is called epigenetics.

DNA methylation is used in some genes to differentiate which copy is inherited from the father and which is inherited from the mother, in a process called imprinting. It can also help to explain why identical twins are not phenotypically identical. In addition, epigenetic control is responsible for X-chromosome inactivation in women that guarantees they have the same number of X-chromosome gene products as do men.[9]

mRNA Processing (Splicing)

Splicing is the pre-mRNA processing mechanism by which introns are removed and exons are joined together to form the mature mRNA. Specific sequences in the pre-mRNA show where introns and exons are located. Splicing is usually constitutive, meaning that all exons are joined together in the same order they occur in the pre-mRNA. Alternative splicing is also observed, however, and the exons are combined in different ways. In alternative splicing, sequences may serve as exons and be included in the final mRNA, but under different conditions the same sequence can be treated as an intron and be removed from the mature mRNA.[10]

Alternative splicing enables a single gene to generate more than 1 mRNA and contributes to the diversity of proteins in eukaryotes. Cells respond to environment modifications by changing gene expression and protein activity, which can also deregulate alternative splicing.[11]

Scientists estimate that many human genetic diseases may involve splicing errors, making better understanding the splicing mechanisms an important area of research.

Other RNA Subtypes—The Noncoding RNA

Human DNA safely and stably stores genetic material in the nuclei of cells. In the meantime, mRNA carries the same information as DNA but is not used for long-term storage and can freely exit the nucleus. Although the mRNA sequence is complementary to the DNA template, it carries uracils instead of thymines and, after splicing, the molecule receives signals to cytoplasmic location.

Other types of RNAs are also transcribed, but they are differently processed and exported to the cytoplasm. Once they do not generate mRNA, they are referred to as bob-coding RNA, because they do not encode proteins.[12] Two of them have been implicated to help mRNA translation:

- Transfer RNA (tRNA) carries the appropriate amino acids into the ribosome for inclusion in the new protein.
- Ribosomal RNA (rRNA) forms the ribosomes.

In addition to rRNA and tRNA, other noncoding RNAs exist in eukaryotic cells. These molecules participate in many essential functions. As a group, these RNAs are frequently referred to as small regulatory RNAs and are divided into different subgroups:

- Small nuclear RNAs (snRNAs) play a critical role in gene regulation by join in RNA splicing. snRNAs are found in the nucleus and are typically tightly bound to proteins in complexes called small nuclear ribonucleoproteins (snRNPs). The most abundant of these molecules are the U1, U2, U5, and U4/U6 particles, which are involved in splicing pre-mRNA to form mature mRNA.[13]
- MicroRNAs (miRNAs) are small regulatory single-stranded RNAs that are approximately 22 to 26 nucleotides in length. Their functions in gene regulation were initially discovered in the nematode *Caenorhabditis elegans*.[14,15] MiRNAs bind to the 3′ untranslated region of their target mRNAs through imperfect base pairing and inhibit translation. Therefore, miRNAs inhibit gene expression in a post-transcription phase. Additional studies indicate that miRNAs also play significant roles in cancer and other diseases.
- Small interfering RNAs (siRNAs) are another class of small RNAs that also inhibit gene expression. Specifically, 1 strand of a double-stranded siRNA molecule can be incorporated into a complex called RNA-induced silencing complex (RISC). This RNA-containing complex can then inhibit transcription of an mRNA that has a sequence complementary to its RNA component.
- Small nucleolar RNAs are abundant in nucleolar extracts. These molecules function to process rRNA molecules, often resulting in the methylation and pseudouridylation of specific nucleosides.

New forms of noncoding RNAs with novel functions continue to be discovered.

Protein Synthesis (Translation and Post-transcriptional Mechanisms of Control—Small Interfering RNA/MicroRNA)

The mature mRNA arrives at the cytoplasm and goes to the ribosome. There, the ncRNAs and a complex of enzymes are responsible for its translation into proteins. In the mRNA, each sequence of three letters (A, C, G, or U) is called a codon. Individual codons code for specific amino acids. After the machinery for translation is ready at the ribosome, tRNAs bring the amino acids and the peptide strands begins to be synthesized.[16]

The presence of miRNAs and siRNAs can inhibit translation by two different mechanisms in association with a complex called RISC. The small interfering RNA (si-RNA) molecule is opened by the RNA-induced silencing complex (RISC) and remain bound to one single strand, which then binds to a sequence-specific region of the mRNA, signaling for another component of RISC, called Slicer, to cut the mRNA in the middle of the binding region. The cells do not recognize the cut mRNA and degrade it.

In the case of miRNA, an miRNA-induced silencing complex associates with the mature miRNA and binds to mRNA on the ribosome, blocking translation. MiRNAs can imperfectly bind complementary mRNA, as opposed to siR-NAs, that require near-perfect binding.

One ncRNA has many different mRNA targets. These two mechanisms of post-transcriptional inhibition of gene expression by ncRNAs are being intensely studied and are associated with many different diseases. Scientists are trying to develop specific target drugs to deliver synthetic and antagonist ncRNAs to sick cells and combat specific pathologies (**Fig. 1**).

MOLECULAR ABNORMALITIES

In normal conditions during cell division, mistakes may happen in DNA replication. The cell has mechanisms to repair or eradicate the error (DNA repair enzymes). If the error is irrecoverable, the cell dies by apoptosis. In cases of

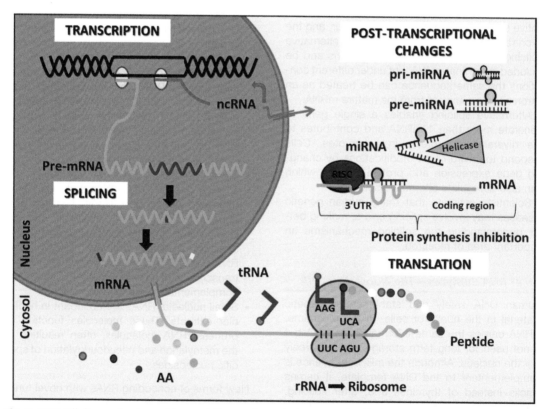

Fig. 1. Intracellular mechanisms of transcription and translation. DNA double helix is opened to propitiate RNA syntheses. Precursor ncRNAs and mRNAs are transcribed in the nucleus. Some ncRNAs stay in the nucleus and act as transcription or epigenetic factors. Others go to the cytosol and participate in cellular activities. Both tRNA and rRNA are crucial for translation. After splicing (constitutive and alternative), the mature mRNA is exported to the cytoplasm and attaches to the ribosomal subunits to start translation. T-RNAs pair with mRNA sequence and add 1 new amino acid (AA) to the new peptide code. Some ncRNAs are responsible for post-transcriptional changes and control of protein synthesis (eg, miRNAs are processed from large precursor - primary-miRNA (pri-miRNA) - to small precursor - pre-miRNA - and finally in the cytosol to mature miRNA, forming a protein complex that pairs imperfectly with mRNA and inhibits translation).

problems in DNA repair/apoptosis mechanisms, cells accumulate genomic abnormalities and pass them through generations of cells. The accumulation of mutations causes diseases and even tumors, by changing transcription of genes or regulatory ncRNAs and by changing gene function.

In diseases like cancer, there are mutations in key genes that control normal cell processes, such as cell cycle, differentiation, and apoptosis. A person has two copies of each gene, one from the mother and one from the father. People with a hereditary predisposition to a disease inherit one copy of the damaged gene but the other copy is still normal. These people are considered heterozygous for the feature determined by that gene. Gene mutations that are inherited occur in the germline, meaning that all a person's cells carry the mutation. During life, a mutation may occur in the other copy of the gene and the pearson starts to present a defective phenotype. Most mutations are not inherited, however; they are acquired by somatic cells during individuals' lives (the mutations occur in one specific type of adult somatic cell, then not all cells carry the mutations; thus these cells cannot be transmitted to the descendants).[17]

Examples of typical abnormalities include polymorphisms, chromosomes aberrations, point mutations that alter coding sequences, and changes on chromatin structure. These phenomena are explained as follows.

Single Nucleotide Polymorphisms

A single nucleotide polymorphism (SNP) is a DNA sequence variation occurring when a single nucleotide of a gene (A, T, C, or G) differs among individuals.

Within a population, SNPs can be referred as the allele of minor frequency, in other words, the less common variant carried by the part of population. SNPs are frequently expressed differently in human populations; therefore, an SNP allele that is common in one region or in one ethnic group may be rare in another.

SNPs may be found in coding and noncoding regions of gene or in the intergenic regions between genes. SNPs within a coding sequence may not change the amino acid sequence due to degeneracy of the genetic code (both sequences led to the same polypeptide). SNPs that change the amino acid in general lead to different phenotypes but do not cause problems to the cell. SNPs that are not in protein coding regions may still have consequences for gene splicing, transcription factor binding, or the sequence of ncRNAs, also implying in change of protein synthesis.

SNPs occur in more than 1% of the population. They are common enough to be considered a normal genetic variation and are responsible for many of the normal differences between people, such as eye color, hair color, and blood type. Although most SNPs do not have negative effects on a person's health, some of them may influence the risk of developing diseases.[18]

Chromosomal Aberrations

There are 2 main types of chromosomal abnormalities: numeric and structural aberrations. Any increases or decreases in chromosomal material interfere with normal development and function.[19]

- Structural aberrations
  Structural aberrations can be intra- or interchromosomal. Intrachromosomal aberrations include deletion, duplication, and inversion. Interchromosomal include translocations. Deletions can happen naturally or be caused by chemical mutagens and radiation. When part of a dominant allele is deleted, it may cause the expression of a recessive character, configuring pseudodominance.
  In turn, duplications occur in a lower frequency than deletions. In inversion, a segment of chromosomes is inverted on reversed by 180°. Translocations involve two nonhomologous chromosomes and position of part of the chromosome is changed, leading to change in arrangement of chromosomes.
  Alteration in chromosome structure has been associated with prognosis and therapy response of many diseases, for example, translocations found in leukemias and lymphomas. Almost all patients with chronic myeloid leukemia carry the fusion gene BCR-ABL, which results from the translocation of chromosome 9 and 22.[20] In solid tumors, individual structural aberrations have not been shown sufficiently prevalent, except for prostate cancer, in which 70% of the patients carry the fusion gene TMPRSS2-ETS.[21]
- Copy number aberrations
  Numeric aberrations are caused by a defect in chromosome division, resulting in cells with extra chromosomes or a deficiency in chromosomes.
  Gametes with these anomalies can result in conditions, such as Down syndrome (47

chromosomes instead of 46) or Turner syndrome (45 chromosomes).

Many regions of amplification and lower-level copy number abnormalities have been identified by comparative genomic hybridization (CGH) in different cancers, for example, *NMYC* in euroblastoma,[22] *EGFR* in glioblastoma,[23] and *RB1* in retinoblastoma.[24]

Point Mutations, Insertions, Deletions, and Duplications

The DNA sequence of a gene can be altered in several ways. Gene mutations have varying effects on health, depending on where they occur and whether they alter the function of resulting proteins. The types of mutations include

- Missense mutation—changes 1 DNA base pair and results in protein changes
- Nonsense mutation—also changes 1 DNA base pair but instead of changing 1 codon for another, the altered sequence signals to stop transcription, resulting in a shortened protein
- Insertion—addiction of bases in the DNA sequence, resulting in a protein that may not work properly
- Deletion—loss of a piece of the DNA sequence; small deletions remove 1 or a few base pairs from a gene, and larger deletions remove an entire gene or nearby genes
- Duplication—part of the DNA sequence is abnormally copied 1 or more times
- Frameshift mutation—when the addition or loss of DNA bases changes a gene's reading frame. A reading frame consists of groups of 3 bases that each code for 1 amino acid. A frameshift mutation shifts the grouping of these bases and changes the code for amino acids. The protein resultant is often nonfunctional. Insertions, deletions, and duplications can all be frameshift mutations.

Epigenetics

Epigenetic silencing is 1 way to turn genes off, and it can contribute to differential protein expression among cells from different tissues. Epigenetics is involved in many normal cellular processes but it has been associated with many diseases. There are 3 epigenetic systems that can interact with each other to silence genes: DNA methylation, histone modifications, and RNA-associated silencing.[25]

In DNA methylation, a methyl group is added to DNA. It is highly specific and always happens in a region in which a cytosine is located next to a guanine linked by a phosphate (called a CpG site). CpG sites

are methylated by 1 of 3 enzymes called DNA methyltransferases. Inserting methyl groups changes the appearance and structure of DNA, modifying a gene's interactions with the machinery within a cell's nucleus that is needed for transcription.

When histones are modified after they are translated into protein, they settle chromatin arrangement, which can determine whether the associated DNA is transcribed. If chromatin is opened, DNA can be transcribed. But if chromatin is condensed (creating a complex called heterochromatin), DNA is not transcribed.

There are 2 ways histones can be modified: by acetylation and by methylation. Acetylation is usually associated with active chromatin, whereas deacetylation is associated with heterochromatin. On the other hand, histone methylation can be a marker for both active and inactive regions of chromatin.[26]

Genes can also be turned off by RNA-associated silencing when it is in the form of antisense transcripts, ncRNAs. RNA might affect gene expression by causing heterochromatin to form or by initiating histone modifications and DNA methylation.

Epigenetic changes are required for normal processes but they can also be involved in some mechanisms of pathogenesis. Disrupting any system that contributes to epigenetic alterations can cause abnormal activation or silencing of genes. Such disruptions have already been associated with cancer, syndromes involving chromosomal instabilities, and mental retardation.

Genome Instability and Loss of Heterozygosity

When the normal mechanisms of epigenetic control are altered, genome instability is lodged in the cell. Genome instability causes nondisjunction during mitosis, segregation during recombination, or deletion of a chromosome segment. This phenomenon provides conditions for the loss of 1 copy of a gene allele (or loss of heterozygosity [LOH]) due to the accumulation of mutations. LOH becomes critical when the remaining allele contains a point mutation that changes protein expression. Then, people who already carry heterozygous mutations in 1 allele of an important gene may have the other allele lost or inactivated. This is a common occurrence in cancers where a tumor suppressor gene is affected.

Telomere Maintenance Mechanism

Telomerase is a ribonucleoprotein that elongates telomeric DNA by adding hexanucleotide repeats to compensate for progressive DNA loss that happens during each cell division. Telomerase consists in a catalytic protein subunit with reverse transcriptase activity (h-TERT), encoded by the hTERT gene and an RNA component (TERC), encoded by TERC gene, that serves as a template for the telomere repeat. Recently, high-expression levels of TERC and *hTERT* were associated with worse survival of children with non-brainstem high-grade gliomas, making telomerase a promising potential therapeutic target in this disease (**Fig. 2**).[27]

TECHNOLOGIES TO IDENTIFY GENETIC ABNORMALITIES
Classic Cytogenetics

Classic cytogenetics by karyotyping has been used in clinical research laboratories for more than 50 years. Chromosomes in metaphase can be identified by using certain staining techniques, called bandings. Banding allows individual chromosomes and their aberrations to be identified with accuracy. The most commonly used technique is Giemsa or G banding (**Fig. 3**). There are limitations to this technique, however, due to the difficulty in obtaining and preparing samples and interpreting results from solid tumors genomes.[28]

Fluorescence In Situ Hybridization

In 1985, thyroglobulin was the first human gene to be mapped using FISH.[29] FISH maps DNA sequences to specific regions of human chromosomes. FISH involves the use of fluorescently labeled DNA probes, which hybridize to complementary chromosomal regions. This technique allows the visualization of chromosomal location of a particular gene or DNA sequence. The result is a fluorescent dot at the chromosomal location

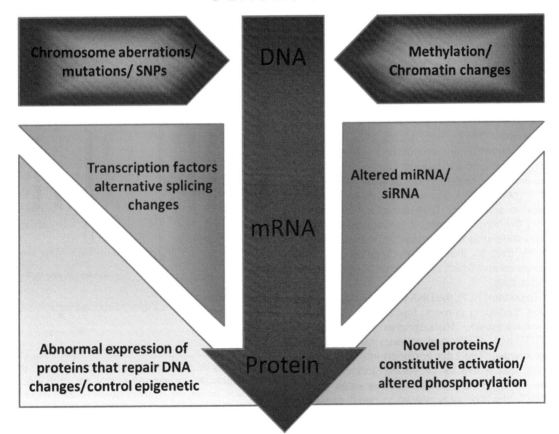

Fig. 2. Schematic illustration of how genetic and epigenetic aberrations may contribute to the pathogenic mechanism of diseases.

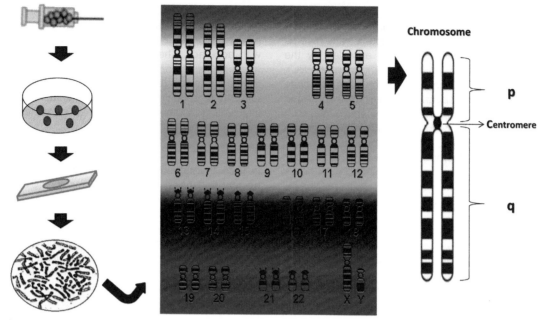

Fig. 3. G banding is one of the most used techniques for chromosome banding. Described in 1971, the treatment with trypsine and Giemsa results in the chromosome band being distinguishable from its adjacent segments by appearing darker or lighter. Cells are collected, cultured for 3 days, fixed, and spread onto slides. The metaphases analysis shows the short (p) and long (q) arms of the chromosome divided in bands.

where the labeled probe binds that can be seen through a microscope (**Fig. 4**).

Polymerase Chain Reaction

Created in 1985 by Kary Mullis, PCR is a rapid, simple, sensitive, and one of the most used techniques in molecular biology laboratories around the world. It consists in the in vitro amplification of a specific DNA sequence. PCR amplification requires some prior DNA sequence information from the target sample. It is used to design 2 small oligonucleotide sequences, named primers, which bind to the start and end of the DNA sequence and which are approximately 20 nucleotides long.

To perform PCR, the DNA template is added to a tube containing primers, free nucleotides (the 4 deoxynucleoside triphosphates: dATP, dCTP, dGTP, and dTTP), and an enzyme called DNA polymerase. The tube is placed into a PCR machine that works by increasing and decreasing the temperature in automatic repeated steps. Initially, the mixture is heated to denature (separate) the double-stranded DNA template into single strands. The mixture is then cooled to provide primers annealing (bind) to the DNA template. Hence, the DNA polymerase begins to synthesize

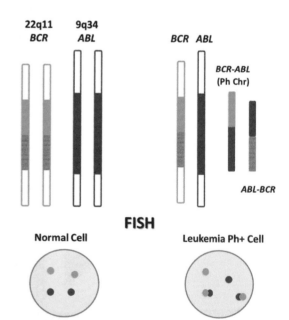

Fig. 4. This is an example of FISH to detect the Philadelphia chromosome (Ph+, *BCR-ABL*) with a double fusion probe, which stains green for *BCR* and red for *ABL*. On the left is a normal interphase and on the right a leukemic cell. The normal genes are 9 and 22 separate, and the fusion on 9q+ and 22q-s what should be a yellow signal (a fused green and red signal).

new strands of DNA starting from the primers. The newly synthesized DNA segments serve as templates in the following PCR cycles, which allow the DNA target to be exponentially amplified millions of times.

Also, with the implementation of reverse transcriptase, it became possible to analyze the expression of a specific mRNA in the sample, after synthesizing a complementary DNA (cDNA) from the target RNA, by reverse transcription–PCR (RT-PCR).[30]

With time, progress was made in PCR technology and it became possible to quantify amplification products. Real-time PCR (RQ-PCR), also called quantitative PCR, became a common lab test. Expression analysis by RQ-PCR is based on continuous fluorescent monitoring of PCR products amplification from a cDNA template.[31] There are different RQ-PCR systems—one uses a specific method to detect the accumulation of

PCR products. Those used most often are SYBR ˙ Green I (Molecular Probes, Eugene, Oregon) and TaqMan Assay (Life Technologies, Carlsbad, California). RQ-PCR provides a quick and low-cost assessment of the expression pattern of several genes in many diseases (**Fig. 5**).

Sequencing

DNA sequencing is a laboratory method used to determine the sequence of nucleotides in a DNA molecule. The method was developed by Frederick Sanger in 1975, who was later awarded a Nobel prize for his discoveries.[32] Consequently, this method has been automated and is referred to as first-generation sequencing. With the development of technical resources, the methods for sequencing are getting more sensitive and cheaper, with higher coverage and better resolution.[33] The evolution has led to the

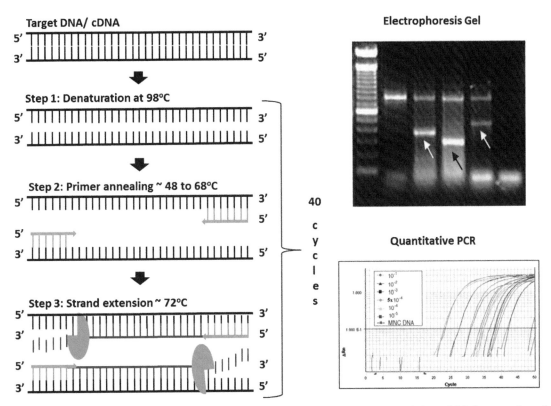

Fig. 5. PCR is performed in at least 40 cycles of 3 different temperature steps, consisting of (1) denaturation of DNA double strands, (2) primer annealing, and (3) new strand extension by polymerase enzyme. The accumulated strands can be visualized on a gel after electrophoresis (eg, agarose gel to detect different isoforms of BCR-ABL transcript amplified by RT-PCR [*arrows*] and a control band that corresponds to the amplification of the constitutive BCR transcript). The quantitative PCR estimates the amount of DNA/cDNA by analyzing melting curves from the fluorescence detection of probe activity during each cycle of strand amplification. A given number of amplification cycles yield a fluorescent signal that can be measured and again applied to a standard curve, used to calculate the number of BCR-ABL transcripts, for example.

second- and third-generation sequencing technologies, described as follows.

- First-generation sequencing

  Automated Sanger sequencing is considered the first generation of DNA sequencing technologies. In Sanger sequencing, the DNA to be sequenced serves as a template for DNA synthesis. A DNA primer is designed to be a starting point for DNA synthesis on the strand of DNA to be sequenced. Four individual DNA synthesis reactions are performed. The four reactions include normal A, G, C, and T deoxynucleotide triphosphates (dNTPs), and each contains a low level of 1 of 4 dideoxynucleotide triphosphates (ddNTPs): ddATP, ddGTP, ddCTP, or ddTTP. When a ddNTP is incorporated into a chain of nucleotides, synthesis terminates. It happens because dideoxynucleotides (ddNTP) molecule lacks 3'-hydroxyl group which is required to form a link with the next nucleotide in the chain. Because the ddNTPs are randomly incorporated, synthesis terminates at many different positions for each reaction.

  After synthesis, the products of the A, G, C, and T reactions are individually loaded into four lanes of a single gel and separated using gel electrophoresis, a method that separates DNA fragments by their sizes. The bands of the gel are detected, and then the sequence is read from the bottom of the gel to the top, including bands in all four lanes. For example, if the lowest band across all four lanes appears in the A reaction lane, then the first nucleotide in the sequence is A. Then, if the next band from bottom to top appears in the T lane, the second nucleotide in the sequence is T and so forth.[34]

  Despite strong availability and accuracy, Sanger sequencing has technical limitations in its workflow because of high costs, it is time consuming, and it has limited coverage. Current estimates suggest a cost of approximately $5 million to $30 million to sequence an entire human genome using this method, and on 1 machine, it would take approximately 60 years to finish the whole task (Fig. 6).

- Next-generation sequencing

  Next-generation sequencing (NGS) refers to the high-throughput DNA sequencing, technologies available since 2007, which are

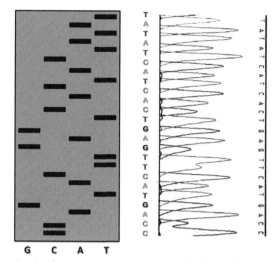

Fig. 6. The Sanger sequencing method is performed using fluorescent labeling instead of radiolabeling. A different fluorescent label is used for each ddNTP and the reactions are run in a capillary gel (left), which is automatically read by a computer to indicate which bases were added in what order. This produces a colorful graph called a chromatogram (right).

capable of sequencing large numbers of different DNA sequences in a single reaction. There are different methods of NGS from different brands, such as Illumina, Roche, and Life Technologies. All NGS technologies monitor the sequential addition of nucleotides to immobilized and spatially arrayed DNA templates but differ substantially in how these templates are designed and how they are analyzed to reveal target sequences.[35,36]

One of the key limitations of NGS is the high volume of data generated: it provides huge sequence results (in the range of megabases to gigabases), and data interpretation requires time and specific knowledge. Moreover, the amount and nature of data produced by all NGS platforms demand a lot of computational technology and biostatistics expertise at all stages of sequencing, including data tracking and quality control (Fig. 7).[37]

Microarray Tools

The microarray is a technique used to detect the expression of thousands of genes at the same time. DNA microarrays are microscope slides, referred as DNA chips, that are printed with thousands of spots in defined positions, each one containing a known DNA sequence. The DNA molecules attached to each chip act as probes to

1977			2007			2012		
Sequencing	**1st Generation**		**Next (2nd) Generation**			**Next Next (3rd) Generation**		
Company	Sanger	AB	Illumina	Life Tech	Roche	Pac Bio	Helicos	Oxford
Sequencing chemistry		By ligation	By synthesis	H+ Ion sensitive	Pyroseq		By synthesis	
Sample preparation			Solid-phase	Emulsion PCR	Emulsion PCR	Single molecule	Single molecule	NA
Read length	800 bp	50 bp	150 bp	200 bp	700 bp	2900 bp	NA	NA
Reads/run	1	$1,2*10^9$	$3*10^9$	$5*10^6$	$1*10^6$	$75*10^5$	NA	NA
Time/run	2 hours	14 days	10 days	2 hours	10 hours	2 hours	1GB/hour	NA
Price \$ ($1*10^6$ bases)	\$2400	\$0.13	\$0.1	\$1	\$10	\$2	NA	NA

Fig. 7. NGS has similar properties to Sanger sequencing but has much higher throughput, meaning that it has the capacity to sequence many more regions at the same time. There are various NGS techniques that differ in the mechanisms used to distinguish the nucleotides, the length of sequences read, and the time and the cost of total sequencing. NGS is used for 3 main purposes: to analyze DNA mutations (genome assembly), to analyze mRNA expression (mRNAseq), and to find DNA sequences that interact with proteins, meaning to find transcription factors or gene expression regulators (chromatin immunoprecipitation). The recent methods available (third-generation sequencing) are capable of sequencing 1 single cell genome. This figure shows most popular platforms currently available in the market. AB, Applied Biosyntems (Carlsbad, California); Illumina, Illumina (San Diego, California); Life Tech, Life Technologies (Carlsbad, California); NA, data not available; Thermo Fisher Scientific (Waltham, Massachusetts); Roche, Roche (Basel, Switzerland); Pac Bio, Pacific Biosciences (Menlo Park, California); Helicos, Helicos BioSciences (Cambridge, Massachusetts); Oxford, OxfordBioMedica (Oxford, United Kingdom).

detect gene expression, what means the amount of mRNA transcripts expressed by a group of genes.[38]

To perform the analysis, it is necessary to use both a target and a reference sample. For example, the reference (control) sample could be from a healthy donor and the experimental sample could be collected from a tumor. The two mRNA samples are then converted into cDNA, and each sample is labeled with a fluorescent probe of a different color (one in green and other in red). The two samples are mixed together and hybridize to the microarray chip. After hybridization, the microarray is scanned to measure the expression of each gene printed on the chip. If the expression of a particular gene is higher in the tumor than in the control sample, then the corresponding spot on the microarray appears red. In contrast, if the expression in the tumor is lower, then the spot appears green. Finally, if there is equal expression in both samples, then the spots are yellow. Microarrays provide the analysis of gene expression profiles, showing changes in the expression of different genes according to a particular condition or therapy (**Fig. 8**).[39]

Array Comparative Genomic Hybridization

The modernization of cytogenetic techniques led to the development of aCGH, which combines CGH with high-throughput microarrays to simultaneously analyze hundreds or thousands of regions of the genome and identify unbalanced karyotypes. aCGH combines the locus-specific nature of FISH with the global genome view of high-resolution chromosomes.

By using microarrays, it is possible to identify unknown chromosomal regions and genes that are amplified or missing. aCGH data can be verified using FISH analysis, but not with the same sensibility. To have the same results derived from one aCGH experiment, thousands of FISH experiments would need to be performed.

A recent study using aCGH to analyze rearrangements of subtelomeric regions (frequent in individuals with idiopathic mental retardation) was able to identify novel common abnormalities that could not be classified previously using only FISH.[40,41] The identification of these sorts of complex rearrangements suggests that chromosomal abnormalities are often more complex than previously thought (**Fig. 9**).

Sample Preparation

Expression Analysis

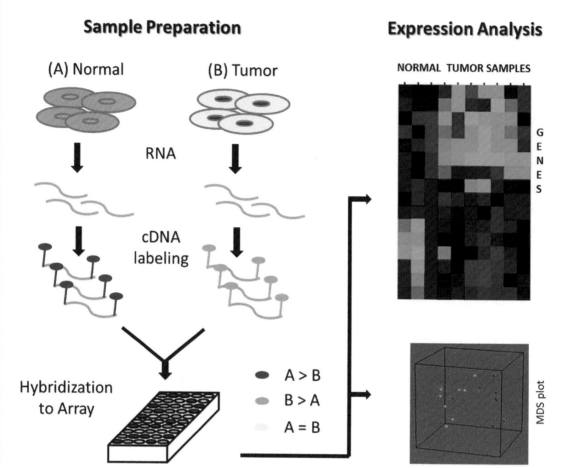

Fig. 8. The microarray approach for expression profiling uses a 2-color cDNA chip. RNA is extracted from the target cells and retrotranscribed to cDNA. Then cDNA molecules are labeled with different fluorescent dyes; the normal sample (healthy donor) is labeled red whereas the tumor is labeled green. The labeled cDNA molecules are hybridized to the DNA on the microarray chip that contains thousands of known fragments of DNA. Each DNA spotted on the chip binds to the complementary strand from the target cDNA. The relative ratio of the gene at each spot is determined by the color after hybridization. Green spots are tumor expression greater than normal, red spots are tumor less than normal, and yellow spots indicate equal amounts. The signal is scanned in for each array and analyzed. The genes can be clustered by expression similarity, and expression can be represented in a multidimensional space (MDS) plot, meaning 2 different groups divided by gene expression profile. The cluster tree also exhibits green and red signals, but this time it refers to the intensity of each gene (green for up-regulated and red for down-regulated; the darker signal is the most intense event).

GENETICS AND EPIGENETICS OF NEUROLOGIC DISORDERS

For many years it has been known that most pathologic conditions result from genetic mutations. Monogenic diseases are usually rare and aggressive. For example, many cases of cystic fibrosis are associated with a mutation in the *CFTR* gene.[42] In contrast, multigenic diseases result from mutations in more than 1 gene. Interaction among the phenotypic effects of different genes, known as epistasis, increases the complexity in studies of the genetic mechanisms of pathogenesis. For instance, epistasis between SNPs within *NRG1* and between *NRG1* and selected protein interaction partners influences the risk of schizophrenia.[43]

In the past 20 years, the development of molecular biology tools for analyses of genomic abnormalities has revealed the mechanism implicated in different diseases. Leukemia and lymphoma were among the cancers that most benefited from genetic advances techniques, and many genes were found to have a role in the pathogenesis. These data led not only to a better stratification of patients during diagnosis, providing better

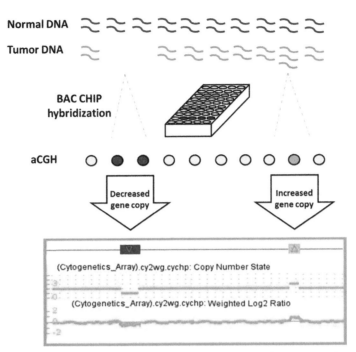

Normal DNA

Tumor DNA

BAC CHIP hybridization

aCGH

Decreased gene copy

Increased gene copy

(Cytogenetics_Array).cy2wg.cychp: Copy Number State

(Cytogenetics_Array).cy2wg.cychp: Weighted Log2 Ratio

Fig. 9. aCGH reveals the loss or gain of chromosomal regions in target samples in comparison to a reference control (eg, tumors and normal cells). DNA in the test and reference samples is labeled with green and red fluorochromes and allowed to compete for hybridization sites on an array of bacterial artificial chromosome (BAC) clones that represent thousands of small DNA segments distributed across the genome. Areas on the chromosome, or spots on the array chip, that are more green than average are present in extra copies in the target sample; those that are more red than average are deleted. The resulting graph shows the exact genome position of the event and allows the identification of copy number variation and LOH.

treatment, but also to the development of targeted therapies that increased patients' overall survival and drastically reduced the death ratios of both malignances.

In the past decade, scientists have begun to study nervous system cancers with molecular tools, and many genetic abnormalities have been found associated with tumor subtypes, adding information and helping in the morphologic classification. To date, however, it has not yet brought much progress to clinics, but new high-throughput techniques associated with modern imaging tools may enable further progress to better delineate disease mechanisms to provide new insights for preventive approaches and therapeutic targets.[44,45]

Other than cancer, many neurologic conditions have been associated with genetic mutations (**Table 1**). This is the case in fragile X syndrome, the most frequently inherited mental disability. Both genders can be affected in this condition, but it is more frequent in males, because they have only one X chromosome. People with this syndrome have severe intellectual disabilities, delayed verbal development, and autistic-like behavior.[46]

It has been demonstrated that the disease is caused by an abnormality in the fragile X mental

retardation 1 (*FMR1*) gene. Healthy people carry 6 to 50 repeats of the trinucleotide CGG in their *FMR1* gene. Individuals who carry an FMR1 mutation express with more than 200 repeats and usually show symptoms of the syndrome. Abundant CGGs causes hypermethylation of *FMR1* gene. This methylation blocks the *FMR1* gene transcription and the production of an important protein, the fragile X mental retardation protein, causing fragile X syndrome. The mechanism by which CGG expansion may be the cause of fragile X, the epigenetic change associated with *FMR1* methylation, was recently discovered to be the real cause for the syndrome.[47]

Epigenetic changes and the presence of highly prevalent germline polymorphisms may also increase the susceptibility to some abnormal behaviors, such as psychosis and aggressiveness, and different diseases that affect the nervous system.

For instance, some genomic and epigenomic abnormalities can help the diagnosis and also can be associated with therapy response and prediction of relapse in glioblastomas, such as expression of the DNA repair gene O-6-methyl-guanine-DNA methyltransferase (*MGMT*). Epigenetic silencing of gene by promoter methylation

Table 1
Summary of the most important genome abnormalities associated with neurologic disorders

Condition	Chromosome	Gene Product	Function	References
Huntington disease	4p16.3	*HTT*	Mutation causes CAG trinucleotide repeat expansion	Huntington's Disease Collaborative Research Group,[50] 1993
Fragile X syndrome	X	*FMR1*	Promoter methylation	Handt et al,[47] 2014
Spinal muscular atrophy	5q.13	*SMN*	Deletion cause loss of protein function	Lefebvre et al,[51] 1995
Tuberous sclerosis	9q34/16p3.3	*TSC1* and 2	Deletion cause novel protein	The TSC1 Consortium,[52] 1997
Multiple sclerosis	6p21	*HLA* complex	Specific haplotypes were strongly associated with MS	Dyment et al,[53] 2005
Schizophrenia	8p12	*NRG1*	SNPs led to increased gene expression	Nicodemus et al,[43] 2010
Alzheimer disease	21/19q12-13/ 14q24/1q42	*βAPP/APOE/ PS1/PS2*	Missense mutations alters βAPP and β-amyloid peptide	George-Hyslop et al,[54] 2014
Glioblastoma	7p11.2/10q26	*EGFR/ MGMT1*	Gene amplification/ promoter methylation	Hatanpaa et al,[23] 2010/Hegi et al,[48] 2005
Glaucoma	1q23-25/2p21	*GLC1A/ CYP1B1*	Mutations	Stone et al,[55] 1997
Inherited epilepsies	17p13.3/ 10q26/Xq28	LIS1/EMX2/ Filamin 1	Mutations	Noebels,[56] 2014
Parkinson	4q21/12q12/ 1p35-36	SNCA/LRRK2/ PINK1/DJ-1	Mutations	Van der Vegt et al,[57] 2009

compromises DNA repair and is associated with better survival rates in patients with glioblastoma who receive alkylating agents, such as temozolomide.[48]

Because so many diseases, such as cancer, involve epigenetic changes, some trials are testing patients with epigenetic treatments. These target drugs benefit from the fact that epigenetic changes are reversible, instead of most of genetic changes where patients carry mutations in DNA sequences. The most popular of these treatments aims to alter either DNA methylation or histone acetylation. Although it looks promising, it is important to have caution in using epigenetic therapy because epigenetic processes and changes happen constantly in normal cells, and drug off-target effects may appear.[49] Scientists are making progress in specifically targeting abnormal cells with minimal damage to normal ones. Nevertheless, the nervous system requires more attention once there are difficulties in drug delivery, but, in the near future, with better elucidation of genetic and pathogenesis, it is expected that patients may benefit from additional therapies.

REFERENCES

1. Alberts B, Bray D, Lewis J, et al. Molecular biology of the cell. 3rd edition. New York; London: Garland Publishing; 1994.
2. Sanger F, Air GM, Barrell BG, et al. Nucleotide sequence of bacteriophage phi X174 DNA. Nature 1977;265(5596):687–95.
3. Mullis K, Faloona F, Scharf S, et al. Specific amplification of DNA in vitro: the polymerase chain reaction. Cold Spring Harb Symp Quant Biol 1986;51:260.
4. Mendelsohn J, Howley PM, Israel MA, editors. The Molecular Basis of Cancer. 3rd edition. Philadelphia: Saunders/Elsevier; 2008.
5. Stankiewicz P, Shaw CJ, Dapper JD, et al. Genome architecture catalyzes nonrecurrent

chromosomal rearrangements. Am J Hum Genet 2003;72:1101–16.

6. Lupski JR, Stankiewicz P. Genomic disorders: molecular mechanisms for rearrangements and conveyed phenotypes. PLoS Genet 2005;1:627–33.

7. Shaffer LG, Bejjani BA, Torchia B, et al. The identification of microdeletion syndromes and other chromosome abnormalities: cytogenetic methods of the past, new technologies for the future. Am J Med Genet C Semin Med Genet 2007;145C:335–45.

8. Clancy S. DNA transcription. Nat Educat 2008; 1(1):41.

9. Shaw CJ, Lupski JR. Implications of human genome architecture for rearrangement-based disorders: the genomic basis of disease. Hum Mol Genet 2004;13: R57–64.

10. Shin C, Manley JL. Cell signalling and the control of pre-mRNA splicing. Nat Rev Mol Cell Biol 2004;5: 727–38.

11. Barash Y, Calarco JA, Gao W, et al. Deciphering the splicing code. Nature 2010;465:53–9.

12. Eddy S. Non-coding RNA genes and the modern RNA world. Nat Rev Genet 2001;2:919–29.

13. Fournier MJ, Maxwell ES. The nucleolar snRNAs: catching up with the spliceosomal snRNAs. Trends Biochem Sci 1993;18:131–5.

14. Lee RC, Feinbaum RL, Ambros V. The C. elegans heterochronic gene lin-4 encodes small RNAs with antisense complementarity to lin-14. Cell 1993; 75(5):843–54.

15. Wightman B, Ha I, Ruvkun G. Posttranscriptional regulation of the heterochronic gene lin-14 by lin-4 mediates temporal pattern formation in C. elegans. Cell 1993;75(5):855–62.

16. Nabavi S, Nazar RN. Nonpolyadenylated RNA polymerase II termination is induced by transcript cleavage. J Biol Chem 2008;283:13601–10.

17. Shaffer LG, Lupski JR. Molecular mechanisms for constitutional chromosomal rearrangements in humans. Annu Rev Genet 2000;34:297–329.

18. Mao X, Young BD, Lu YJ. The application of single-nucleotide polymorphism microarrays in cancer research. Curr Genomics 2007;8(4):219–28.

19. Moore CM, Best RG. Chromosomal genetic disease: structural aberrations. Encyclopedia of Life Sciences. Nature Publishing Group; 2001. p. 1–8.

20. Wong S, Witte ON. BCR-ABL story: bench to bedside and back. Annu Rev Immunol 2004;22:247–306.

21. Tomlins SA, Rhodes DR, Perner S. Recurrent fusion of TMPRSS2 and ETS transcriptor factor genes in prostate cancer. Science 2005;310:644–8.

22. Maris JM, Matthay KK. Molecular biology of neuroblastoma. J Clin Oncol 1999;17:2264–79.

23. Hatanpaa KJ, Burma S, Zhao D, et al. Epidermal growth factor receptor in glioma: signal transduction, neuropathology, imaging, and radioresistance. Neoplasia 2010;12(9):675–84.

24. Lohmann DR. RB1 gene mutations in retinoblastoma. Hum Mutat 1999;14(4):283–8.

25. Simmons D. Epigenetic influence and disease. Nat Education 2008;1(1):6.

26. Egger G, Liang G, Aparicio A, et al. Epigenetics in human disease and prospects for epigenetic therapy. Nature 2004;429(6990):457–63.

27. Dorris K, Prog Sobo M, Onar-Thomas A, et al. Prognostic significance of telomere maintenance mechanisms in pediatric high-grade gliomas. J Neurooncol 2014;117:67–76.

28. Bates SE. Classical cytogenetics: karyotyping techniques. Methods Mol Biol 2011;767:177–90.

29. Landegent JE, Jansen in de Wal N, van Ommen GJ, et al. Chromosomal localization of a unique gene by non-autoradiographic in situ hybridization. Nature 1985;317(6033):175–7.

30. Liang P, Pardee AB. Differential display of eukaryotic messenger RNA by means of the polymerase chain reaction. Science 1992;257:967.

31. Schena M, Shalon D, Davis RW, et al. Quantitative monitoring of gene expression patterns with a complementary DNA microarray. Science 1995;270:467.

32. Pettersson E, Lundeberg J, Ahmadian A. Generations of sequencing technologies. Genomics 2009; 93(2):105–11.

33. Niedringhaus TP, Milanova D, Kerby MB, et al. Landscape of Next-Generation Sequencing Technologies. Anal Chem 2011;83(12):4327–41.

34. Prober JM, Trainor GL, Dam RJ, et al. A system for rapid DNA sequencing with fluorescent chain-terminating dideoxynucleotides. Science 1987; 238(4825):336–41.

35. ten Bosch JR, Grody WW. Keeping up with the next generation. J Mol Diagn 2008;10(6):484–92.

36. Liu L, Li Y, Li S, et al. Comparison of next-generation sequencing systems. J Biomed Biotechnol 2012;1–11.

37. Tucker T, Marra M, Friedman JM. Massively parallel sequencing: the next big thing in genetic medicine. Am J Hum Genet 2009;85(2):142–54.

38. Brown PO, Botstein D. Exploring the new world of the genome with DNA microarrays. Nat Genet 1999;21:33.

39. Cheung VG, Morley M, Aguilar F, et al. Making and reading microarrays. Nat Genet 1999;21:15.

40. Shaw-Smith C, Redon R, Rickman L, et al. Microarray based comparative genomic hybridisation (array-CGH) detects submicroscopic chromosomal deletions and duplications in patients with learning disability/mental retardation and dysmorphic features. J Med Genet 2004;41:241–8.

41. Subramonia-Iyer S, Sanderson S, Sagoo G, et al. Array-based comparative genomic hybridization for investigating chromosomal abnormalities in patients with learning disability: systematic review meta-analysis of diagnostic and false-positive yields. Genet Med 2007;9(2):74–9.

42. Cheng SH, Gregory RJ, Marshall J, et al. Defective intracellular transport and processing of CFTR is the molecular basis of most cystic fibrosis. Cell 1990;63(4):827–34.

43. Nicodemus KK, Law AJ, Radulescu E, et al. Biological validation of increased schizophrenia risk with NRG1, ERBB4, and AKT1 epistasis via functional neuroimaging in healthy controls. Arch Gen Psychiatry 2010;67(10):991–1001.

44. Schadt EE, Turner S, Kasarskis A. A window into third-generation sequencing. Hum Mol Genet 2010;19(2):R227–40.

45. Bigos KL, Weinberger DR. Imaging genetics - days of future past. Neuroimage 2010;53:804–9.

46. Knight SJ, Regan R, Nicod A, et al. Subtle chromosomal rearrangements in children with unexplained mental retardation. Lancet 1999;354:1676–81.

47. Handt M, Epplen A, Hoffjan S, et al. Point mutation frequency in the FMR1 gene as revealed by fragile X syndrome screening. Mol Cell Probes 2014. [Epub ahead of print].

48. Hegi ME, Diserens AC, Gorlia T, et al. MGMT Gene Silencing and Benefit from Temozolomide in Glioblastoma. N Engl J Med 2005;352:997–1003.

49. Zhaurova K. Genetic causes of adult-onset disorders. Nat Education 2008;1(1):49.

50. Huntington's Disease Collaborative Research Group. A novel gene containing a trinucleotide repeat that is expanded and unstable on Huntington's disease chromosomes. Cell 1993;72:971.

51. Lefebvre S, Bürglen L, Reboullet S, et al. Identification and characterization of a spinal muscular atrophy-determining gene. Cell 1995;80:155.

52. The TSC1 Consortium. Identification of the tuberous sclerosis gene TSC1 on chromosome 9q34. Science 1997;277:805.

53. Dyment DA, Herrera BM, Cader MZ, et al. Complex interactions among MHC haplotypes in multiple sclerosis: susceptibility and resistance. Hum Mol Genet 2005;14:2019–26.

54. George-Hyslop PH, Farrer LA, Goedert MM. Alzheimer disease and the frontotemporal dementias: diseases with cerebral deposition of fibrillar proteins. In: Valle D, Beaudet AL, Vogelstein B, et al, editors. OMMBID - the online metabolic and molecular bases of inherited diseases. New York: McGraw-Hill; 2014.

55. Stone EM, Fingert JH, Alward WL, et al. Identification of a gene that causes primary open angle glaucoma. Science 1997;275:668.

56. Noebels JL. The inherited epilepsies. In: Valle D, Beaudet AL, Vogelstein B, et al, editors. OMMBID - the online metabolic and molecular bases of inherited diseases. New York: McGraw-Hill; 2014.

57. Van der Vegt JP, Van Nuenen BF, Bloem BR, et al. Imaging the impact of genes on Parkinson's disease. Neuroscience 2009;164:191–204.

Molecular Imaging in Genetics

José Leite, MD, MBA, MSc[a],*, Roberta Hespanhol, MD[a], Carlos Alberto Buchpiguel, MD, PhD[b]

KEYWORDS

- Alzheimer disease • Parkinson disease • Genetics • PET imaging • Molecular imaging

KEY POINTS

- The effect of genes is not expressed at the level of mental behavior, but is mediated by molecular and cellular effects; therefore, molecular imaging is important.
- There is a need to shift from late intervention to prevention, targeting at-risk asymptomatic patients with disease-modifying drugs, when the potential for preservation of function is the greatest.
- Fluoro-[18F]-deoxyglucose positron emission tomography (FDG-PET) and amyloid PET imaging can be a marker of Alzheimer disease risk in patients carrying genetic related mutations.
- In Parkinson disease, prospective longitudinal assessment of nonmanifesting genetic at-risk patients will provide fundamental information about the natural history of the disease and possibly halt its progression.

INTRODUCTION

In recent years, with important advances in molecular genetics, neuroimaging has emerged as a potentially valuable tool to link individual differences in the human genome to structure and functional variation into brain system. This allows narrowing the gaps in the casual chain from a given genetic variation to a brain disorder. Considering that the effect of genes are not usually expressed directly at the level of mental behavior, but rather are mediated by their molecular and cellular effects, molecular imaging could play a key role on this regard.

This article reviews the literature using molecular imaging as an intermediate phenotype and/or biomarker for illness related to certain genetic alterations. Focus is on the two most common neurodegenerative disorders, Alzheimer's disease (AD) and Parkinson disease (PD).

ALZHEIMER'S DISEASE

AD is the most important cause of dementia and affects 1 in 10 individuals over the age of 65. By 2050, there will be an estimated 1 million new cases per year in the United States, increasing health care costs by around 85%.[1] Even if a prevention therapy has only a modest effect, it could provide an extraordinary public health benefit. For instance, a therapy that delays by 5 years the onset of this disorder could reduce the risk of it by one half.[2] It is estimated that in almost 50 years, a treatment modestly helpful, could reduce the prevalence of AD from 16 to 9 million cases and reduce costs from $750 to $425 billion per year.[3]

Amyloid plaques and neurofibrillary tangles are the most common neuropathologic hallmarks of AD and occur decades before symptoms. It is well known that the clinical diagnosis is not possible until a more advanced pathologic stage

The authors have nothing to disclose.
a PET/CT, Clínica de Diagnóstico Por Imagem (CDPI), Rio de Janeiro, Rio de Janeiro, Brazil; b Department of Nuclear Medicine and Molecular Imaging, São Paulo University (USP), São Paulo, Brazil
* Corresponding author. Clínica de Diagnóstico Por Imagem (CDPI & Multi-Imagem), Av. das Américas, 6205, Loja G, Barra da Tijuca, Rio de Janeiro, Brazil.
E-mail address: leite_jose@yahoo.com

of disease is reached.[4] Therefore, there is a need to shift the paradigm from late intervention (where treatment comes too late in the course of the disease) to prevention, targeting at-risk asymptomatic patients with disease-modifying drugs, when the potential for preservation of function is the greatest, and before irreversible synaptic and neuronal injury. Thus, it is necessary to identify individuals who are still cognitively normal, or who present mild symptoms (mild cognitive impairment) and have either a high risk for developing AD or are in a presymptomatic stage of disease.

Over one half of the risk for developing AD is owing to genetic factors, with heritability estimates in the range of 58% to 74%.[5] Case-control genome-wide association revealed a large number of genetics variants that have now been consistently associated with AD, and have been disclosed by meta-analyses of large number of studies worldwide.[6] Molecular neuroimaging, especially with fluoro-[18F]-deoxyglucose positron emission tomography (FDG-PET) and with amyloid-β peptides (Aβ) PET ligands have provided evidence for phenotypic differences in cognitively normal individuals under some genetics or heritable risks for AD. For instance, FDG-PET has been successfully used to demonstrate signs of AD pathology, predicting patients with mild cognitive impairment who will decline in cognition.[7] The FDG-PET pattern in AD demonstrates specific reductions in the cerebral metabolic rate of glucose (CMRglc) in the parietotemporal areas, posterior cingulate cortex (PCC) and medial temporal lobe, whereas cerebellum, striatum, basal ganglia, and primary visual and sensorimotor remain preserved.[8] AD can be divided into 2 groups by age of onset: Early onset, at less than 65 years (EOAD) and late onset, at greater than 65 years (LOAD), each having some known gene mutations.

Molecular Imaging and Early Onset Alzheimer's Disease

EOAD is very rare, accounting for approximately 1% of AD in the general population. Different autosomal-dominant genetic mutations located in 3 different genes have been firmly linked to this form: Amyloid precursor protein on chromosome 21, presenilin (PSEN1) on chromosome 14, and presenilin 2 (PSEN2) on chromosome 1. Although rare, these mutations have full penetrance in early age of onset, usually before 65 years old.[9] Some FDG-PET studies on cognitively normal individuals carrying these genetic mutations showed a slightly different AD pattern, characterized by global reductions of CMRglc, being more pronounced on parietotemporal, PCC, and medial temporal lobe (Table 1).

In addition to the typical AD pattern on FDG-PET, cognitively normal individuals carrying amyloid precursor protein mutations also present additional prefrontal CMRglc impairment (mild intensity).[10] The reductions in CMRglc in cognitively normal individuals carrying PSEN1 mutations not only precede clinical symptoms and structural brain changes, but also can be present up to 13 years before the onset of symptoms (Fig. 1).[12]

In symptomatic or cognitively normal individuals carrying amyloid precursor protein or PSEN mutations, Pittsburg Compound B (PiB) retention is

Table 1
FDG-PET studies on normal individuals carrying genetic mutations

Author, Year	N	Gene	Clinical Characteristics	Imaging Findings
Kennedy et al,[10] 1995	24	APP PSEN1	Mean MMSE, 29/30 (range, 25–30) Mean age, 44.7 y (range, 31–60)	↓CMRglc parietotemporal with additional minor dorsolateral prefrontal
Perani et al,[11] 1997	7	APP	Mean age, 34.6 y (range, 18–55) All subjects APOE 3/3	Significant ↓CMRglc parietotemporal and additional to dorsolateral prefrontal Thalamic impairment was seen
Mosconi et al,[12] 2006	7	PSEN1	Age range, 35–49 y MMSE range, 25–30 (5/7 with 30)	AD ↓CMRglc pattern preceding MRI signs of atrophy
Nikisch et al,[13] 2008	1	PSEN2	3-Year follow-up of a 48-year-old woman who had MMSE dropping from 28 to 0	At first presentation, MRI showed subtle changes, whereas FDG-PET showed marked ↓CMRglc on left parietal and precuneus cortex

Abbreviations: AD, Alzheimer's disease; APOE, apolipoprotein E; APP, amyloid precursor protein; CMRglc, cerebral metabolic rate of glucose; FDG-PET, fluoro-[18F]-deoxyglucose positron emission tomography; MMSE, Minnesota Mini Mental State Examination; PSEN, presenilin.

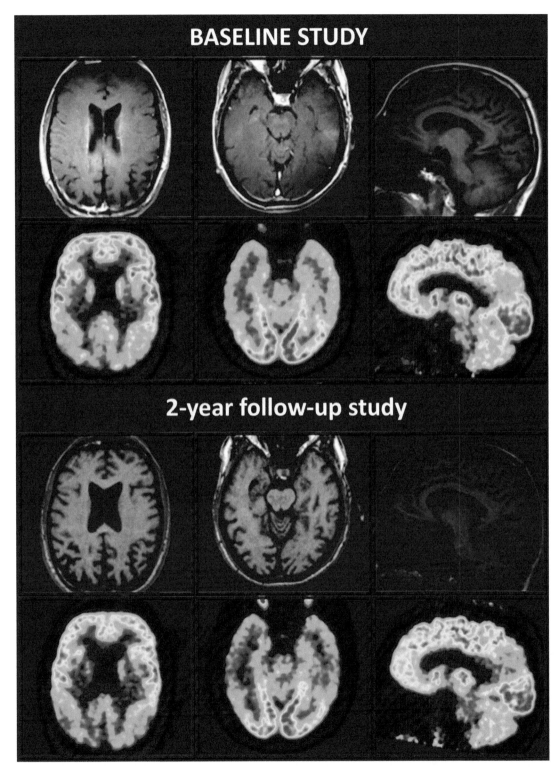

Fig. 1. A 56-year-old male, presenilin carrier presented with subjective memory complaint but not meeting criteria for mild cognitive impairment. The fluoro-[^{18}F]-deoxyglucose positron emission tomography image shows severe hypometabolism in the parietal, temporal, precuneus, and posterior cingulate cortex at the baseline study. No MRI signs of atrophy are identified on the corregistered images at this time. The same plane slices in a 2-year follow-up show greater glucose metabolism impairment of these cortex regions in addition to structural signs of sulci enlargement on MRI.

seen predominately in the striatum and PCC.[14] Unlike the situation in sporadic AD, these patients do not have as much as Aβ burden in the frontal and parietotemporal lobes, as well as the PCC (Table 2).

Molecular Imaging and Late-Onset Alzheimer's Disease

The evidence from EOAD individuals with genetic mutation studies provided not only important data about preclinical AD-related brain impairment, for instance, supporting the key role for Aβ in this disease, as well served as resource for studying the relationship between genetic and phenotypic expression of this disorder.

Different from the EOAD, LOAD represents the majority of the AD cases (99%) and does not seem to be associated with clearly discernible genetic mutations. LOAD has a complex polygenic (risk alleles), and nongenetic background (sociodemographic background [education level], lifestyle [diet, environmental], and medical history [medication, vascular disease], etc), which modifies not only age at onset, but also the course of disease. In most cases, genetic influence seems to be predominant.[18]

Molecular Imaging and apolipoprotein E ε4–associated genetic risk for late-onset Alzheimer's disease

The epsilon 4 allele (ε4) of apolipoprotein E (APOE) gene located in chromosome 19, is a well-recognized risk factor for LOAD, and not only accounts for the majority of LOAD cases, but is associated with an earlier age of onset compared with other genotypes.[19] Indeed, the ε4 gene dose

(ie, number of alleles in a person's APOE genotype) is associated with higher risk for developing AD. Individuals with a double dose of the ε4 have a 35-fold increase risk of developing the disease.[20]

Several FDG-PET studies have demonstrated the association between metabolic impairment in cognitively normal individuals carrying at least 1 ApoE ε4 allele compared with ε4 noncarriers. This metabolic impairment is characterized by a significant reduction on CMRglc in PCC/precuneus, parietotemporal, and prefrontal regions, the same as clinically affected AD patients.[21] Moreover, APOE ε4 homozygote carriers have significantly lower CMRglc in each of these brain regions, when compared with APOE ε4 heterozygotes and noncarriers, which shows that gene dose is a putative risk for brain metabolism impairment as well.[22] Even young adults (20–39 years old) who are ε4 carries have been detected to have low rates of CMRglc bilaterally in the posterior cingulate, parietotemporal, and prefrontal cortex, which may be the earliest brain abnormalities described, several decades before the possible onset of dementia.[23] Longitudinal studies showed that in cognitively normal late-middle-aged ε4 carries, the CMRglc impairment is progressive and correlates with future cognitive decline.[24,25] From a prevention research perspective, this leads to a paradigm for testing the potentials of treatment to prevent this disorder, without having to study thousands of subjects or wait many years to determine whether or when treated individuals develop symptoms.

Imaging Aβ burden PET ligands through PiB in middle-aged to old cognitively normal individuals revealed that fibrillar Aβ is significantly associated

Table 2
Symptomatic or normal individuals carrying APP or PSEN mutations

Author, Year	N	Gene	Clinical Characteristics	Imaging Findings
Klunk et al,[14] 2007	5	PSEN1	Age range, 35–45 y None of the patients were symptomatic	Increased striatum uptake with a relative lack of PiB retention in cortical areas
Remes et al,[15] 2008	2	APP	49-year-old man with MMSE 22/30 and 60-year-old woman with MMSE 17/30	Increased striatum and PCC uptake
Koivunen et al,[16] 2008	4	PSEN1	One woman and 3 men (mean age ± SD, 53.0 ± 5.5 y) MMSE were 14, 16, 24, and 27/30	Increased striatum, PCC and anterior cingulate gyrus
Knight et al,[17] 2011	7	PSEN1	Presymptomatic and mildly affected (MMSE ≥20)	Increased thalamus uptake; increased striatum uptake were seen, but in a minor intensity compared with previous studies

Abbreviations: AD, Alzheimer's disease; APP, amyloid precursor protein; MMSE, Minnesota Mini Mental State Examination; PCC, posterior cingulate cortex; PiB, Pittsburg Compound B; PSEN, presenilin.

with the APOE ε4 carrier status and ε4 gene dose in AD-affected mean cortical, frontal, temporal, PCC, precuneus, and basal ganglia (Fig. 2). Of interest, the homozygote ε4 carriers with mild cognitive impairment had an even greater fibrillar Aβ burden, comparable with the average in patients with probable AD.[26]

Molecular Imaging and family history risk for late-onset Alzheimer's disease

After advanced aged, family history (FH) is the second greatest risk factor for LOAD, even in the absence of known genetic mutations. Children of affected parents are especially at high risk of AD.[27] Although having one parent with AD is per se a major risk factor for developing AD in the offspring, maternal transmission may have a major impact than the paternal transmission.[28]

Recent FDG-PET studies showed phenotypic differences in CMRglc between cognitively normal individuals with a maternal FH (FHm), paternal FH (FHp), or negative FH for AD.[29] Reductions in

CMRglc were seen in the medial temporal lobe, parietotemporal, PCC, and frontal cortex, similar to the findings detected in clinical AD patients. Interestingly, this difference in CMRglc remained significant after accounting for potential risk factors, such as APOE ε4 genotype or the presence of subjective memory complaints. AD glucose metabolism pattern was found within the group of FHm subjects, irrespective of their APOE status. APOE ε4 FHm noncarriers had CMRglc reductions compared with the APOE ε4 noncarriers with an AD father and those with no parents affected. Moreover, FHm subjects have a progressive decline on CMRglc in the parietotemporal, PCC, and MTC as compared with FHp and no FH.[30] Again, this decline remained significant after accounting for potential risk factors as APOE ε4 genotype or the presence of subjective memory complaints. These findings on FHm raise the hypothesis that a combination of defective mitochondrial function, increased oxidative stress, and possible mitochondrial DNA mutations leads

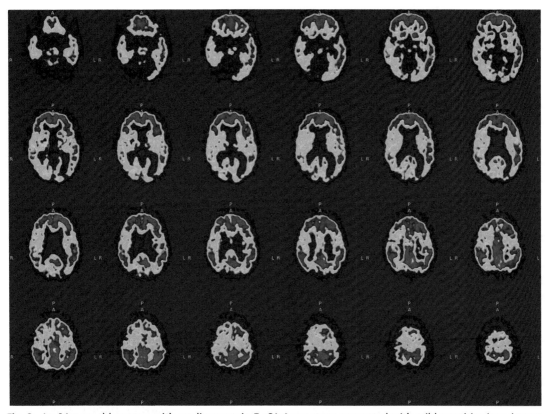

Fig. 2. An 84-year-old woman with apolipoprotein E e3/e4 genotype presented with mild cognitive impairment. The Pittsburgh compound B positron emission tomography axial slices through the brain show high amyloid burden in the anterior and posterior cingulate cortex, parietotemporal, and frontal cortices. (*Courtesy of* Dr G.K. von Schulthess and Dr F. Buck, Nuclear Medicine, University Hospital Zurich, Zurich, Switzerland; and Dr C. Hock, Psychiatry, University Hospital Zurich, Zurich, Switzerland.)

to the CMRglc alterations. The fact that mitochondrial DNA is entirely maternally inherited in humans support this hypothesis.[31]

A PiB-PET study showed that cognitively normal subjects with LOAD parents have high Aβ burden in brain regions typically affected in clinical AD, such as anterior and PCC, precuneus, parieto-temporal, occipital, and frontal cortices compared with cognitively normal subjects with no FH.[32] However, FHm subjects have increased and more widespread PiB retention than FHp subjects. Moreover, although both the FHp and FHm subjects showed increased PiB retention in the PCC and medial frontal gyrus, only FHm showed PiB retention in the lateral neocortex, which according to Braaks's neuropathologic staging[33] seems to be a sign of a more advanced stage of brain amyloidosis than FHp subjects.

PARKINSON DISEASE

Parkinson's disease (PD) is the second most common neurodegenerative disorder. Disease prevalence is age associated, with approximately 1% of the population being affected at 65 years, increasing to 4% to 5% at 85 years old.[34] The mean age of onset is about 70 years, although 4% of patients develop early-onset disease before the age of 50.[35]

The patients present some combination of motor symptoms, such as tremor at rest, bradykinesia, rigidity, and postural instability; the onset of PD is insidious, asymmetrical, and progressive. The most important pathologic finding in PD is the loss of dopaminergic neurons in the substantia nigra that project to the striatum, a central component of the basal ganglia, which is responsible for the initiation and control of movement. However, clinical symptoms only emerge when around 70% to 80% of nigrostrial nerve terminals have undergone degeneration.[36] The logical implication is that, for most patients, the neurodegenerative process has likely started well in advance of the first overt clinical motor symptoms, although the length of this presymptomatic period remains unknown.[37]

Although a heritable basis was originally thought unlikely, recent progress in neurogenetics of this disease provided evidence that genetic factors play a relevant role in the etiology of PD, beyond the influence of environmental factors, which are associated with an increased risk of PD.[38–40] The discovery of mutations in single genes that can cause autosomal-dominant (α-synuclein [SNCA]) and leucine-rich repeat kinase 2 (LRRK2) gene or recessive (Parkin, PTEN-induced putative kinase 1 [PINK1], DJ-1, and ATP13A2 gene) forms of PD

has provided advances in the molecular pathogenesis of PD, which has also benefited the neuroimaging area.

In symptomatic mutation carriers (ie, those with overt disease), brain mapping can help to link the molecular pathogenesis of PD more directly with functional and structural changes. In addition, neuroimaging of presymptomatic (ie, nonmanifesting) mutation carriers has emerged as a valuable tool to identify mechanisms of adaptive motor reorganization at the preclinical stage that may prevent or delay clinical manifestation.[37]

Monogenic Forms of Parkinson's Disease

Dominantly inherited mutations

The genes and chromosomal locus linked to familial autosomal dominant forms of PD include PARK 1(=4), 3, 5, 8, 11, and 13 (Table 3). Herein, we confine the explanation of genetic forms PARK 1 (SNCA) and 8 (LRRK2). Genetic studies of PD began with the discovery of pathogenic missense mutations in the gene *SNCA* that encodes α-synuclein, a protein that is expressed throughout the brain and believed to participate in the maturation of presynaptic vesicles and to function as a negative co-regulator of neurotransmitter release.

A number of families with Parkinsonism have been identified as carriers of single allele triplications (initially assigned as PARK4) or duplications of the wild type SNCA gene.[41] Penetrance has been described to be as low as 33%[42] and it implies that many carriers of a pathogenic genetic abnormality remain asymptomatic. It is believed also that neuroimaging may provide some of the answers and help to clarify the pathophysiologic substrate for this variable penetrance. For many of the SNCA-linked cases, the severity of the phenotype seems to depend on gene dosage, and patients with SNCA duplications clinically resemble "idiopathic" PD patients more than those with triplications, although the phenotypic spectrum can be remarkably broad.[37]

The genetic form PARK 1 has the early-onset Parkinsonism (around 40 years of age) and it is associated with cognitive decline, autonomic dysfunction, and dementia. The progression is more rapid in SNCA triplication cases.

Leucine-rich repeat kinase 2 (*LRRK2*) has been added to the list of genes that are implicated in PD. As for PARK 1, penetrance is incomplete and age dependent, so it has the same implications for neuroimaging as PARK1. Mutations in the LRRK2 gene are mostly associated with late-onset disease and the clinical phenotype is associated with dystonia, amyotrophic signs, gaze palsy, and occasionally dementia.

Table 3
Summary of well-established genetic forms of Parkinson disease

Locus (Chromosomal Position)	Gene	Mode of Inheritance	Age of Onset	Main Clinical Features	Pathology
PARK1/PARK4 (4q21-q23)	SNCA (alpha-Synuclein)	Autosomal dominant	38–65 y (duplications) and 24–48 y (triplications)	Cognitive decline, autonomic dysfunction and dementia	Diffuse Lewy bodies disease, with prominent nigral and hippocampal loss
PARK8 (12q12)	LRRK2	Autosomal dominant	Between 50–70 y	Parkinsonism consistent with sporadic; classical parkinsonism	Predominantly Lewy bodies, rare cases have only neurofibrillary tangles and/or nigral neuronal loss
PARK2(6q25.2-q27)	Parkin	Autosomal recessive	~30–40 y	Often presenting with dystonia, with diurnal fluctuations and sleep benefit; exquisite responsive to L-DOPA, slow disease progression	Predominantly nigral neuronal loss; compound heterozygotes with Lewy bodies or tau pathology are described
PARK6(1p35-p36)	PINK1 PTEN-induced putative kinase 1	Autosomal recessive	~30–40 y	Exquisite responsive to L-DOPA, slow disease progression	Undetermined
PARK7(1p36)	DJ-1	Autosomal recessive	~30–40 y	Slow disease progression, occasionally with behavioral or psychiatric disturbance	Undetermined

Abbreviation: L-DOPA, L-dopamine.

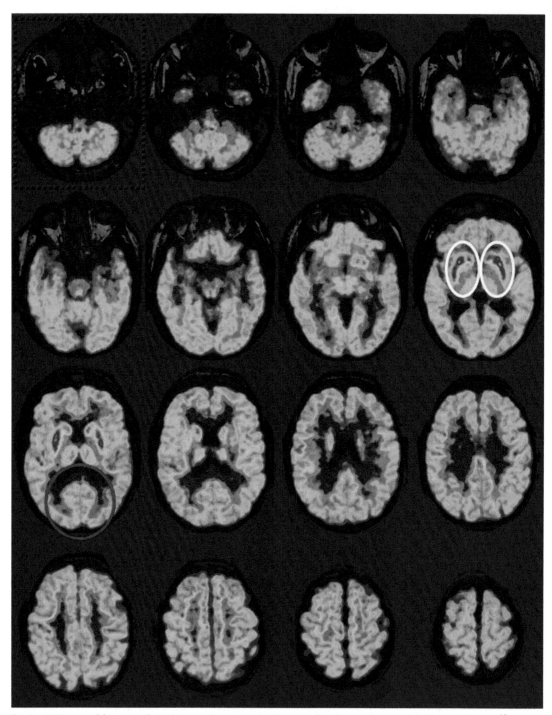

Fig. 3. A 64-year-old man with Parkinson disease and a history of hallucinations. Axial slices of fluoro-[18F]-deoxyglucose positron emission tomography (FDG-PET) and MR brain fused images show intense FDG uptake in the striatum (*white circle*). Reduced cerebral metabolic rate of glucose is seen in the parietotemporal cortex as well as the occipital (*red circle*).

LRRK2 is expressed in most brain regions, including the substantia nigra, caudate nucleus, and the putamen,[43] and it is unclear how LRRK2 substitutions result in neuropathology. Then, further genetic and functional studies are necessary to identify LRRK2 disease modifiers, either genetic or environmental, which influence age of onset and the disparate clinical and pathologic presentations.[41]

Recessively inherited mutations
Three recessive forms of Parkinsonism have been identified, including homozygous and compound heterozygous mutations in the genes that encode Parkin, oncogene DJ1, and PTEN-induced kinase 1 (*PINK1*).[44–46] All are relatively rare, present early (around 40 years of age), respond to L-dopamine (L-DOPA), and show slow clinical progression. These forms of Parkinsonism tend to result in a more selective loss of dopaminergic neurons than that associated with sporadic, late-onset PD.[41]

Molecular Imaging of Dopaminergic Neurotransmission in Monogenetic Forms of Parkinsonism

PD is typically associated with increased glucose metabolism or blood flow in the basal ganglia and thalamus coupled with reductions in the supplementary motor, premotor, and temporo–parietal–occipital cortex. Involvement of the occipital cortex may be related to the occurrence of hallucinations (Fig. 3). Glucose metabolism and blood flow are also increased in the pons and cerebellum.[47] This pattern is distinct from those seen in other disorders resulting in Parkinsonism, such as multiple system atrophy (basal ganglia and cerebellar hypometabolism), progressive supranuclear palsy (brainstem and medial frontal cortical hypometabolism), and corticobasal degeneration (asymmetric cortical and basal ganglia hypometabolism).[48]

Because the changes on structural imaging are limited, the abnormalities of symptomatic and nonsymptomatic mutation carriers of PD can be detected with imaging techniques such as PET or single photon emission computed tomography, beside functional MRI. Some radiotracers have been used to evaluate the presynaptic and postsynaptic nigrostriatal integrity (Table 4).[37]

Radiotracers and changes in symptomatic patients
Studies in symptomatic mutation carriers that have used 6-[18F]fluoro-L-3,4-dihydroxyphenyla-lanine ([18F]F-DOPA) showed significant reduction of presynaptic [18F]-F-DOPA uptake (Fig. 4). Symptomatic patients with the sporadic form of PD also show a reduction in striatal [18F]F-DOPA uptake, as well as a marked reduction in striatal vesicular monoamine transporter type 2 (VMAT2) and dopamine transporter (DAT) binding, beside a caudorostral gradient with a stronger impairment of presynaptic dopaminergic function in putamen compared with the caudate nucleus. However, the presynaptic changes in Parkin and PINK1 mutation carriers tend to be symmetric pattern and in Parkin mutation carriers the [18F]F-DOPA PET revealed a slower progression in presynaptic dysfunction compared with sporadic PD.

The postsynaptic function can be studied using several radiolabeled agonist or antagonist ligands. Some ligands have been developed to study the dopamine D2 receptor. High-affinity antagonists, such as spiperone (labeled with either 11C or

Table 4
Radiotracer presynaptic and postsynaptic nigrostriatal integrity of positron emission tomography (PET) and single photon emission computed tomography (SPECT)

	Presynaptic Nigrostriatal Integrity	Postsynaptic Nigrostriatal Integrity
PET	[18F]-fluoro-L-DOPA [11C]-dihydrotetrabenazine (DTBZ) [11C]-2-β-carbomethoxy-3-β-[4-fluorophenyl]tropane [11C]-d-threomethylphenidate [18F]-N-3-fluoropropyl-2-β-carboxymethoxy-3-β- (4-iodophenyl) ortropane ([18F] FPCIT)	[11C]-raclopride [18F]-benperidol [18F]/[11C]-spiperone [11C]-PHNO [11C]N-propyl-norapomorphine
SPECT	[123I]FP-CITc [2-[[2-[[[3-(4-chlorophenyl)-8-methyl-8-azabicyclo [3.2.1]octyl]methyl](2-mercaptoethyl)amino]ethyl] amino]ethanethiolato-(3-)-N2,N2=,S2,S2=] oxo- [1R-(exo-exo)]-[99mTc]technetium ([99mTc]TRODAT-1)	[123I]-iodobenzamide (IBZM)

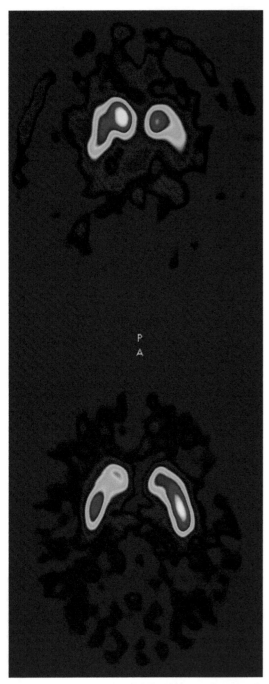

Fig. 4. A 62-year-old man with tremor predominantly on the right side. *Top*: Fluorodopa (FDOPA), imaging 80 to 90 minutes, shows reduced uptake in the left striatum, predominantly in the putamen. *Bottom*: C-11 raclopride, imaging 40 to 50 minutes, shows increased uptake in the left putamen. The findings are consistent with Parkinson disease. (*Courtesy of Dr G.K. von Schulthess and Dr F. Buck, Nuclear Medicine, University Hospital Zurich, Zurich, Switzerland; and Dr C. Hock, Psychiatry, University Hospital Zurich, Zurich, Switzerland.*)

18F) or 18F-labeled benperidol,[49] bind equally to high- and low-affinity states of the receptor and are not sensitive to occupancy by endogenous dopamine. In contrast, [11C]raclopride has a lower affinity, and its binding is accordingly affected by changes in the availability of synaptic dopamine (see **Fig. 4**).[50,51] Agonists such as [11C]N-propyl-norapomorphine or [11C]-labeled PHNO may be used to estimate changes in synaptic dopamine.[47]

Because patients with mutations in PARK 1, 6, and 8 were subjected to studies with [11C] raclopride, the postsynaptic function resulted within normal range. The postsynaptic function was also preserved in patients with mutation in PARK6 the single photon emission computed tomography using [123I]-IBZM. However, patients with mutation in PARK2 and treated with levodopa showed a decrease in striatal raclopide binding.

Therefore, the results of PET in patients with monogenic forms of PD, similar to those found in sporadic forms, have shown loss of presynaptic dopaminergic nigrostriatal integrity without accompanying postsynaptic neurodegeneration.

Radiotracers and changes in asymptomatic patients

There are few studies of PET and single photon emission computed tomography in this context, although functional imaging can detect dopamine dysfunction in asymptomatic individuals. The first demonstration of this was done in subjects exposed to the nigral toxin N-methyl-4-phenyl-1,2,3,6-tetrahydropyridine, in whom [18F]F-DOPA uptake was reduced in subjects who were clinically normal.[52]

Consistent presynaptic abnormalities in striatal dopaminergic neurotransmission were demonstrated in nonmanifesting carriers of single heterozygous mutations in PARK2 and PARK6, as indexed by a mild decrease in striatal DAT binding[53] or presynaptic [18F]F-DOPA uptake.[54] In LRRK2 mutations (PARK8), PET imaging with multiple tracers showed reduced striatal DAT binding in 2 nonmanifesting mutation carriers, whereas another 2 were initially normal but later developed a decrease in DAT binding after 4 years of follow-up.[55] The reduction in striatal DAT binding occurred in the absence of any change in striatal [18F]F-DOPA uptake, suggesting that mapping striatal DAT binding is more sensitive to a subclinical loss of nigrostriatal dopaminergic afferents than mapping regional [18F]F-DOPA uptake.

It was also noted that, in Parkin nonmanifesting mutation carriers, an inverse relationship is seen between PET and MRI findings. MRI showed a bilateral increase in the volume of gray matter in the posterior putamen and internal globus pallidus, and [18F]F-DOPA PET showed regional decreases in the same regions. This "hypertrophy" can be maintained only partially in the symptomatic stage of PD, but regression analyses revealed bilateral gray matter decreases in the basal ganglia in symptomatic Parkin mutation carriers, suggesting that the basal ganglia are subject to a progressive atrophy, which gradually increases with disease severity and duration.[37] In asymptomatic individuals, the postsynaptic dopaminergic function of the basal ganglia seems to be different from the presynaptic, which seems to be normal.

The presence of a mutation in 1 gene of the PD may lead to changes in presynaptic dopaminergic function, without leading to clinical manifestation. It is suggested that there are mechanisms of adaptive presynaptic and apparently not present on postsynaptic that compensate for the loss of dopamine in the striatum.

SUMMARY

Because the effect of genes are not expressed directly at the level of behavior, but rather are mediated by their molecular and cellular effects, molecular imaging can play a key role on narrowing the gaps in the casual chain from a given genetic variation to a brain disorder. The well-established FDG-PET pattern of reduced parietotemporal, PCC, precuneus, and prefrontal cortex CMRglc has high accuracy in distinguishing AD from controls, as well as in discriminating individuals at higher versus lower AD risk. For individuals carrying EOAD mutations, this same pattern appears in presymptomatic subjects and is a well-established biomarker of disease. Moreover, for at-risk LOAD subjects, more longitudinal studies have to be conducted to understand where the subtle line is that divides this pattern as an endophenotype or a biomarker of disease. Nonetheless, this pattern can be seen as a marker of AD risk.

Despite some patterns differences in EOAD and LOAD at-risk subjects, increased brain Aβ burden is seen using amyloid plaque ligands, and can be a promising strategy, to combine the sensitivity of FDG-PET with pathology-specific Aβ measurements. Once available, these molecular imaging techniques can be of great value for detecting the earliest signs of AD, before symptoms appear. Therefore, in the future one might be able to interfere in the natural history of the disease.

For PD, the prospective longitudinal assessment of patients nonmanifesting mutation carriers and manifesting mutation carriers will provide fundamental information of the natural history of the disease and possibly to halt the progression of it.

REFERENCES

1. Brookmeyer R, Johnson E, Ziegler-Graham K, et al. Forecasting the global burden of Alzheimer's disease. Alzheimers Dement 2007;3:186–91.
2. Khachaturian Z. The five-five, ten-ten plan for Alzheimer's disease. Neurobiol Aging 1992;2:197–8.
3. Brookmeyer R, Gray S, Kawas C. Projections of Alzheimer's disease in the United States and the public health impact of delaying disease onset. Am J Public Health 1998;88(9):1337–42.
4. Larson EB, Shadlen MF, Wang L, et al. Survival after initial diagnosis of Alzheimer disease. Ann Intern Med 2004;140(7):501–9.
5. Braskie MN, Ringman JM, Thompson PM. Neuroimaging measures as endophenotypes in Alzheimer's disease. Int J Alzheimers Dis 2011;2011:490140.
6. Nussbaum RL. Genome-wide association studies, Alzheimer disease, and understudied populations. JAMA 2013;309(14):1527–8.
7. Anchisi D, Borroni B, Franceschi M, et al. Heterogeneity of brain glucose metabolism in mild cognitive impairment and clinical progression to Alzheimer disease. Arch Neurol 2005;62(11):1728–33.
8. Silverman DH, Small GW, Chang CY, et al. Positron emission tomography in evaluation of dementia: Regional brain metabolism and long-term outcome. JAMA 2001;286(17):2120–7.
9. Tanzi RE, Bertram L. New frontiers in Alzheimer's disease genetics. Neuron 2001;32(2):181–4.
10. Kennedy AM, Frackowiak RS, Newman SK, et al. Deficits in cerebral glucose metabolism demonstrated by positron emission tomography in individuals at risk of familial Alzheimer's disease. Neurosci Lett 1995; 186(1):17–20.
11. Perani D, Grassi F, Sorbi S, et al. PET study in subjects from two Italian FAD families with APP717 Val to Ileu mutation. Eur J Neurol 1997;4:214–20.
12. Sorbi S, de Leon MJ, de Leon MJ, et al. Hypometabolism exceeds atrophy in presymptomatic early-onset familial Alzheimer's disease. J Nucl Med 2006;47(11):1778–86.
13. Nikisch G, Hertel A, Kiessling B, et al. Three-year follow-up of a patient with early-onset Alzheimer's disease with presenilin-2 N141I mutation - case report and review of the literature. Eur J Med Res 2008;13(12):579–84.
14. Klunk WE, Price JC, Mathis CA, et al. Amyloid deposition begins in the striatum of presenilin-1 mutation carriers from two unrelated pedigrees. J Neurosci 2007;27(23):6174–84.
15. Remes AM, Laru L, Tuominen H, et al. Carbon 11-labeled Pittsburgh compound B positron emission tomographic amyloid imaging in patients with APP locus duplication. Arch Neurol 2008;65(4):540–4.
16. Koivunen J, Pirttilä T, Kemppainen N, et al. PET amyloid ligand [11C]PIB uptake and cerebrospinal

fluid beta-amyloid in mild cognitive impairment. Dement Geriatr Cogn Disord 2008;26(4):378–83.

17. Knight WD, Okello AA, Ryan NS, et al. Carbon-11-Pittsburgh compound B positron emission tomography imaging of amyloid deposition in presenilin 1 mutation carriers. Brain 2011;134:293–300.

18. Gatz M, Reynolds CA, Fratiglioni L, et al. Role of genes and environments for explaining Alzheimer disease. Arch Gen Psychiatry 2006;63(2):168–74.

19. Laws SM, Hone E, Gandy S, et al. Expanding the association between the APOE gene and the risk of Alzheimer's disease: possible roles for APOE promoter polymorphisms and alterations in APOE transcription. J Neurochem 2003;84(6):1215–36.

20. Genin E, Hannequin D, Wallon D, et al. APOE and Alzheimer disease: a major gene with semi-dominant inheritance. Mol Psychiatry 2011;16(9):903–7.

21. Reiman EM, Caselli RJ, Yun LS, et al. Preclinical evidence of Alzheimer's disease in persons homozygous for the epsilon 4 allele for apolipoprotein E. N Engl J Med 1996;334(12):752–8.

22. Reiman EM, Chen K, Alexander GE, et al. Correlations between apolipoprotein E epsilon4 gene dose and brain-imaging measurements of regional hypometabolism. Proc Natl Acad Sci U S A 2005;102(23):8299–302.

23. Reiman EM, Chen K, Alexander GE, et al. Functional brain abnormalities in young adults at genetic risk for late-onset Alzheimer's dementia. Proc Natl Acad Sci U S A 2004;101(1):284–9.

24. Small GW, Ercoli LM, Silverman DH, et al. Cerebral metabolic and cognitive decline in persons at genetic risk for Alzheimer's disease. Proc Natl Acad Sci U S A 2000;97(11):6037–42.

25. Reiman EM, Caselli RJ, Chen K, et al. Declining brain activity in cognitively normal apolipoprotein E epsilon 4 heterozygotes: A foundation for using positron emission tomography to efficiently test treatments to prevent Alzheimer's disease. Proc Natl Acad Sci U S A 2001;98(6):3334–9.

26. Reiman EM, Chen K, Liu X, et al. Fibrillar amyloid-beta burden in cognitively normal people at 3 levels of genetic risk for Alzheimer's disease. Proc Natl Acad Sci U S A 2009;106(16):6820–5.

27. Green RC, Cupples LA, Go R, et al. Risk of dementia among white and African American relatives of patients with Alzheimer disease. JAMA 2002;287(3):329–36.

28. Gómez-Tortosa E, Barquero MS, Barón M, et al. Variability of age at onset in siblings with familial Alzheimer disease. Arch Neurol 2007;64(12):1743–8.

29. Mosconi L, Brys M, Switalski R, et al. Maternal family history of Alzheimer's disease predisposes to reduced brain glucose metabolism. Proc Natl Acad Sci U S A 2007;104(48):19067–72.

30. Mosconi L, Mistur R, Switalski R, et al. Declining brain glucose metabolism in normal individuals with a maternal history of Alzheimer disease. Neurology 2009;72(6):513–20.

31. Lin MT, Beal MF. Mitochondrial dysfunction and oxidative stress in neurodegenerative diseases. Nature 2006;443(7113):787–95.

32. Mosconi L, Rinne JO, Tsui WH, et al. Increased fibrillar amyloid-{beta} burden in normal individuals with a family history of late-onset Alzheimer's. Proc Natl Acad Sci U S A 2010;107(13):5949–54.

33. Braak H, Braak E. Neuropathological staging of Alzheimer-related changes. Acta Neuropathol 1991;82(4):239–59.

34. Fahn S. Description of Parkinson's disease as a clinical syndrome. Ann N Y Acad Sci 2003;991:1–14.

35. Van Den Eeden SK, Tanner CM, Bernstein AL, et al. Incidence of Parkinson's disease: variation by age, gender, and race/ethnicity. Am J Epidemiol 2003;157(11):1015–22.

36. Bernheimer H, Birkmayer W, Hornykiewicz O, et al. Brain dopamine and the syndromes of Parkinson and Huntington. Clinical, morphological and neurochemical correlations. J Neurol Sci 1973;20(4):415–55.

37. van der Vegt JP, van Nuenen BF, Bloem BR, et al. Imaging the impact of genes on Parkinson's disease. Neuroscience 2009;164(1):191–204.

38. Firestone JA, Smith-Weller T, Franklin G, et al. Pesticides and risk of Parkinson disease: a population-based case-control study. Arch Neurol 2005;62(1):91–5.

39. Jankovic J. Searching for a relationship between manganese and welding and Parkinson's disease. Neurology 2005;64(12):2021–8.

40. Priyadarshi A, Khuder SA, Schaub EA, et al. Environmental risk factors and Parkinson's disease: a metaanalysis. Environ Res 2001;86(2):122–7.

41. Farrer MJ. Genetics of Parkinson disease: paradigm shifts and future prospects. Nat Rev Genet 2006;7(4):306–18.

42. Nishioka K, Hayashi S, Farrer MJ, et al. Clinical heterogeneity of alpha-synuclein gene duplication in Parkinson's disease. Ann Neurol 2006;59(2):298–309.

43. Zimprich A, Biskup S, Leitner P, et al. Mutations in LRRK2 cause autosomal-dominant parkinsonism with pleomorphic pathology. Neuron 2004;44(4):601–7.

44. Valente EM, Abou-Sleiman PM, Caputo V, et al. Hereditary early-onset Parkinson's disease caused by mutations in PINK1. Science 2004;304(5674):1158–60.

45. Kitada T, Asakawa S, Hattori N, et al. Mutations in the parkin gene cause autosomal recessive juvenile parkinsonism. Nature 1998;392(6676):605–8.

46. Bonifati V, Rizzu P, van Baren MJ, et al. Mutations in the DJ-1 gene associated with autosomal recessive early-onset parkinsonism. Science 2003;299(5604):256–9.

47. Stoessl AJ. Neuroimaging in Parkinson's disease. Neurotherapeutics 2011;8(1):72–81.

48. Eckert T, Barnes A, Dhawan V. FDG PET in the differential diagnosis of parkinsonian disorders. Neuro-image 2005;26(3):912–21.

49. Moerlein SM, Perlmutter JS, Markham J, et al. In vivo kinetics of [18F](N-methyl)benperidol: a novel PET tracer for assessment of dopaminergic D2-like receptor binding. J Cereb Blood Flow Metab 1997; 17(8):833–45.

50. Seeman P, Guan HC, Niznik HB. Endogenous dopamine lowers the dopamine D2 receptor density as measured by [3H]raclopride: implications for positron emission tomography of the human brain. Synapse 1989;3(1):96–7.

51. Laruelle M. Imaging synaptic neurotransmission with in vivo binding competition techniques: a critical review. J Cereb Blood Flow Metab 2000; 20(3):423–51.

52. Calne DB, Langston JW, Martin WR. Positron emission tomography after MPTP: observations relating to the cause of Parkinson's disease. Nature 1985; 317(6034):246–8.

53. Pellecchia MT, Varrone A, Annesi G, et al. Parkinsonism and essential tremor in a family with pseudo-dominant inheritance of PARK2: an FP-CIT SPECT study. Mov Disord 2007;22(4):559–63.

54. Hilker R, Klein C, Ghaemi M, et al. Positron emission tomographic analysis of the nigrostriatal dopaminergic system in familial parkinsonism associated with mutations in the parkin gene. Ann Neurol 2001;49(3):367–76.

55. Adams JR, van Netten H, Schulzer M, et al. PET in LRRK2 mutations: comparison to sporadic Parkinson's disease and evidence for presymptomatic compensation. Brain 2005;128(Pt 12): 2777–85.

Brain Imaging and Genetic Risk in the Pediatric Population, Part 1
Inherited Metabolic Diseases

Maria Gabriela Longo, MD[a], Filippo Vairo, MD, MSc[b,c],
Carolina Fischinger Souza, MD[b], Roberto Giugliani, MD, PhD[b,d],
Leonardo Modesti Vedolin, MD, PhD[a,e],*

KEYWORDS

- Brain imaging • MRI • Magnetic resonance • Inborn errors of metabolism • Genetics
- Metabolic disorder

KEY POINTS

- Inherited metabolic diseases (IMD) form a group of disorders, mostly genetically inherited, caused by abnormal protein formations.
- One strategy to increase the accuracy of neuroimaging in IMD is to compare the genetic information (genotype) with the imaging phenotype detected by MRI (MR phenotype).
- Some MR phenotypes are related to specific gene mutations, such as bilateral hypertrophy of inferior olives in patients harboring POLG and SURF1 mutations, and central lesions in the cervical spinal cord in nonketotic hyperglycinemia patients harboring GLRX5 gene mutation.
- From a neuroimaging point of view, a desirable scenario of the future could be using brain imaging, such as advanced MRI, as a biomarker (MR phenotype) to predict the most probable genetic abnormality of a specific neurologic disease (genotype).

INTRODUCTION

Significant advances in imaging of the structure and function of the brain, brainstem, and cerebellum have been made in the last decades.[1–6] High-resolution MRI and diffusion tensor imaging have been extensively used in both clinical and neurosciences settings, expanding and redefining the applications of modern neuroimaging techniques. An example of this issue can be clearly found in the malformation of the cerebral cortex, in which development of MRI technology associated with a better understanding of embryology, neurodevelopment, and neurogenetics has dramatically changed the way researchers classified these diseases.[7–10]

Equal achievements occurred in our understanding of the human genome and its role in normal and abnormal development of the central nervous system (CNS).[11–15] From a biological perspective, the identification of a genetic abnormality can improve our understanding of the mechanism of specific diseases. From a clinical

The authors have nothing to disclose.
[a] Radiology Service, Hospital de Clínicas de Porto Alegre, Porto Alegre, Rio Grande do Sul, Brazil; [b] Medical Genetics Service, Hospital de Clínicas de Porto Alegre, Porto Alegre, Rio Grande do Sul, Brazil; [c] Post Graduation Program on Genetics and Molecular Biology, Universidade Federal do Rio Grande do Sul, Porto Alegre, Rio Grande do Sul, Brazil; [d] Department of Genetics, Universidade Federal do Rio Grande do Sul, Porto Alegre, Rio Grande do Sul, Brazil; [e] Post Graduation Program on Medical Sciences: Medicine, Department of Internal Medicine, Universidade Federal do Rio Grande do Sul, Porto Alegre, Rio Grande do Sul, Brazil
* Corresponding author. Rua Carlos Trein Filho, 909 ap 502, Porto Alegre, Rio Grande do Sul 90450-120, Brazil.
E-mail address: lvedolin@hcpa.ufrgs.br

neuroimaging.theclinics.com

perspective, a genetic diagnosis could optimize diagnosis, prognosis, and treatment of neurologic disorders.

In this context, imaging and genetic studies have been predominant in the investigation of many pediatric neurologic disorders, particularly congenital malformations of the CNS (CMCNS) and inherited metabolic disorders (IMD).[6,16–21] Linking genetic data and neuroimaging phenotype is an emerging approach in neuroscience to better understand the complex imaging appearance of these disorders. From a neuroimaging point of view, a desirable scenario of the future could be using brain imaging, such as advanced MRI, as a biomarker (MR phenotype) to predict the most probable genetic abnormality of a specific neurologic disease (genotype). This approach could be useful to both neuroscientists (better genetic-neuroimaging integration) and clinical physicians (better approach to neurologic diseases), making imaging a better diagnostic tool for more effective treatment and prognosis definition.

In this article, the genotype-MR phenotype correlation of the most common or clinical relevant IMD and CMCNS in the pediatric population are reviewed. Although many disorders could be included in this review, the data focus on the most commonly diagnosed diseases and those in which the neuroimaging abnormalities are better defined. The PubMed/Medline database was searched with a combination of key words such as "genotype-phenotype correlation," "genotype-imaging correlation", and "neuroimaging-genetic correlation" in both IMD and CMCNS. The searches were limited to articles in English and those with abstracts. After the searches were conducted, the abstracts of the returned articles were examined, to determine their applicability for review. Relevant studies were defined liberally to be those that included any discussion about correlation of neuroimaging and a genetic abnormality in both IMD (part 1) and CMCNS (part 2 elsewhere in this issue). A review of the general rules of genotype-phenotype correlation is included in this review (part 1), because we believe that knowledge of the principles of medical genetics is essential for every neuroscientist (including radiologists).

GENOTYPE-PHENOTYPE CORRELATION

In neurosciences, few topics have advanced as fast as neurogenetics.[11–15] Data from the last 20 years in recombinant DNA technology and polymerase chain reaction (PCR) linkage studies significantly increase the number of neurologic disease genes identification, but identifying genes for both autosomal dominant and recessive diseases has been challenging. However, the advent of next-generation sequencing (NGS) with the whole genome sequencing (WGS), target sequencing, and whole exome sequencing (WES) has dramatically changed this scenario. These new techniques are emerging as a tool to facilitate cost-effective molecular diagnoses in routine clinical care of these disorders.

As a rule, most genes have been identified by defining a candidate gene by both its chromosomal location and its proprieties. Gene identification was based on methods in which the chromosomal location of the disease locus was not required (positional-independent strategies) and those that depended on this knowledge (positional cloning). In the former, gene identification was achieved based on thorough knowledge of the protein product, DNA sequence, or its normal function. In the latter, disease genes were identified using only knowledge of their approximate chromosomal location. Although both strategies are separate in principle, most commonly, geneticists and neuroscientists use a combination of both sets of information to identify a potential genetic variation. The most often used tool is based on NGS (as WGS and WES) and genome-wide association studies. There are some bioinformatics tools that help researchers to predict if a genomic variation could be damaged, but all variations should be tested with functional studies to ensure that they are related to a good candidate gene consistent with the disease phenotype.

In this context, the association between the presence of a certain mutation or mutations (genotype) and the resulting physical trait, abnormality, or pattern of abnormalities (phenotype) has been studied as a promising investigational tool. Several general principles have emerged as a result of the intensive study of causative variations in genetic disorders.

According to the Mendelian paradigm, a specific disease is caused by mutations in a single gene. Because there are 2 alternative forms of any given gene (alleles), a genetic disease can occur if a mutated allele was inherited from the father or from the mother (autosomal dominant transmission) or if both mutated alleles were inherited from the parents (autosomal recessive transmission). However, even single gene (monogenic) diseases can manifest with a wide range of symptoms, severity, and prognostic issues, which is called variable expressivity.

However, most neurologic disorders are complex (multifactorial) and not monogenic disorders. There are variations in the genome that are more frequent in the population (polymorphisms) and that can play a role in several common diseases, whenever they occur in a particular combination with an overall effect that causes a biochemical/biological pathologic condition. Environmental effects can also contribute to the pathophysiology of some neurologic diseases.

There are several limitations for the genotype-phenotype correlation. For example, mutations in the same gene may be responsible for more than 1 disease. In the same context, mutations in a single gene (allelic heterogeneity) can cause different and distinct clinical phenotypes and, on the other hand, there are many similar clinical phenotypes caused by mutations in different genes (nonallelic heterogeneity or genetic heterogeneity). Also, mutations in more than 1 gene may be required to express a given clinical phenotype (digenic inheritance or triallelic inheritance), and different mutations in the same gene may give rise to distinct dominant and recessive forms of the same disease. The definition of the phenotype is mostly qualitative, being either present or absent, which could be a confounder in establishing a genotype-phenotype correlation of a specific disease.

NEUROIMAGING IN INHERITED METABOLIC DISORDERS

IMD are a group of diseases caused by abnormal protein formations as a result of a gene mutation. These anomalous proteins disrupt the function of 1 or more metabolic pathways. The diagnosis of these disorders is a challenge, and usually, the clinical presentation is variable. As a result, most patients do not receive a diagnosis, despite the investigation. Although most IMD cannot be treated, a specific diagnosis is critical for some treatable metabolic diseases and also for proper genetic counseling.

Because of its high sensitivity in detecting changes in myelination, structural damage, and specific patterns of brain involvement, MRI techniques (structural imaging, diffusion imaging, and proton spectroscopy) are the modalities of choice to investigate patients with inborn errors of metabolism (IEM). However, imaging interpretation is complex. As a rule, it demands the knowledge of many radiologic signs, age of onset of the disease, genetic pattern, and recognition of the most important clinical findings.

Strategies to increase the accuracy of neuroimaging in IEM, such as systematic analysis of the pattern of CNS involvement and the discriminating MRI pattern approach, have been described.[19,22,23] With recent advance in genetic and neuroimaging technology, it is becoming possible to compare the genetic information

(genotype) with the imaging phenotype detected by MRI (MR phenotype).[24–27] The goal is to identify specific MRI phenotypic changes related to a particular genetic abnormality. Although difficult to achieve, there is a potential benefit of this strategy to reduce the differential diagnosis, guide clinical decisions, and reduce cost of additional tests, including imaging and genetic tools.

MR PHENOTYPE-GENOTYPE CORRELATION IN DISORDERS INVOLVING ENERGY METABOLISM

This group includes disorders with clinical findings related to a deficiency in energy production or utilization, such as mitochondrial defects, disorders of glycolysis, glycogen metabolism, gluconeogenesis, and creatine metabolism. Most of the genotype-MR phenotype of this group is related to mitochondrial respiratory chain defect disorders.

The mitochondrion is a highly specialized organelle occurring in almost all eukaryotic cells producing cellular energy through oxidative phosphorylation (OXPHOS). Its role depends on a complex relationship between the mitochondrial genome (mtDNA) and the nuclear genome (nDNA), and the nDNA has a fundamental role for most of the OXPHOS system, for maintaining and replicating mtDNA and also for the organelle network proliferation and destruction. Almost 100 structural OXPHOS subunit genes have been identified, and approximately 80% are encoded by the nuclear genome, including the complex I-V subunits.

Defects in either the mtDNA or nDNA are responsible for mitochondrial diseases (a group of genetically and phenotypically diverse disorders). With a prevalence of 1 in 10,000 newborns, the diagnosis should be considered when a patient presents with a progressive course involving seemingly unrelated organs.[28] A wide variety of neurologic manifestations such as optic atrophy, seizures, strokelike episodes, ataxia, and neuropathy can be present. A detailed family history is important; a clear maternal inheritance (without male transmission) indicates a primary mtDNA defect, whereas an autosomal inheritance pattern indicates nDNA interaction.

Neuroimaging of patients with mitochondrial diseases usually shows focal or diffuse lesions in the cerebral cortex, white matter, basal ganglia, and brainstem.[22,23] Restricted diffusion and lactate peak on MR spectroscopy are also common (Figs. 1 and 2). Cerebral and cerebellar atrophy appears in patients with longer disease duration. In many cases, blood or cerebrospinal fluid (CSF) lactate concentration, cardiac evaluation, and muscle biopsy for histologic or

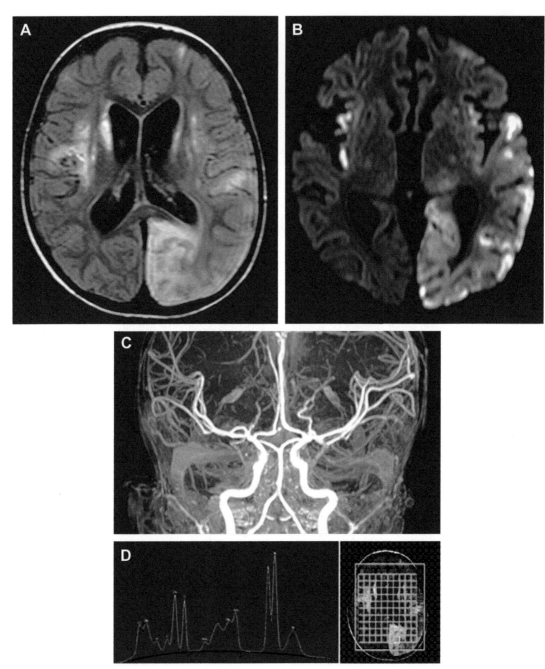

Fig. 1. Mitochondriopathy related to deficiency of complex IV. (*A*) Axial FLAIR MRI shows abnormal hyperintensity signal lesions in basal ganglia and left cortical occipital and parietal lobes, brain atrophy, and ventriculomegaly. (*B*) Diffusion-weighted MRI shows restricted diffusion at the same location. (*C*) Magnetic resonance angiography shows no vascular occlusion or stenosis. (*D*) Magnetic resonance spectroscopy with lactate peak in the cortex.

histochemical evidence can indicate mitochondrial disease. However, establishing a molecular genetic diagnosis is preferred.

Specific genes are known to be responsible for some mitochondrial respiratory chain defect disorders, although different mutations in the same gene can cause a variety of diseases (Table 1). A genetic review of all genes related to mitochondrial disorders, including mutations associated with complex I-V deficiencies, is beyond the scope of this article, but a review of 1 gene (POLG) is useful to understand the complexity of this issue.

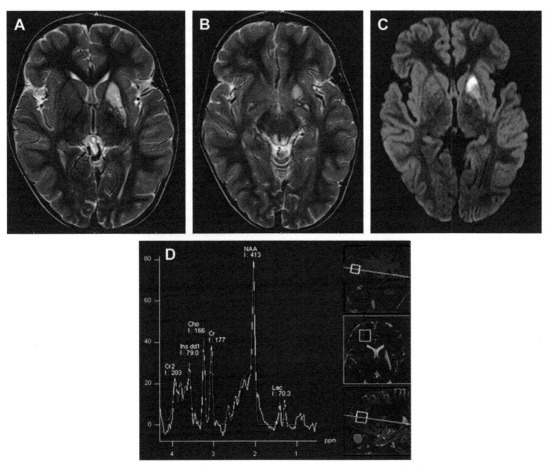

Fig. 2. Mitochondriopathy related to deficiency of complex I. (A, B) Axial T2-weighted MRI shows abnormal hyperintensity signal lesions in basal ganglia, especially in the putamen. (C) Diffusion-weighted MRI shows restricted diffusion at the same location. (D) Magnetic resonance spectroscopy with lactate peak in the cortex.

Table 1
Mitochondrial respiratory chain defect disorders, loci gene, and the associated disease

Mutation Site	Disease or Syndrome
POLG (15q25)	KSS
	PEO
	Alpers disease
	Ataxia-neuropathy syndrome
	MNGIE (without CNS commitment)
SURF1 (3q34)	Leigh syndrome
TYMP (22q13.32)	MNGIE (with CNS commitment)
Multiple deletion of mtDNA	MELAS

Abbreviations: KSS, Kearns-Sayre syndrome; MELAS, mitochondrial encephalomyopathy, lactic acidosis, and strokelike episodes; MNGIE, mitochondrial neurogastrointestinal encephalopathy; PEO, progressive external ophthalmoplegia.

POLG (polymerase DNA directed γ) located on 15q23 region is the gene that codes for the catalytic subunit of the mtDNA polymerase. Mutations in the POLG gene are an important cause of pediatric mitochondrial disease, such as Kearns-Sayre syndrome (KSS) and Alpers syndrome. Studying patients with A467T and W748S POLG mutations, Tzoulis and colleagues[29] reported lesions in the occipital cortex, deep cerebellar structures, and the thalamus, which spare the basal ganglia. An additional potential neuroimaging discriminator feature is a pattern of involvement of the inferior olivary nuclei. Kinghorn and colleagues[30] studied 3 patients, 2 of whom were heterozygous (p.Ala467Thr and p.Trp748Ser) for POLG gene mutations. Both of them had bilateral signal abnormality and hypertrophy of the inferior olives. However, these alterations are not pathognomonic for POLG mutations, because they were also described in patients with SURF1 gene mutations with Leigh syndrome (LS) phenotype. Also, at least 150 mutations (see http://www.hgmd.org) in the POLG have been described and were associated with several phenotypes of neurodegenerative diseases.

Leber Hereditary Optic Neuropathy

Leber hereditary optic neuropathy (LHON) is a common cause of inherited blindness, which typically presents with bilateral, painless, subacute visual failure in young adult men. Clinical diagnosis is usually confirmed by molecular genetic analysis showing a mtDNA mutation affecting genes coding for complex I subunits of the respiratory chain, such as m.3460G>A, m.11778G>A, and m14484T>C. MRI is usually normal or shows increased T2 signal changes in the optic tract and chasm. Swelling and enhancement of the optic nerves/chiasm on gadolinium-enhanced imaging with signal changes in the optic tracts have been described.[31,32] LHON associated with cerebellum and inferior olivary nucleus atrophy can suggest a specific mtDNA pattern related to G11778A and T3394C mutations.[33]

Leigh Syndrome

LS, also known as subacute necrotizing encephalomyelopathy, refers to a symptom complex, characterized by progressive neurodegeneration, with variable clinical and pathologic manifestations. The classic pathologic abnormalities are microcystic cavitation, vascular proliferation, neuronal loss, and demyelination in the midbrain, basal ganglia, cerebellar dentate nuclei, and cerebral white matter.[34]

Several mutations of both mtDNA and nDNA are responsible for the LS, involving genes coding for proteins in respiratory chain complexes I, II, III, IV, and V, mitochondrial transfer RNA (tRNA), pyruvate dehydrogenase complex, and coenzyme Q10. All of them were divided into 4 groups: defects of the pyruvate dehydrogenase complex; cytochrome oxidase deficiency; patients with apparently mutation on the mitochondrial adenosine triphosphatase 6 gene; and complex I deficiency. The group of cytochrome C oxidase complex (respiratory chain complex IV) deficiency is believed to be the most common cause of LS.

Studies have tried to identify a homogeneous neuroimaging pattern associated with SURF1 mutations. The characteristic lesion distribution of patients harboring any mutation was along the brainstem, thalamus, and basal ganglia. However, it seems that LS caused by SURF1 mutations presents a peculiar MRI pattern of bilateral involvement of the subthalamic nuclei. Farina and colleagues[35] performed a study with 22 patients with LS, 8 with SURF1 mutations and 14 with mutations in other genes. All of the patients with SURF1 mutations presented subthalamic nuclei abnormality, compared with 2 patients in the other group. These results were confirmed in other studies shown in Table 2.[36–40] The involvement of the basal ganglia, which used to be considered the hallmark of LS, is not essential for the diagnosis. The basal ganglia spared seem to be more common in patients harboring SURF1 mutations.

Mitochondrial Encephalomyopathy, Lactic Acidosis, and Strokelike Episodes

Mitochondrial encephalomyopathy, lactic acidosis, and strokelike episodes (MELAS) refers to a group of disorders with recurrent strokelike events, with either permanent or reversible neurologic deficits. The classic presentation is strokelike cortical lesions (hyperintense on T2/fluid-attenuated inversion recovery [FLAIR] images with restricted diffusion), crossing vascular territories with shifting spread (appearance, disappearance, reappearance elsewhere).[41] The involvement of the parieto-occipital lobe is usually more extensive, and intracranial calcification (usually in the basal ganglia) is also common, as shown in Table 3.[42–46]

MELAS is caused by mtDNA mutations, especially in the MTTL1 gene, which encodes tRNAleu in about 80% of the cases.[47] The most common

Table 2
Patients with LS harboring SURF1 mutation

Studies	Total Number of Patients	MRI Findings (Number of Patients with Affected Brain Region)				
		Brainstem	Cerebellar	Subthalamic Nuclei	Thalami	Basal Ganglia
Farina et al,[35] 2002	8	8	6	8	2	2
Xie et al,[36] 2009	8	3	3	3	1	2
Rossi et al,[37] 2003	3	3	3	3	0	1
Sonam et al,[38] 2014	4	4	4	0	0	2
Bruno et al,[39] 2002	1	1	0	1	0	0
Salviati et al,[40] 2004	1	1	1	0	0	0

Table 3
Patients with MELAS harboring m.3243A>G mutation: clinical reports

Studies	BG Calcification	CT and MRI Findings (Affected Brain Region)			
		Hyperintensity Lesion in T2			
		Occipital	Temporal	Parietal	Frontal
Bi et al,[42] 2006	+	+	+	+	–
Karkare et al,[43] 2009	–	+	+	+	–
Chung et al,[44] 2005	+	+	+	+	–
Liu et al,[45] 2013	+	+	+	–	–
Casimiro et al,[46] 2012	0	–	+	+	–
Total	3/5	4/5	5/5	4/5	0/5

Abbreviations: +, present; –, absent; 0, CT not performed; BG, basal ganglia; CT, computed tomography.

mutation is m.3243A>G. In 1998, Sue and colleagues[48] studied 26 patients with MELAS, 22 of whom harbored the m.3243A>G mutation. The most common neuroimaging finding was basal ganglia calcification (seen in both young and adult patients), which was present in 14 patients (11 with the m.3243A>G mutation). Globus pallidus was seen in 12 patients.

Alpers Disease

Alpers disease is an autosomal recessive disorder characterized by rapid progressive cerebral and hepatic degeneration caused by mutations in the POLG gene. CNS compromise is characterized by progressive degeneration of the cerebral and cerebellar cortex, thalamus, and basal ganglia, usually in the first years of life. MRI of patients with Alpers can be normal in the early stages, but the classic imaging findings are T2/FLAIR hyperintensity in the cortex, subcortical white matter, and basal ganglia, with cortical thinning, especially in the frontal, posterior temporal, and occipital lobes. In a recent retrospective study of 66 children with mitochondrial disorders,[49] 10 patients with Alpers disease were evaluated. All of them had POLG mutations (p.A467T/ R574W, p.A467T/G303R, and p.W748S–7p.Q497H–4p.E1143G/ R852C). The most prevalent finding was cerebral cortex atrophy, which presented in 70% of the patients. Basal ganglia involvement, considered a classic feature, was presented just in 30%.

Progressive External Ophthalmoplegia and Kearns-Sayre Syndrome

Progressive external ophthalmoplegia (PEO) can appear isolated or in association with KSS. In addition to PEO, KSS consists of retinal dystrophy and at least 1 of the following features appearing before 20 years old: heart block, cerebellar ataxia or increased protein in CSF. MRI of patients with PEO and KSS is similar, showing T2/FLAIR hyperintensities in the white matter, with early involvement of the subcortical U fibers and sparing of periventricular areas. Later in the course of the disease, deep cerebral white matter and the deep gray matter nuclei, particularly the dorsal

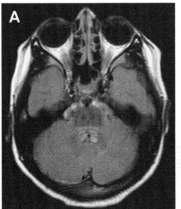
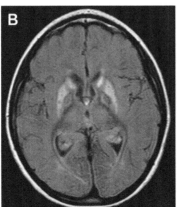
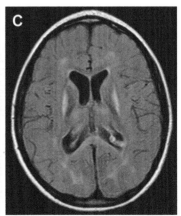

Fig. 3. KSS. (*A–C*) Axial FLAIR MRI shows symmetric and bilateral hyperintensity signal in the white matter, basal ganglia, thalamus, and midbrain.

Table 4
IEM related to intoxication symptoms

Disease	Genetic (Inheritance/ Gene Locus)	Suggestive Clinical Findings	MRI	Basic Defect and Diagnostic Tests
Aminoacidopathies				
Phenylketonuria	AR/PAH (12q24,1)	Severe mental retardation	T2 hyperintensity PV WM, mainly posterior portions. Later involvement of subcortical WM and corpus callosum	Increased plasma phenylalanine levels
MSDU	AR/BCKDHA (19q13.2), BCKDHB (6q14.1) and DBT (1p21.2)	Vomiting, dystonia, opisthotonic posturing, and seizure with onset during the first week of life	Edema in the deep cerebellar white matter, brainstem, cerebral peduncles, posterior limb of the internal capsule, and sensorimotor tracts in the centrum semiovale	Accumulation of BCAAs, alloisoleucine, and branched-chain ketoacids in plasma
Homocystinuria	AR/CBS (21q22,3)	Mental retardation and thromboembolic events	Small foci of T2 hyperintensity cerebral WM, cortical infarct and sinovenous thrombosis	Increased homocysteine plasma levels
Organic aciduria				
Methylmalonic acidemia	AR/MUT (6p21)	Metabolic acidosis, vomiting, tachypnea, lethargy, and seizure, leading to death Survivors are small with small heads, with quadriparesis, movement disorder, and psychomotor retardation	Increased water, mainly in the WM and globi pallidi Cystic changes of the globi pallidi. T2 hyperintensity may be present in PV WM	Ketoacidosis and excretion of methylmalonic acid in the urine
Propionic acidemia	AR/PCCA (13q32) and PCCB (13q21-23)	Like methylmalonic academia	Increased water, mainly in putamina and caudate Cystic changes of the globi pallidi. T2 hyperintensity may be present in PV WM	Ketoacidosis and excretion of propionic acid in the urine

Disease	Inheritance/Gene	Clinical features	Imaging	Biochemistry
Isovaleric acidemia	AR/IVD (15q14-15)	Neonatal form: metabolic acidosis characterized by vomiting, dehydration, and restlessness, leading to rapid death. Chronic form: periodic attacks of severe ketoacidosis after a trigger	T2 hyperintensity in the bilateral globi pallidi	Excretion of isovaleric acid in the urine
Glutaric aciduria type I	AR/GCDH (19p13.2)	Initially normal development. Acute encephalopathy, seizures, dystonia, choreathetosis, and mental retardation. Episodic crises follow trigger (infection, surgery). Age at onset: first year	T2 hyperintensity caudate, putamina and globus pallidus. Sylvian fissure cystlike spaces isointense to CSF and subependymal pseudocysts	Measurement of urine organic acids. Accumulation of glutaric, glutaconic, and 3-OH-glutaric acid
Urea cycle defects				
Ornithine transcarbamylase deficiency	XR/OTC (Xp21.1)	Progressive irritability, lethargy, poor feeding, hypothermia, and seizure. Age at onset: neonatal form (with poor neurodevelopmental outcome) and later onset	T2 hyperintensity and swelling in the insular cortex (posterior more than anterior), perirolandic cortex, and BG (particularly the globi pallidi)	Orotic aciduria. No citrulline in plasma
Citrullinemia	AR/ASS1 (9q34.1)	Like ornithine transcarbamylase deficiency	Like ornithine transcarbamylase deficiency	High plasma citrulline, ammonia, alanine. High urinary orotic acid
Intolerance to sugars				
Galactosemia	AR/GALT (9p13)	Severe liver disease, profound mental retardation, epilepsy and choreoathetosis.	Delayed myelination in the subcortical WM and consequent blurring of the cortical-WM junction	Measurement of total plasma galactose and erythrocyte GALT. Chromatography of carbohydrates in urine

Abbreviations: AR, autosomal recessive; BCAA, branched-chain amino acids; BG, basal ganglia; GALT, galactose-1-phosphate uridyl transferase; MSDU, maple syrup urine disease; PV, periventricular; WM, white matter; XR, X-linked recessive.

midbrains, medial and posterior thalami, and the globus pallidus, show T2 hyperintesity (**Fig. 3**).[34] PEO and KSS can be caused by POLG mutations, but other genes, such as PEO1, OPA1, and RRM2B, are associated with this condition.

Mitochondrial Neurogastrointestinal Encephalomyopathy

Mitochondrial neurogastrointestinal encephalomyopathy (MNGIE) is a progressive and multisystemic disorder characterized by severe gastrointestinal dysmotility, intestinal pseudo-obstruction, cachexia, PEO, peripheral neuropathy, leukoencephalopathy, and lactic acidosis. It is usually related to mutations in the gene encoding thymidine phosphorylase (TYMP, located on the 22q13.32-qter region). In addition, there is an MNGIE form without CNS involvement caused by POLG mutation. MRI shows diffuse T2/FLAIR hyperintensity in the periventricular and deep cerebral white matter, with or without basal ganglia and thalami involvement, typically sparing the corpus callosum and subcortical fibers. In some patients, the hyperintensity extends caudally into the internal and external capsules and brainstem.[34,50] Some case reports described a novel TYMP mutation (c112 G>T), which had CNS involvement of brainstem and cerebellum predominantly.[51]

Myoclonus Epilepsy with Ragged Red Fibers

Myoclonus epilepsy with ragged red fibers (MERRF) is typically characterized by myoclonus, ataxia, generalized seizures, and ragged red fibers in muscular biopsy caused by m.8344A>G mutation. Clinical severity is correlated with patient heteroplasmy, with high levels of mutant mtDNA, often causing severe complex I or IV deficiency and occasionally a combined complex I and IV deficiency.[52] Much like MELAS, the genotype-phenotype correlation of m.8344A>G can be extended beyond MERRF. Neuroimaging of patients with MERRF shows atrophy of the superior cerebellar peduncles, cerebellum, and brain stem. However, the severity of MRI findings is not related to clinical disability.[53]

MR PHENOTYPE-GENOTYPE CORRELATION IN DISORDERS NOT RELATED TO ENERGY METABOLISM: INHERITED INTOXICATION AND LARGE MOLECULES DISEASES

Neuroimaging of patients with IEM not involving energy metabolism is related to the intoxication and large molecules subgroups, as described in the genetic literature. Genotype-MR phenotype correlation in both groups is not well understood,

and the role of structural neuroimaging is restricted to diagnosis, imaging follow-up, and to measuring treatment efficacy. Genetics, clinical findings, and neuroimaging are reviewed to guide the reader to a better understanding of these disorders.

IEM related to intoxication symptoms present with a wide range of abnormalities (**Table 4**). This group includes IEM that cause acute symptoms and progressive intoxication caused by accumulation of toxic compounds. Examples are aminoacidopathies (phenylketonuria, tyrosinemia, homocystinuria, maple syrup urine disease) (**Fig. 4**), organic acidurias (propionic, isovaleric, methylmalonic acidurias), urea cycle disorders (which cause ammonia accumulation), sugar intolerances (hereditary fructose intolerance, galactosemia), metal accumulation (hemochromatosis, Wilson disease, Menkes disease, neuroferritinopathy), porphyries, and inborn errors of neurotransmitter synthesis and catabolism (such as γ-aminobutyric acid, glycine, serine, and glutamine). There are restricted data about genetic-MR phenotype correlation in this group. An exception is nonketotic hyperglycinemia (NKH). NKH is a disorder biochemically characterized by increased glycine levels in serum and CSF. Patients with classic NKH present neonatally with lethargy evolving to coma, apnea, and myoclonic jerks. Patients with a mild phenotype present in infancy with developmental delay, seizures, hyperactivity, and chorea. In classic NKH, most patients have a causative mutation in the GLDC and AMT genes. Recent data showed that patients with variant phenotypes presented with preserved cognition, progressive spasticity, and neurodegeneration after an initially normal early development. These variant phenotypes are related to mutations in the LIAS, BOLA3, and GLRX5 genes. Brain MRI of this variant NKH showed central lesions in the cervical spinal cord (GLRX5 gene mutation) and neurodegeneration after normal development (BOLA3 gene mutation). These MRI findings are not present in classic NKH.[54]

IEM related to large molecule abnormalities include diseases caused by abnormalities in the synthesis or catabolism of molecules that accumulate in cellular organelles.[20,22,55,56] Examples are lysosomal disorders (such as Gaucher disease and mucopolysaccharidosis [MPS]), peroxisomal disorders (such as X-linked adrenoleukodystrophy and Zellweger disease), disorders of intracellular trafficking and processing (such as mucolipidosis), and congenital disorders of glycosylation. Over time, excessive storage can cause permanent cellular and tissue damage. The brain is particularly sensitive to lipid storage, and any

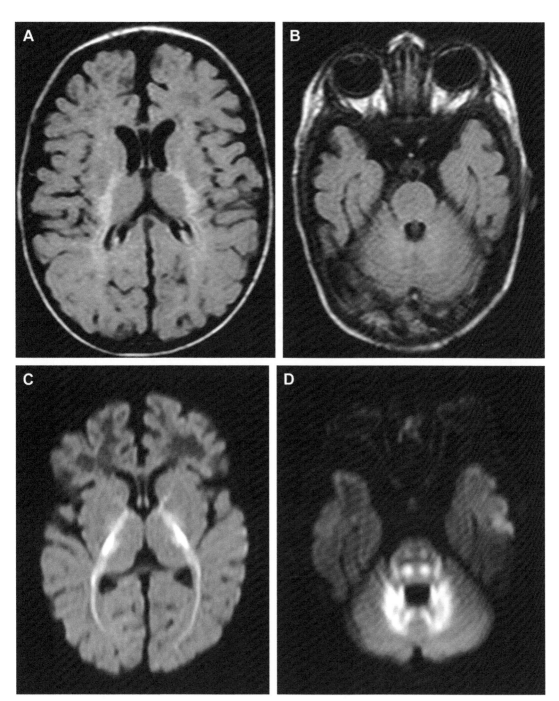

Fig. 4. Maple syrup urine disease. (*A*, *B*) Axial FLAIR MRI shows hyperintensity signal with corresponding areas of restriction to diffusion-weighted imaging (*C*, *D*), at the posterior limb of the internal capsule, midbrain, cerebellar white matter, and corticospinal tracts.

increases in fluids or deposits lead to pressure changes and interference with normal neurologic function. Symptoms are permanent, progressive, and unrelated to food intake (Table 5). Neuroimaging of these disorders shows a range of abnormalities, including leukodystrophy MR pattern (metachromatic leukodystrophy and X-linked adrenoleukodystrophy), hydrocephalus associated with brain atrophy and perivascular spaces enlargement (MPS), cranial nerve enhancement associated with thalamic hyperdensities (Krabbe disease), bone marrow infiltration (Gaucher

Table 5
IEM related to large molecules

Disease	Genetic (Inheritance/Gene Locus)	Suggestive Clinical Findings	MRI	Basic Defect and Diagnostic Tests
Lysosomal disorders				
Fabry disease	XR/GLA (Xq2)	Intermittent burning pain in extremities. angiokeratomas, corneal opacifications Age of onset: adolescents	Cerebrovascular alterations, small hyperintense WM changes in T2, T1 hyperintensity in the pulvinar	Deficiency of leukocytes α-galactosidase enzyme
Tay-Sachs disease	AR/HEXA (15q23-q2) (high in Ashkenazi Jews)	Hyperacusis, arrest in intellectual development, macular cherry-red spots; convulsion Age of onset: 3–10 mo	MRI findings change during evolution Mainly gray matter changes Late in the course marked brain atrophy and diffuse WM lesions	Deficiency of leukocyte enzymatic hexosaminidases A
MLD with arylsulfatase A deficiency	AR/ARSA (22q13.31-qter)	Slowly progressive motor problems: ataxia, spasticity, dystonia, peripheral neuropathy; followed by mental decline	Demyelination begins in central and PV WM; tigroid pattern; U fibers tend to be spared; corpus callosum is early affected; atrophy is a late sign; cerebellar white matter is affected in later course	Deficient activity of leukocytes arylsulfatase A enzyme, urine chromatography sulfatide levels increased, CSF protein levels increased, nerve conduction velocity decreased
MLD with activator defect	AR/PSAP (10q22.1)	Similar to MLD with arylsulfatase A deficiency	Symmetric T2 hyperintensity in cerebral and cerebellar WM	Deficiency of saposin B; arylsulfatase A activity normal, urinary sulfatide levels increased
MLD with multiple sulfatase deficiency	AR/SUMF1 (3p26)	Similar to MLD, dysmorphic signs as in mucopolysaccharidoses, ichthyosis Age of onset: neonatal, infantile and juvenile forms	Not specific pattern. Progressive WM hyperintensity on T2, initially spating of subcortical U fibers	Low activities of several sulfatases, abnormal granules in leukocytes, urinary glucosaminoglycan levels increased

Krabbe disease	AR/GALC (14q3)	Combination of symptoms of central and peripheral nervous system Initially, patients may have increased or decreased muscle stretch reflexes Classic infantile form that begins with 4–6 mo and the late onset form, which begins in children	T2 hyperintensity in WM, notably in parietal and central lobes; pattern of radial stripes; dental nucleus hyperintense in T2	Deficient activity of leukocyte galactocerebrosidase enzyme CSF protein levels may be increased
GM1 gangliosidosis type 1	AR/GLB1 (3p21.33)	Variable degrees of neurodegeneration and skeletal abnormalities, dysmorphies, hepatosplenomegaly, macular cherry-red pots; acoustic startle; ataxia and spasticity Age of onset: infancy	Hypomyelination; thalamus hypointense in T2	Deficiency of leukocytes β-galactosidase
Mucopolysaccharidosis and mucolipidoses	Genes related to deficient enzyme	May show typical dysmorphic stigmata	Perivascular spaces may appear enlarged	Urinary glucosaminoglycan levels increased (not in mucolipidoses)
NCL (types 1–14)	AR/some: PPT1 (1p32), TPP1 (11p15.5), CLN3 (16p12), CLN5 (13q22), CLN6 (15q21) and CLN8 (8p23)	Depends on the type of NCL and the age of presentation Infantile forms: deceleration of head growth and muscular hypotonia after the age of 6 mo Ataxia, irritability, sleep disturbance, and visual failure	Infantile form: variable cerebral and cerebellar atrophy associated with T2 hyperintense rims around the ventricles and T2 hypointensity in the thalami and globi pallidi	
Sialuria, Finnish type	AR/SLC17A5 (6q14-q15)	Slowly progressive psychomotor deficitts, hypotonia, cerebellar ataxia, mental retardation; visceromegaly and coarse features may develop Age of onset: late infancy	Hypomyelination/demyelination, may have thin corpus callosum	Deficiency of a carrier-mediated transport system in the lysosome

(continued on next page)

Table 5
(continued)

Disease	Genetic (Inheritance/Gene Locus)	Suggestive Clinical Findings	MRI	Basic Defect and Diagnostic Tests
Free sialic acid storage disease (infantile type)	AR/SLC17A5 (6q14-q15) (allelic variant)	Progressive neurologic deterioration, coarse facial features, dysostosis multiplex; variable phenotypes reported	Hypomyelination of supratentorial and infratentorial WM; T2 pallidum hypointense	Deficiency of leukocytes α-L-fucosidase
Peroxisomal diseases				
X-linked adrenoleukodystrophy	XR/ABCD1(ALDP) (Xq28)	Variable: it may cause cerebral degeneration, adrenomyeloneuropathy, or Addison disease only The childhood cerebral form typically begins subacutely with loss of mental and emotional performance, followed by loss of motor performance and spasticity	T2 hyperintensity of PV WM; starts mostly in parieto-occipital WM; internal capsule early affected MRS: choline-containing compound levels increased early Lesions frequently show a strong inflammatory component (contrast enhancement)	Deficient ATP-binding-cassette protein (ABC protein) VLCFA levels increased, electrolyte imbalance, and endocrinologic findings of adrenocortical failure
Refsum disease	AR/PHYH (10p13) and PEX7 (6q23.3)	Peripheral polyneuropathy, cerebellar ataxia, retinitis pigmentosa, and ichthyosis Age at onset: childhood to adolescence	Symmetric signal change involving the corticospinal tracts, cerebellar dentate nuclei, and corpus callosum	VLCFA levels increased
Zellweger syndrome	AR/several different PEX genes involved in peroxisome biogenesis	Typical face and skull anomalies (high forehead, huge fontanelle), severe hypotonia, visual and hearing loss, liver disease	Diffuse WM hyperintensity on T2; cortical abnormalities such as polymicrogyria	
Neonatal adrenoleukodystrophy	AR/several different genes	Dysmorphic features, hearing deficit, hypotonia, hepatomegaly, seizures, retinopathy Age of onset: 1–3 mo	Central and PV WM hyperintense on T2; cerebellum, BG, thalamus, corpus callosum may be affected; polymicrogyria	

Oxidation defects	AR/ACOX1 (17q25)	Cranial dysmorphies, liver disease, developmental regression in later infancy	Mostly cerebellar WM involved	VLCFA levels increased
Defects in protein glycosylation				
Congenital disorders of glycosylation (CDG syndromes)	Molecular analysis of genes related, exome sequencing	A group of mostly multisystem disorders; some patients have dysmorphies	Cerebellar hypoplasia and hypomyelination may be present	Atypical transferrins in serum
Disorders of cholesterol				
Cerebrotendinous xanthomatosis	AR/CYP27A1 (2q33-qter)	Cataracts, chronic diarrhea, neurologic deficit, and tendinous or tuberous xanthomas beginning in childhood Cerebellar ataxia beginning after puberty	T2 hyperintensity in cerebral WM, particularly in globi pallidi, and cerebellar WM	Increased levels of plasma cholestanol
Smith-Lemli-Opitz syndrome	AR/DHCR7 (11q12-13)	Distinctive facial features, small head size (microcephaly), intellectual disability or learning problems, and behavioral problems (autism spectrum)		Increased levels of serum 7-dehydrocholesterol
Niemann-Pick type C	AR/NPC1 (18q11-q12) and NPC2 (14q24.3)	Highly variable, symptoms include vertical supranuclear gaze palsy, liver disease, psychiatric symptoms; late infantile course leads to spasticity	Central WM changes mild and later in course	Cholesterol esterification; skin biopsy for Filipin staining

Abbreviations: AR, autosomal recessive; ATP, adenosine triphosphate; BG, basal ganglia; MLD, metachromatic leukodystrophy; MRS, magnetic resonance spectroscopy; NCL, neuronal ceroid lipofuscinosis; PV, periventricular; VLCFA, very-long fatty acids; WM, white matter; XR, X-linked recessive.

Table 6
Leukodystrophies with known genetic inheritance in pediatric population

Disease	Genetics (Inheritance/ Gene Locus)	Suggestive Clinical Findings	MRI	Basic Defect and Diagnostic Tests
With intracerebral cysts or calcifications				
Megalencephalic leukodystrophy with cysts	AR/MLC1 (22q13.33) and HEPACAM (11q24)	Megalencephaly, slowly progressive spasticity and dementia Age at onset: infancy to 10 y High incidence in Asian Indians	Complete absence of myelin in the subcortical WM, sparing some central WM Subcortical cysts in the anterior temporal and frontoparietal lobes	
Aicardi-Goutières syndrome	AR/AGS1-4 (13q14.3)	Severe postnatal encephalopathy, suggestive of intracranial infection	Intracerebral calcifications, especially in BG; PV and central WM hyperintensity on T2; later atrophy	Cell count and interferon levels in CSF increased
Mainly hypomyelinating disorders				
PMD	XR/PLP1 (Xq22)	Early symptoms are nystagmus, stridor, muscular hypotonia; later spasticity Initially, not a progressive disorder Age at onset: infancy	Global hypomyelination sparing or not corticospinal tracts	Defective proteolipid protein
PMD-like disease	AR/type 1: GJA12 (1q41-q4)	PMD-like Age at onset: infancy	Delayed myelination of central WM Type 2 has almost complete absence of myelin	Type 1: connexin (gap junction protein) defect Type 2: increased N-acetylaspartylglutamate in CSF
3-Phosphoglycerate dehydrogenase deficiency	AR/PHGDH (1q12jkmio)	Microcephaly, severe psychomotor retardation, intractable seizures Age of onset: newborn	Hypomyelination, reversible attenuation of cerebral WM	Low concentrations of the amino acid serine in plasma and CSF
Hypomyelination and congenital cataract	AR/DRCTNNB1A (7p21.3- p15.3)	Cataract, developmental delay, and slowly progressive spasticity, ataxia, tremor, mild to moderate mental retardation, peripheral neuropathy Age of onset: infancy	Diffuse supratentorial hypomyelination	Motor nerve conduction velocity reduced

18q-syndrome	Deletion of chromosome 18	Variable malformations mental retardation, short stature, hypotonia, hearing impairment, foot deformities Age of onset: congenital	T2: poor differentiation of gray matter and WM	
Allan-Herndon-Dudley syndrome	XR/MCT8 (Xq13.2)	Hypotonia, weakness, reduced muscle mass, delay of development Age of onset: infancy	Hypomyelinated WM	Thyroid anomalies (T3 resistance)
With other neuroradiologic features				
Leukoencephalopathy with brainstem and spinal cord involvement and elevated lactate	AR/DARS2 (1q25)	Slowly progressive, variable mental deficits, pyramidal and cerebellar dysfunction Age of onset: early childhood to adolescence	Diffuse or spotty WM abnormalities, involvement of pyramidal tract, sensory tracts and cerebellar peduncles MRS: increased lactate	
Leukoencephalopathy with hydrocephalus	AD?	Macrocephaly, nystagmus, spasticity, nonprogressive Age of onset: infancy	Obstructive hydrocephalus caused by enlarged cerebellum, abnormal cerebellar WM, progresses to atrophy	
Leukoencephalopathy with vanishing white matter	AR/EIF2B1-5 or AD form	Symptoms triggered by stress (head trauma, high fever), coursing with progressive spasticity, ataxia, dementia	T2 hyperintensity of central hemispheric WM; central WM signal becomes similar to that of CSF; U fibers affected, atrophy later in disease course	Mutations in genes coding for 1 of 5 subunits of translation initiation factor EIF2B
With prominent features outside the nervous system				
Leukoencephalopathy with metaphyseal	XR/Xq25-q27	Slowly progressive spastic paraplegia, later tremor, ataxia, optic atrophy, and tetraparesis; broad wrist sand knees without significant contractures Age of onset: 2–3 y	Diffuse leukoencephalopathy	Radiograph: bone and cartilage show mild metaphyseal chondrodysplasia
Giant axonal neuropathy type 1	AR/GAN (16q24.1)	Chronic polyneuropathy, kinky or curly hair, typical posture of legs Age of onset: childhood	Progressive cerebral WM degeneration	Longitudinal grooves in hair

(continued on next page)

Table 6
(continued)

Disease	Genetics (Inheritance/Gene Locus)	Suggestive Clinical Findings	MRI	Basic Defect and Diagnostic Tests
Trichothiodystrophy	AR/XPD (19q13.2-q13.3), XPB (6p25.3,2q21) and	Ichthyosiform skin, abnormal hair and nails, mental and growth retardation Age of onset: infancy	Lack of myelination in the supratentorial WM	
Sjögren-Larsson syndrome	ALDH3A2 (17p11.12)	Ichthyosiform skin, slowly progressive dementia, spasticity, retinal abnormalities Age of onset: infancy	Retarded myelination, mild persistent myelin deficit MRS: lipid peak in WM	Defect of fatty aldehydehydrogenase, detectable in fibroblasts
Miscellaneous genetic disorders				
Biotinidase deficiency	AR/BTD (3p25)	Seizures, hypotonia, ataxia, sensorineural deafness Cutaneous features (erythematous exudative dermatitis, alopecia) Age of onset: infancy	Delayed myelination, pronounced WM damage possible	Deficient recycling of biotin, a cofactor of multiple carboxylases Lactate levels may be increased in serum and CSF
Glucose transporter 1 deficiency syndrome	AD/GLUT1 (1p35-p31.3)	Seizures, developmental delay, ataxia, dystonia Age of onset: infancy	Delayed myelination	Low glucose ratio in CSF/blood
Infantile neuroaxonal dystrophy	AR/PLA2G6 (22q13.1)	Psychomotor regression, relentlessly progressive to spasticity, visual impairment (optic atrophy) Age of onset: infancy	Cerebellar atrophy. T2 hyperintensity of cerebellar cortex, some have marked cerebral WM hyperintensity	Fast EEG rhythms (β EEG) Axonal spheroids on skin biopsy
Cockayne syndrome type A	AR/ERCC8 (5q1)	Progerialike symptoms, light sensitivity, short stature, peripheral neuropathy, retinopathy; progressive symptoms typically apparent after the age of 1 y	Patchy central and subcortical WM changes; BG calcification	

Abbreviations: AD, autosomal dominant; AR, autosomal recessive; BG, basal ganglia; EEG, electroencephalography; MRS, magnetic resonance spectroscopy; PMD, Pelizaeus-Merzbacher disease; PV, periventricular; WM, white matter; XR, X-linked recessive.

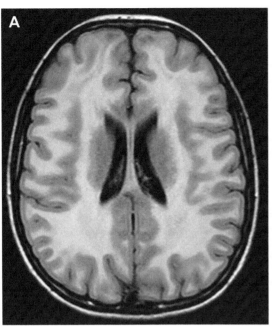
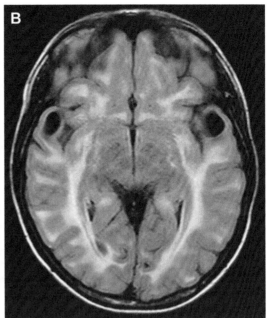

Fig. 5. MLC. (*A*) Axial FLAIR MRI shows diffusely increase signal intensity of periventricular, deep and subcortical white matter. (*B*) Axial FLAIR MRI shows subcortical cysts in the temporal lobes.

disease), vascular abnormalities (Fabry disease), and cortical dysplasia (Zellweger disease).

Recently, leukodystrophies have emerged as an additional group of IMD (Table 6). The goal of this review is not to describe all MRI findings related to white matter disorders, but a review of megalencephalic leukoencephalopathy with subcortical cysts (MLC) is an example of how imaging has been used recently. MLC is an autosomal recessive disorder characterized by macrocephaly, deterioration of motor functions with ataxia, and spasticity, eventuating in mental decline. The classic MRI is swollen diffuse subcortical white matter, with enlargement of the gyri in affected regions and the invariable presence of subcortical cysts, which initially develop in the anterior temporal lobes and may arise in the frontal and parietal lobes. Some central white matter is spared, particularly in the corpus callosum, internal capsules, brainstem, and the occipital lobes (Fig. 5). Mutations in 2 genes (MLC1 [located on the 22q13.33 chromosome, 75% of patients] or HEPACAM [located on the 11q24 chromosome, 20% of patients]) are associated with the disease. In our small review with clinical reports, we found congruent features in the MRI of patients with MLC1 mutations, but not related with a specific mutation. As described previously in the literature, all of the 12 patients had subcortical cysts that involved mainly temporal lobes (12 patients) and then the frontal lobe (7 patients). All patients had corpus callosum or occipital lobe spared.[57–64]

SUMMARY

Variable clinical presentation and considerable overlap of phenotypes among IMDs made their diagnosis a challenge. Because of the rarity of the sample that this review aimed to study, finding trials with good statistical power is difficult. However, some genotype-MR phenotype correlation of IMDs has been shown to be a relevant tool for improving the approach to these patients. For some diseases, it is possible to speculate if a specific imaging finding suggests a particular gene mutation. It is hoped that this article may guide neuroscientists to find new correlations between neuroimaging and genetics, especially in diseases with variable and nonspecific clinical manifestations.

REFERENCES

1. Miller JA, Ding SL, Sunkin SM, et al. Transcriptional landscape of the prenatal human brain. Nature 2014;508(7495):199–206.
2. Xue H, Inati S, Sørensen TS, et al. Distributed MRI reconstruction using gadgetron-based cloud computing. Magn Reson Med 2014. [Epub ahead of print].

3. Sun H, Fessler JA, Noll DC, et al. Steady-state functional MRI using spoiled small-tip fast recovery imaging. Magn Reson Med 2014. [Epub ahead of print].

4. Dinse J. A histology-based model of quantitative T1 contrast for in-vivo cortical parcellation of high-resolution 7 Tesla brain MR images. Med Image Comput Comput Assist Interv 2013;16(Pt 2):51–8.

5. Lefranc M. High-resolution three-dimensional T2 star weighted angiography (HR 3-D SWAN): an optimized 3T MRI sequence for targeting the subthalamic nucleus. Neurosurgery 2014;74(6):615–26.

6. Tymofiyeva O. A DTI-based template-free cortical connectome study of brain maturation. PLoS One 2013;8(5):e63310.

7. Doherty D, Millen KJ, Barkovich AJ. Midbrain and hindbrain malformations: advances in clinical diagnosis, imaging, and genetics. Lancet Neurol 2013; 12(4):381–93.

8. Barkovich J. Complication begets clarification in classification. Brain 2013;136(Pt 2):368–73.

9. Barkovich AJ. A developmental and genetic classification for malformations of cortical development: update 2012. Brain 2012;135(Pt 5):1348–69.

10. Barkovich AJ, Millen KJ, Dobyns WB. A developmental and genetic classification for midbrain-hindbrain malformations. Brain 2009; 132(Pt 12):3199–230.

11. Cox MJ, Cookson WO, Moffatt MF. Sequencing the human microbiome in health and disease. Hum Mol Genet 2013;22(R1):R88–94.

12. Halldorsson BV, Sharan R. Network-based interpretation of genomic variation data. J Mol Biol 2013; 425(21):3964–9.

13. DeYoung CG, Clark R. The gene in its natural habitat: the importance of gene-trait interactions. Dev Psychopathol 2012;24(4):1307–18.

14. Foo JN, Liu JJ, Tan EK. Whole-genome and whole-exome sequencing in neurological diseases. Nat Rev Neurol 2012;8(9):508–17.

15. Schofield PN, Hoehndorf R, Gkoutos GV. Mouse genetic and phenotypic resources for human genetics. Hum Mutat 2012;33(5):826–36.

16. van der Knaap MS. New syndrome characterized by hypomyelination with atrophy of the basal ganglia and cerebellum. AJNR Am J Neuroradiol 2002; 23(9):1466–74.

17. van de Kamp JM. Phenotype and genotype in 101 males with X-linked creatine transporter deficiency. J Med Genet 2013;50(7):463–72.

18. Schicks J. Teaching neuroimages: MRI guides genetics: leukoencephalopathy with brainstem and spinal cord involvement (LBSL). Neurology 2013; 80(16):e176–7.

19. van der Knaap MS. MRI as diagnostic tool in early-onset peroxisomal disorders. Neurology 2012; 78(17):1304–8.

20. Steenweg ME. Novel hypomyelinating leukoencephalopathy affecting early myelinating structures. Arch Neurol 2012;69(1):125–8.

21. Vairo F, Vedolin L. The basis of inborn errors of metabolism for neuroradiologists. Top Magn Reson Imaging 2011;22(5):209–14.

22. Vedolin L. Inherited white matter disorders of childhood: a magnetic resonance imaging-based pattern recognition approach. Top Magn Reson Imaging 2011;22(5):215–22.

23. Barkovich AJ. An approach to MRI of metabolic disorders in children. J Neuroradiol 2007;34(2):75–88.

24. Cellini E. Periventricular heterotopia with white matter abnormalities associated with 6p25 deletion. Am J Med Genet A 2012;158A(7):1793–7.

25. Vedolin L. Inherited cerebellar ataxia in childhood: a pattern-recognition approach using brain MRI. AJNR Am J Neuroradiol 2013;34(5):925–34. S1–2.

26. Gonzalez G. Location of periventricular nodular heterotopia is related to the malformation phenotype on MRI. AJNR Am J Neuroradiol 2013;34(4):877–83.

27. Takanashi J. Neuroradiologic features of CASK mutations. AJNR Am J Neuroradiol 2010;31(9):1619–22.

28. Schaefer AM. Prevalence of mitochondrial DNA disease in adults. Ann Neurol 2008;63(1):35–9.

29. Tzoulis C. The spectrum of clinical disease caused by the A467T and W748S POLG mutations: a study of 26 cases. Brain 2006;129(Pt 7):1685–92.

30. Kinghorn KJ. Hypertrophic olivary degeneration on magnetic resonance imaging in mitochondrial syndromes associated with POLG and SURF1 mutations. J Neurol 2013;260(1):3–9.

31. Ong E. Teaching neuroimages: chiasmal enlargement and enhancement in Leber hereditary optic neuropathy. Neurology 2013;81(17):e126–7.

32. van Westen D, Hammar B, Bynke G. Magnetic resonance findings in the pregeniculate visual pathways in Leber hereditary optic neuropathy. J Neuroophthalmol 2011;31(1):48–51.

33. Nakaso K. Leber's hereditary optic neuropathy with olivocerebellar degeneration due to G11778A and T3394C mutations in the mitochondrial DNA. J Clin Neurol 2012;8(3):230–4.

34. Raybaud C, Barkovich AJ. Pediatric neuroimaging. 5th edition. Philadelphia: 2012.

35. Farina L. MR findings in Leigh syndrome with COX deficiency and SURF-1 mutations. AJNR Am J Neuroradiol 2002;23(7):1095–100.

36. Xie S. Heterogeneity of magnetic resonance imaging in Leigh syndrome with SURF1 gene 604G–>C mutation. Clin Imaging 2009;33(1):1–6.

37. Rossi A. Leigh syndrome with COX deficiency and SURF1 gene mutations: MR imaging findings. AJNR Am J Neuroradiol 2003;24(6):1188–91.

38. Sonam K. Clinical and magnetic resonance imaging findings in patients with Leigh syndrome and SURF1 mutations. Brain Dev 2014;36(9):807–12.

39. Bruno C. A novel mutation in the SURF1 gene in a child with Leigh disease, peripheral neuropathy, and cytochrome-c oxidase deficiency. J Child Neurol 2002;17(3):233–6.

40. Salviati L. Novel SURF1 mutation in a child with subacute encephalopathy and without the radiological features of Leigh syndrome. Am J Med Genet A 2004;128A(2):195–8.

41. Osborns S, Barkovich AJ. Diagnostic imaging brain. 2nd edition. 2010.

42. Bi WL, Baehring JM, Lesser RL. Evolution of brain imaging abnormalities in mitochondrial encephalomyopathy with lactic acidosis and stroke-like episodes. J Neuroophthalmol 2006;26(4): 251–6.

43. Karkare S. MELAS with A3243G mutation presenting with occipital status epilepticus. J Child Neurol 2009;24(12):1564–7.

44. Chung SH. Symmetric basal ganglia calcification in a 9-year-old child with MELAS. Neurology 2005; 65(9):E19.

45. Liu XL. Clinical, pathological and molecular biological characteristics of mitochondrial encephalomyopathy with lactic acidosis and stroke-like episode in children. Zhonghua Er Ke Za Zhi 2013;51(2): 130–5 [in Chinese].

46. Casimiro C. Conventional and diffusion-weighted magnetic resonance imaging and proton spectroscopy in MELAS. Acta Med Port 2012;25(Suppl 1): 59–64 [in Portuguese].

47. Uusimaa J. Prevalence, segregation, and phenotype of the mitochondrial DNA 3243A>G mutation in children. Ann Neurol 2007;62(3):278–87.

48. Sue CM. Neuroradiological features of six kindreds with MELAS tRNA(Leu) A2343G point mutation: implications for pathogenesis. J Neurol Neurosurg Psychiatry 1998;65(2):233–40.

49. Sofou K. MRI of the brain in childhood-onset mitochondrial disorders with central nervous system involvement. Mitochondrion 2013;13(4):364–71.

50. Reeve AK, Krishnan KJ, Duchen MR, et al. Mitochondrial dysfunction in neurodegenerative disorders. London: Springer-Verlag; 2012. p. 242.

51. Baris Z. Mitochondrial neurogastrointestinal encephalomyopathy (MNGIE): case report with a new mutation. Eur J Pediatr 2010;169(11):1375–8.

52. Mancuso M. Phenotypic heterogeneity of the 8344A>G mtDNA "MERRF" mutation. Neurology 2013;80(22):2049–54.

53. Ito S. Clinical and brain MR imaging features focusing on the brain stem and cerebellum in patients with myoclonic epilepsy with ragged-red fibers due to mitochondrial A8344G mutation. AJNR Am J Neuroradiol 2008;29(2):392–5.

54. Baker PR 2nd. Variant non ketotic hyperglycinemia is caused by mutations in LIAS, BOLA3 and the novel gene GLRX5. Brain 2014;137(Pt 2):366–79.

55. Finn CT. Magnetic resonance imaging findings in Hunter syndrome. Acta Paediatr Suppl 2008;97(457): 61–8.

56. Vedolin L. Brain MRI in mucopolysaccharidosis: effect of aging and correlation with biochemical findings. Neurology 2007;69(9):917–24.

57. Koyama S. A Japanese adult case of megalencephalic leukoencephalopathy with subcortical cysts with a good long-term prognosis. Intern Med 2012; 51(5):503–6.

58. Yis U. Two cases with megalencephalic leukoencephalopathy with subcortical cysts and MLC1 mutations in the Turkish population. Turk J Pediatr 2010; 52(2):179–83.

59. Mancini C. Megalencephalic leukoencephalopathy with subcortical cysts type 1 (MLC1) due to a homozygous deep intronic splicing mutation (c.895-226T>G) abrogated in vitro using an antisense morpholino oligonucleotide. Neurogenetics 2012;13(3):205–14.

60. Tinsa F. Megalencephalic leukoencephalopathy with subcortical cysts in a Tunisian boy. J Child Neurol 2009;24(1):87–9.

61. Miles L. Megalencephalic leukoencephalopathy with subcortical cysts: a third confirmed case with literature review. Pediatr Dev Pathol 2009;12(3):180–6.

62. Morita H. MR imaging and 1H-MR spectroscopy of a case of van der Knaap disease. Brain Dev 2006; 28(7):466–9.

63. Koussa S. Megalencephalic leucoencephalopathy with subcortical cysts: a study of a Lebanese family and a review of the literature. Rev Neurol (Paris) 2005;161(2):183–91 [in French].

64. Tsujino S. A common mutation and a novel mutation in Japanese patients with van der Knaap disease. J Hum Genet 2003;48(12):605–8.

Brain Imaging and Genetic Risk in the Pediatric Population, Part 2
Congenital Malformations of the Central Nervous System

Maria Gabriela Longo, MD[a,b], Themis Maria Félix, MD, PhD[c],
Patricia Ashton-Prolla, MD, PhD[c,d],
Leonardo Modesti Vedolin, MD, PhD[a,e],*

KEYWORDS

- Brain imaging • MRI • Magnetic resonance • Congenital malformations • Genetics

KEY POINTS

- Structural abnormalities of the central nervous system (CNS) are increasingly recognized by applying high-resolution imaging techniques, particularly MRI.
- As the number and complexity of recognized congenital malformations of the CNS have increased significantly, a multidisciplinary approach is mandatory, involving experts from neuroembryology, neurogenetics, neurochemistry, pediatric neurology, and pediatric neuroradiology.
- The MRI pattern recognition approach evolved, and integrated classifications of congenital malformations have been proposed based on embryology, genetics, and neuroimaging findings. As a result, different neuroimaging phenotypes have been observed, guiding genetic analysis and, frequently, resulting in the identification of causative genes.
- It is essential for every pediatric neuroradiologist to be aware of potential genotype-MR phenotype in congenital disorders of the CNS.

INTRODUCTION

Congenital malformations (CM) of the central nervous system (CNS) are commonly encountered in daily neuroimaging practice, and the significant and continuous development of the various imaging techniques, particularly MRI, has revolutionized the analysis and understanding of these disorders.[1–6] Because the number and complexity of recognized CMCNS have increased significantly, a multidisciplinary approach is mandatory, involving experts from neuroembryology, neurogenetics, neurochemistry, pediatric neurology, and pediatric neuroradiology.

The MRI pattern recognition approach evolved, and integrated classifications of congenital

The authors have nothing to disclose.
[a] Radiology Service, Hospital de Clínicas de Porto Alegre, Porto Alegre, Rio Grande do Sul, Brazil; [b] Post Graduation Program on Medical Sciences, Medicine, Department of Internal Medicine, Universidade Federal do Rio Grande do Sul, Porto Alegre, Rio Grande do Sul, Brazil; [c] Medical Genetics Service, Hospital de Clínicas de Porto Alegre, Porto Alegre, Rio Grande do Sul, Brazil; [d] Post Graduation Program on Genetics and Molecular Biology, Department of Genetics, Universidade Federal do Rio Grande do Sul, Porto Alegre, Rio Grande do Sul, Brazil; [e] Radiology Service, Hospital de Clínicas de Porto Alegre and Hospital Moinhos de Vento, Rio Grande do Sul, Brazil
* Corresponding author. Rua Carlos Trein Filho, 909 ap 502. 90450-120, Porto Alegre, Rio Grande do Sul, Brazil.
E-mail address: lvedolin@hcpa.ufrgs.br

malformations have been proposed based on embryology, genetics, and neuroimaging findings.[1] As a result, different neuroimaging phenotypes have been observed guiding genetic analysis and, frequently, resulting in the identification of causative genes. In this context, it is essential for every pediatric neuroradiologist to be aware of potential genotype-MR phenotype in congenital disorders of the CNS.

Understanding the embryology of the CNS is crucial for every neuroscientist. Although an extensive review about this topic is not presented in this article, some concepts are important to discuss. The CNS appears in the middle of the third week of development as a thickened area of the embryonic ectoderm, the neural plate. At the onset of gastrulation, there is induction of the neural plate, which folds into the neural tube in a process called neurulation. The fusion of the neural tube occurs in a zippering process at 5 different sites in humans.[7] By neurulation, the CNS is subdivided into its major transverse parts: prosencephalon, mesencephalon, rhombencephalon, and spinal cord. Modern neuroembryology integrates descriptive morphogenesis about these parts of the CNS with more recent insights into molecular genetic programming and data enabled by cell-specific tissue markers.[8]

In this article, the genotype-MR phenotype correlation of the most common or clinically relevant CMCNS in the pediatric population is reviewed. The data focus on the most commonly diagnosed diseases and those in which the neuroimaging abnormalities are better defined. The PubMed/Medline database was searched using a combination of key words such as "genotype-phenotype correlation," "genotype-imaging correlation," and "neuroimaging-genetic correlation." Relevant studies were defined based on current knowledge. For a more comprehensive review, the congenital disorders were divided based on an embryologic pattern, in which malformations were classified in 3 groups: ventral induction disorders, cortical malformations, and congenital malformations of the posterior fossa. In this review, malformations of the dorsal induction and spinal congenital disorders are excluded.

MALFORMATIONS OF THE VENTRAL INDUCTION

Malformations of the ventral induction represent a defect in the rostral closure and may result in disorders of formation, cleavage and midline development of the prosencephalon. Genetically, holoprosencephaly (HPE) and commissural abnormalities (including agenesis of the corpus callosum) are the most relevant disorders.

Holoprosencephaly

HPE is the most common developmental defect of the forebrain, with an estimated prevalence of 1 in 10 to 16,000 live births and 1 in 250 human conceptions.[9,10] Children with HPE have a failure of differentiation and midline cleavage of the prosencephalon. Therefore, in the more severe and prevalent form of HPE, called alobar HPE, these patients present a crescent-shaped and single ventricle, which occupies most of the volume of the skull, fusion of the hypothalamic and basal ganglia, and no commissural structures identified.[9,10] The poor prognosis in the most severe forms justifies the importance of genetic counseling in affected families.

The cause of HPE is heterogeneous: teratogens, chromosomal abnormalities, and single gene mutations can be involved. Most genes that have been implicated in HPE belong to the sonic hedgehog signaling pathway. Mutation of at least 12 different loci in 11 chromosomes has been implicated in the development of familial HPE, such as *SHH*, *GLI2*, *PTCH1*, *TGIF*, *ZIC2*, *TDGF1*, and *SIX3*.[9,11,12]

Recent data suggest specific genotype-phenotype correlations in HPE. *SHH* mutations result in a milder disease than mutations in the other common HPE genes.[6,12] Such microforms of HPE are represented by hypotelorism, solitary central maxillary incisor, and cleft lip/palate. Mutations in *ZIC2* (located on 13q32 chromosome) and *SIX3* (located on 2p21 chromosome), for instance, have a high prevalence in more severe HPE types (generally, alobar subtype).[10,13,14] *ZIC2* is also associated to neuronal tube defects, mainly rachischisis, and neuronal migration abnormalities. HPE-related gene mutations in the *SHH* and *TGIF* genes have been correlated with the cause of the pituitary stalk interruption syndrome and isolated pituitary hypoplasia.[15]

Agenesis of the Corpus Callosum

Agenesis of corpus callosum (ACC) is the most common type of commissural agenesis. Recent neonatal and prenatal imaging studies suggest that ACC occurs in at least 1 in 4000 live births[16,17] and up to 3% to 5% of individuals assessed for neurodevelopmental disorders by neuroimaging.[18,19] Complete and partial ACC can result from genetic, infectious, vascular, or toxic causes. Recently, Edwards and colleagues[20] described a comprehensive classification of the clinical and genetic features of syndromes associated with ACC.

Current evidence[21,22] suggests that a combination of genetic mechanisms, including single gene Mendelian, single gene sporadic mutations, and complex genetics (which may have a mixture of inherited and sporadic mutations) may be involved in the cause of ACC. For approximately 40% of individuals with ACC, the cause is identifiable (<10% have chromosomal anomalies and the remaining 30% have recognizable genetic syndromes).[23] Genetically, it can occur either isolated or in association with congenital syndromes. The callosal anomalies are an important feature described in more than 180 syndromes.[5] In a meta-analysis, O'Driscoll and colleagues[22] identified 12 loci with 6 or more individuals with ACC, spread over 10 chromosomes, which is considered a high penetrance according with classification of critical region. Several of these regions are associated with common deletion or duplication syndromes in humans. The 2 ACC causative gene identified from 1 of these regions are *AKT3* (located on 1q43-q44 chromosome) and *FOXG1* (located on 14q12 chromosome). No phenotypic association with other CNS malformations was identified in this cohort of 374 individuals.[22]

The ACC diagnosis is based on a finding of absent callosal fibers as visualized through neuroimaging (ultrasonography, computed tomography, or magnetic resonance [MR]). ACC is typically accompanied by a characteristic dilatation of posterior lateral ventricles (colpocephaly) associated with atypical fiber bundles (Probst bundles), which run anterior to posterior just lateral to the interhemispheric fissure.[24] Neuroimaging can also suggest a specific syndrome based on additional imaging features.

Aicardi syndrome (AS) is the most studied syndrome associated with ACC. This syndrome is an X-linked dominant disorder (loci gene is on Xp22 chromosome). AS should be considered when ACC is related to periventricular nodular or subcortical heterotopia, polymicrogyria, cerebellar hypoplasia, posterior fossa cysts, papillomas in the choroid plexus, and microphthalamia.[12]

ACC associated with classic lissencephaly (LIS) and perisylvian pachygyria with dysgenesis of the brainstem and cerebellum has recently been described in patients with tubulin-related cortical phenotypes. MR with these findings should be a clue to the diagnosis of *TUBA1A* mutation.[25,26]

ACC with abnormal genitalia can be associated with *ARX* gene mutation. *ARX* gene mutation is the second most common cause of X-linked mental retardation (after fragile X syndrome) and has been associated with hydrocephaly with abnormal genitalia, LIS with abnormal genitalia, Partington syndrome, X-linked infantile spasms, myoclonic epilepsy with spasticity and mental retardation, and nonspecific mental retardation.[27]

X-linked hydrocephalus has an incidence of 1 in 30,000 male births and is characterized by intellectual disability, spastic paraplegia, adducted thumbs, and ACC, or corticospinal tract. Most cases are ascribed to loss of function mutations L1 cell adhesion molecule (*L1CAM*) gene. L1 protein plays a key role in neurite outgrowth, axonal guidance, and pathfinding during the development of the nervous system.[28,29]

Additional genetic mutations can be better studied using neuroimaging features. ACC associated with anophthalmia/microphthalmia, for example, has been described in patients with *Vax1/Vax2* mutations. *Vax1* and *Vax2* have been implicated in eye development and the closure of the choroid fissure in animal models.[30] Neuroimaging showing ACC in a patient with a history of a motor-sensory neuropathy has been described in Andermann syndrome, an autosomal recessive disorder caused by mutations of the *KCC3* gene.[31]

MALFORMATIONS OF THE CORTICAL DEVELOPMENT
Microcephaly

Microcephaly can be isolated or associated with other anomalies (often termed syndromic). When present at birth, it has been termed primary microcephaly, as opposed to secondary microcephaly, which develops later. The crucial difference between these groups is that primary microcephaly is usually a static developmental anomaly, whereas secondary microcephaly indicates a progressive neurodegenerative condition.[32–34] Patients born with normal to slightly small head size (≤2 standard deviations [SD] lower than the mean) and developing severe microcephaly in the first 1 to 2 years after birth form a separate group, designated postmigrational microcephaly, because brain growth seems to slow during late gestation or the early postnatal period after normal early development.

Clinically, patients have a reduction in head circumference (HC) during pregnancy (usually at 32 weeks) or at birth. Subsequent head growth is slow, and HC worsens during infancy (<−3 SD at 6 months). Nonprogressive intellectual impairment, delay in early motor milestones, speech delay, and hyperactive behavior are common.

Pathogenesis of microcephaly is heterogeneous. Genetic and environmental factors are potential causes, and these factors may act prenatally, perinatally, or postnatally to inhibit brain growth. Genetically, isolated microcephaly is mostly Mendelian autosomal dominant, recessive, or X-linked genes. Most genes known to cause primary microcephaly compromise pathways and disturb processes such as cell cycle length, spindle positioning, or DNA repair efficiency involved in neurogenesis and, in particular, the cell cycle phases of mitosis. Ten subtypes based on the 11 genes have been differentiated (*MCPH1*, *WDR62*, *CDK5RAP2*, *CEP152*, *ASPM*, *CENPJ*, *STIL*, *CEP63*, *CEP135*, *CASC5*, and *PHC1*).[35–37]

Neuroimaging of patients with autosomal recessive primary microcephalies (MCPH) shows grossly normal, proportionately small-sized brain with some degree of gyral simplification and small normal brainstem and cerebellum. A simplified gyral pattern is frequently described in patients with MCPH5, caused by mutation in the *ASPM* gene (chromosome 1q31).[35,38,39] MCPH2 caused by mutations of *ARFGEF2* has associated periventricular nodular heterotopia.[40–43]

From an imaging point of view, 2 additional diseases are important to discuss: X-linked postmigrational microcephaly associated with mutations of *CASK* (calcium/calmodulin-dependent serine protein kinase) and pontocerebellar hypoplasia (PCH).

Mutations of the *CASK* gene at Xp11.4 have recently been reported to have a wide phenotypic spectrum, ranging from a severe form in female patients (mental retardation and microcephaly with disproportionate brainstem and cerebellar hypoplasia) to a milder form in male patients with congenital nystagmus and mental retardation. MR has been shown to be useful, showing microcephaly with disproportionate cerebellar and brainstem hypoplasia.[44,45] The volume of the corpus callosum is normal in patients with *CASK* mutations, a finding not observed in other microcephalic patients with brainstem/cerebellum hypoplasia such as PCH, PEHO syndrome (Progressive encephalopathy with Edema, Hypsarrhythmia and Optic atrophy), 5p-syndrome, trisomy of chromosome 18, and other complex chromosomal abnormalities.[45] *CASK* is a protein that induces transcription of genes containing *TBR1* binding sequences, such as *RELN*, required for normal development of the cerebrum, brainstem, and cerebellum.

PCH caused by mutations in transfer RNA splicing endonuclease subunit genes (*TSEN54*, *TSEN2*, *TSEN34*) is a prenatal onset neurodegenerative disorder, in which significant microcephaly develops after birth.[46,47] Recently, MR data showed that the common homozygous mutation in *TSEN54* can be predicted reliably from the PCH type 2 MR phenotype, described as a dragonflylike cerebellar hemisphere and a flat pons associated clinically with dyskinesia or dystonia, neonatal irritability, central visual impairment, absence of optic atrophy, and severe cognitive and motor impairment.

Megaloencephaly

A practical approach to patients with macrocephaly divides the megaloencephaly (MEG) syndromes in 2 groups: (1) MEG with normal cortex and (2) MEG with cortical dysplasia.[1,48]

Examples of genetically defined MEG syndromes with a normal cortex are Cowden syndrome, Bannayan-Riley-Ruvalcaba syndrome (BRRS), Proteus syndrome, autism spectrum disorders with macrocephaly (ASDM), and Sotos syndrome. These disorders are also named PTEN hamartoma tumor syndromes and refer to a group of clinical syndromes of aberrant growth caused by mutations in the PTEN tumor suppressor gene.

Neuroimaging of patients with Cowden syndrome can show dysplastic gangliocytoma of the cerebellum (Lhermitte-Duclos disease), and patients with BRRS can present with white matter cysts,[49] complex dural arteriovenous fistula,[50] and progressive spinal epidural lipomatosis.[51] Brain abnormalities are not common in Proteus syndrome; when present, hemimegalencephaly and migrational disorders are typically seen, commonly with an associated seizure disorder. Maxillary and mandibular dysmorphism may occur, including unilateral condylar hyperplasia. Subcutaneous fatty, fibrous, lymphangiomatous masses commonly seen in this syndrome may involve the neck and face, leading to disfigurement and potential airway compromise.[52] Imaging of patients with ASDM with mutation of the *PTEN* gene shows a suggestive pattern of multifocal white matter lesions associated with perivascular spaces.[53] MR studies of patient with Sotos syndromes show ventricular abnormalities, extracerebral fluid spaces, midline abnormalities and migrational abnormalities.[54]

MEG syndromes with cortical dysplasia have been noted to arise as sporadic overgrowth disorders, and recent data from the literature led to the characterization of 2 MEG syndromes by physical and neuroimaging anomalies: megaloencephaly-capillary malformations syndromes (MCAP) and megaloencephaly-polymicrogyriapolydactyly-hydrocephalus syndrome (MPPH). Riviere and colleagues[55] identified a striking correlation between MCAP and MPPH, with mutations in *PIK3CA*, *PIK3R2*, and *AKT3* genes. Neuroimaging of patients with MEG syndromes shows ventricular enlargement, cortical dysplasia (usually polymicrogyria), cerebellar tonsillar ectopia, thickening of the corpus callosum, and cranial asymmetry.[56]

Cortical Dysgenesis with Abnormal Cell Proliferation but Without Neoplasia

Cortical dysgenesis with abnormal cell proliferation can be diffuse, focal, or multifocal. Focal cortical dysplasia (FCD) represents a diverse group of neuron structural abnormalities and can be classified in subtypes I to III, by histopathologic criteria. Evidence has suggested that FCD is unlikely to be associated with a single gene mutation and is probably related to polymorphism mutations in the regulatory elements or to involve multiple genes such as *TSC1* and notch/Wnt signaling pathways. Regarding hemimegaloencephaly, data suggest that somatic mutations of the *PI3K-AKT-mTOR* pathway limited to the brain may represent a potential cause of asymmetric enlargement of the brain.[57,58]

Malformations with Neuroependymal Abnormalities: Periventricular Heterotopia

Periventricular heterotopia (PVH) has been classified in 2 groups based on the location of the nodules: anterior or posterior.[1] Genetically defined anterior PVH with an autosomal dominant inheritance has been described in patients with mutations on chromosomes 1 and 5.[59,60] Mutations of filamin A (*FLNA*), a protein that crosslinks actin filaments into orthogonal networks in cortical cytoplasm, has been described in patients with an X-linked inheritance associated with bilateral PVH.[61,62]

Malformations Caused by Generalized Abnormal Transmantle Migration

LIS and subcortical band heterotopia (SBH) are examples of congenital malformations related to generalized abnormal transmantle migration. Neuroimaging with anterior predominant or diffuse classic (4-layered) LIS and SBH has been shown in patients with *DCX* mutation at Xq22.3–q23.[63] In addition, a frontal predominant mild LIS with severe hippocampal and cerebellum hypoplasia has been associated with *RELN* mutation[64] and *VLDLR* mutation.[65] For the posterior predominant or diffuse classic (4-layered) and 2-layered (without cell-sparse zone) LIS and SBH, *TUBA1A* mutations,[66,67] Miller-Dieker syndrome (4-layered) with deletion at 17p13.3 (YWHAE telomeric to LIS1),[68] and posterior or diffuse LIS (isolated LIS sequence, 4-layered) or posterior SBH with LIS1 deletions or mutations at 17p13.3 have been reported.[63,68] Mutations in *ARX* at Xp22.13 have been shown in patients with X-linked LIS (3-layered, without cell-sparse zone) with callosal agenesis and ambiguous genitalia (XLAG).[69]

Malformations Caused by Abnormal Terminal Migration and Defects in Pial Limiting Membrane

Cobblestone malformation (former type 2 LIS) is a severe neuronal migration disorder characterized by protrusions of neurons beyond the first cortical layer at the pial surface of the brain. It is usually associated with eye anomalies and congenital muscular dystrophy (CMD). Cobblestone malformations occur in a graded series of CMDs, with brain involvement associated with reduced glycosylation of α-dystroglycan, which, from least to most severe, include CMD with mental retardation and microcephaly without obvious cortical malformation; CMD with mental retardation and isolated cerebellar hypoplasia and dysplasia; Fukuyama CMD (FCMD); muscle-eye-brain disease (MEB); and Walker-Warburg syndrome (WWS).

For the genetically defined cobblestone malformations (WWS, MEB, or FCMD) with frontal predominant abnormalities, *POMT1* mutation,[70–74] *FKTN* mutation associated with retinal abnormality (MEB-like),[75–79] and *LARGE* mutation[80] have been shown. Frontal predominant cobblestone has also been shown with *GPR56* mutations (bilateral frontoparietal polymicrogyria [BFPP]).[81]

For the genetically defined cobblestone malformations (WWS, MEB, or FCMD) with posterior predominant abnormalities, *LAMA1A* and *LAMC3* mutation (lacks CMD) has been reported.[82] Cobblestone malformations associated with congenital disorders of glycosylation (CDG) have been reported in patients with *SRD5A3* mutation.[83]

Polymicrogyria

Genetic heterogeneity is expected in polymicrogyria, because many types seem to be inherited as single gene disorders. In some cases, inheritance is multifactorial or complex, with interaction of several modifying genes, each with a small additive effect, and environmental factors (**Fig. 1**).[5,84,85]

Polymicrogyria, including the most common perisylvian subtype, has been associated with several chromosomal deletion and duplication syndromes, including the common deletion at 22q11.2 (DiGeorge syndrome). Multiple observations of familial polymicrogyria have been reported. Three loci of interest for the most common bilateral perisylvian form of polymicrogyria have been identified on the X chromosome, yet only 1 patient has been identified with a mutation in a gene at 1 of these loci, the *SRPX2* gene at Xq22. Other recessive pedigrees show a frontoparietal distribution, with mutations of the *GRP56* gene or a diffuse distribution associated with peroxisomal disorders. Mutations in the *TUBB2B*

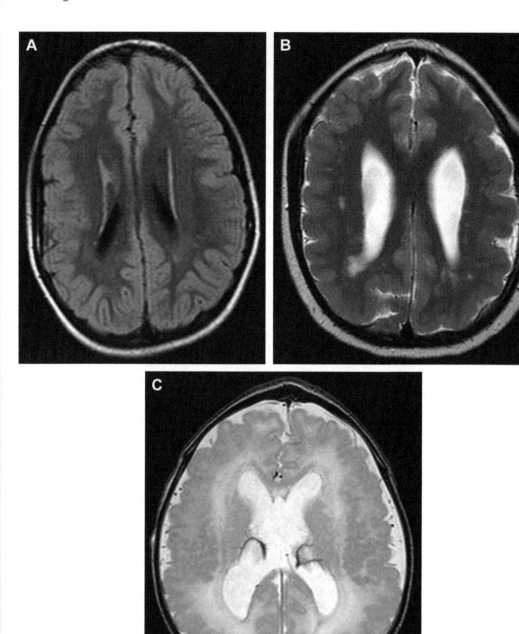

Fig. 1. Examples of polymicrogyria (PMG) in different patients. (*A*) Axial T1-weighted MR shows a patient with right frontoparietal PMG. This unilateral pattern has no gene related. (*B*) Axial T2-weighted MR shows an example of frontoparietal PMG with white matter lesions (pattern described in patients with GPR56 mutation). (*C*) Axial T2-weighted MR shows an example of perisylvian PMG with delayed myelinization and trigonocephaly.

gene have recently been identified in 4 patients with asymmetric polymicrogyria, and functional studies suggest that this gene is required for neuronal migration.[5]

For BFPP, previous studies[86,87] have indicated a gene, *GPR56*, on chromosome 16. Analysis of the *GPR56* gene expression pattern suggests an essential role in regional patterning of the frontoparietal cortex. For perisylvian polymicrogyria, different patterns of inheritance, including X-linked dominant, X-linked recessive, autosomal recessive, autosomal dominant with reduced penetrance, autosomal recessive with pseudodominance, and autosomal dominant have been suggested, showing the genetic heterogeneity of BFPP.[88–91] A unilateral or bilateral polymicrogyria associated with a velocardiofacial syndrome, DiGeorge syndrome, or conotruncal heart malformations has been described in patients with deletion of chromosome 22.[92]

MIDBRAIN AND HINDBRAIN MALFORMATIONS
Dandy-Walker Malformation

The Dandy-Walker malformation (DWM) is a heterogeneous disorder that has been associated with several malformation syndromes and cytogenetic abnormalities (Fig. 2). Over the past decade, several genetic loci have been implicated in the pathogenesis of DWM and other linked disorders, such as cerebellar vermis hypoplasia (CVH) and megacisterna magna (MCM), including the ZIC1, ZIC4, FOXC1, PAX3, NDUFA4, and PHF14 genes.[93–95]

DWM, CVH, and MCM are generally classified as different disorders; however, they share similarities in appearance, and it is not known whether they represent distinct entities or share a common pathogenesis.[94] The low empirical recurrence rate shown in nonsyndromic DWM suggests a polygenic model for the malformation.[95]

Rhombencephalosynapsis

Rhombencephalosynapsis (RES) is a congenital malformation that consists of cerebellar

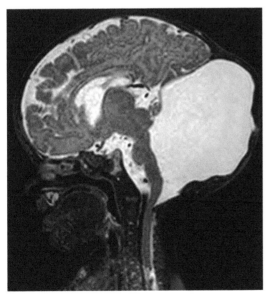

Fig. 2. DWM. Sagittal T2-weighted MR shows cystic dilatation of the fourth ventricle and developmental failure of the vermal primordial. Several genetic loci have been implicated with this MR phenotype.

hemisphere continuity, usually in the dentate nuclei and superior cerebellar peduncles caused by total or partial agenesis of the vermis. The classic MR findings are fusion of the cerebellar hemispheres, with continuous white matter tract crossing midline, fourth ventricle in a diamond shape, and absence of primary fissure. It might be related to aqueductal stenosis (causing hydrocephalus) or dysgenesis of the corpus callosum, mainly the posterior portion (Fig. 3).[96]

Most cases of RES are sporadic, although there are a few recurrent family cases, which suggests an autosomal recessive inheritance.[97,98] Mutations on several genes have been blamed on the isthmic organizer, which is responsible for the abnormal cerebellar patterning in RES, such as En1, En2, Pax2, Lmx1a, Lmx1b, FGF8, and Wnt1.[99,100] In animal models, homozygous mutation of Lmx1a resulted in agenesis of the vermis and fusion of the cerebellar hemisphere, making this mutation a strong candidate for genetic cases of RES.[101]

Joubert Syndrome

The radiologic hallmark of Joubert syndrome (JS) is the molar tooth sign, because of the appearance of the midbrain malformation in axial images on MR caused by CVH with prominent superior cerebellar peduncles. This finding is not pathognomonic of JS, and there are other syndromes with this abnormality: JS-related disorders (JSRD). Other MR findings related to JSRD are ventriculomegaly, polymicrogyria, hippocampal malformations, corpus callosum defects, absence of the pituitary gland, and other brainstem abnormalities, mainly in the midbrain and tectum (Fig. 4).[12,102]

All patients with JSRD clinically present hypotonia progressing to ataxia, development delay, oculomotor apraxia, and episodic hyperpnea (or other breathing abnormalities). In addition, subsets of patients also can have multiorgan involvement, such as retinal dystrophy, chorioretinal coloboma, cystic kidney disease, liver fibrosis, and postaxial polydactyly. JS is an autosomal recessive disorder, with a heterogeneous genetic profile. Twenty-one genes have been identified related, including AHI1, NPHP1, CEP290, TMEM67 (MKS3), RPGRIP1L, ARL13B, CC2D2A, INPP5E, KIF7, OFD1, TCTN1, TCTN2, and TMEM216.[102]

CC2D2A is one of the most prevalent mutations, and data have shown an association between this specific mutation and ventriculomegaly.[103] In addition, mutation in TMEM67 (MKS3) has been described in patients with liver disease,[104] and nephropathy is related to mutations in AHI1 and

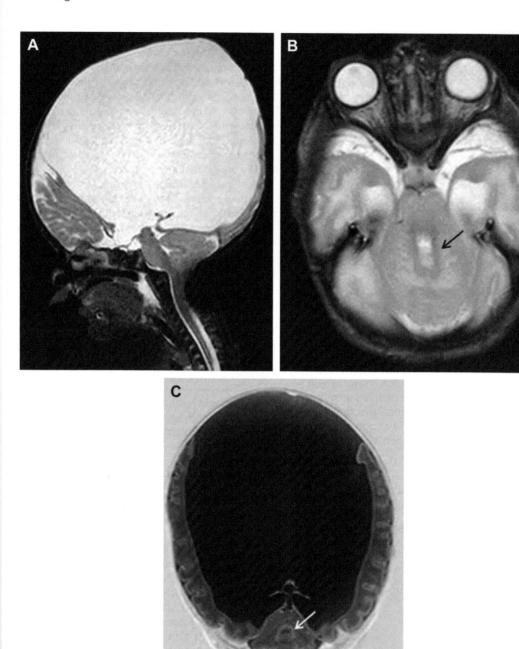

Fig. 3. RES. (*A*) Sagittal T2-weighted MR shows ACC, aqueduct stenosis, and tonsil herniation. Axial T2-weighted MR (*B*) and coronal T1 MR (*C*) show the keyhole sign (*arrow*) caused by the fusion of the dentate nuclei and the folia across the midline. Supratentorial hydrocephalus secondary to the aqueduct stenosis is common in patients with RES. Most cases of RES are sporadic, although there are a few recurrent family cases.

NPHP1.[105,106] *NPHP1* homozygous deletions seem to have thinner superior cerebellar peduncles, although this association needs to be further studied.[107]

Axon Guidance Disorders of the Hindbrain

Axon pathfinding is essential for the establishment of proper neuronal connections during

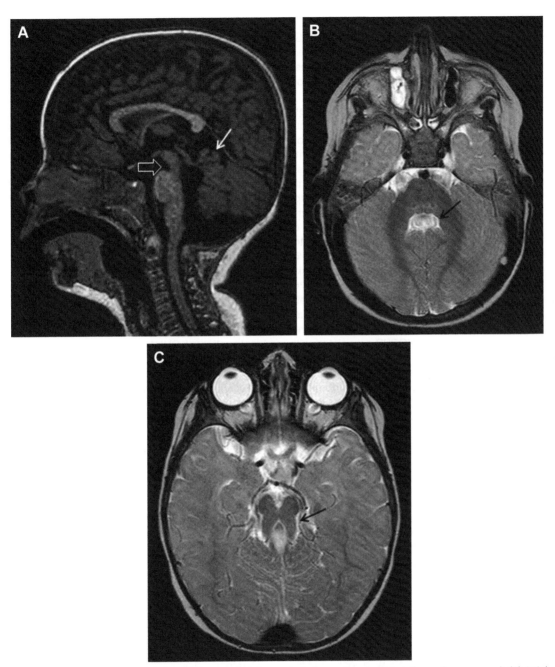

Fig. 4. JS and JSRD. (*A*) Sagittal T1 MR shows vermis hypoplasia (*arrow*) and a thin isthmus (*open arrow*). (*B*) Axial T2-weighted MR shows the classic batwing sign of the fourth ventricle (*arrow*) caused by the absence of vermis with apposed cerebellar hemispheres. (*C*) Axial T2-weighted MR shows the classic molar tooth appearance of midbrain with prominent superior cerebellar peduncles (*arrow*). JSRD are autosomal recessive disorders, with at least 21 genes already described.

development of the brainstem and cerebellum. Axon guidance disorders refers to an increasingly recognized group of diseases related to abnormal guidance or target innervations of axonal processes during neurodevelopment. These subtle morphologic anomalies have been studied recently by advanced MR techniques, including high-resolution MR and diffusion tensor imaging (DTI). The MR findings and genotype of horizontal gaze palsy with progressive scoliosis (HGPPS), congenital fibrosis of the extraocular muscles (CFEM), and pontine tegmental cap dysplasia

(PTCD), Duane syndrome (DS), HOXA1 and HOXB1 syndromes, Kallmann syndrome (KS), and Moebius syndrome (MS) are discussed. Some investigators have described some of these entities as congenital cranial dysinnervation disorders (CCDD).[108,109]

HGPPS is a rare disorder that results from axonal midline crossing defects of specific populations of neurons in the hindbrain and possibly spinal cord. Affected individuals are born with restricted horizontal gaze and develop scoliosis within the first decade of life. Normally, patients are intellectually and physically normal. This autosomal recessive disorder was described as early as 1970,[110] but it was not until 2004 that loss of function mutations in the axon guidance receptor *ROBO3* was found to underlie HGPPS.[111] MR of patients with HGPPS shows pontine hypoplasia, absent facial colliculi, butterfly configuration of the medulla, and a deep midline pontine cleft, whereas DTI maps showed absence of decussating pontocerebellar fibers and superior cerebellar peduncles.[6,112,113] HGPPS associated with bilateral polymicrogyria without *ROBO3* mutation has recently been described in the literature.[114]

CFEM refers to at least 7 autosomal dominant genetically defined strabismus syndromes, including *CFEM1A*, *CFEM1B*, *CFEM2*, *CFEM3A*, *CFEM3B*, *CFEM3C*, and Tukel syndrome. Patients present with nonprogressive ophthalmoplegia affecting part or all of the oculomotor nucleus and nerve and its innervated muscles.[115,116] Intellectual disability, social disability, facial weakness, or a progressive axonal peripheral neuropathy has been described in patients with CFEM3A, and patients with Tukel syndrome also have postaxial oligodactyly or oligosyndactyly of the hands. The diagnosis of CFEM is based on ophthalmologic features and genetic findings, such as *KIF21A* mutations (CFEM1), *PHOX2A* mutations (CFEM2), and *TUBB3* mutations (CFEM3).[117,118] MR of patients with CFEM shows hypoplasia of the oculomotor nerve and the muscles innervated by its superior branch, the levator palpebrae superioris and superior rectus. In patients with social and intellectual disabilities, MR shows agenesis or hypoplasia of the anterior commissure and corpus callosum, as well as malformed basal ganglia.[116,119,120] Congenital ophthalmoplegia associated with hypoplasia of extraocular muscles and intraorbital cranial nerves has also been described in patients with RYR1 mutations and malignant hyperthermia.[121]

PTCD is a newly described brainstem malformation with distinct neuroimaging findings, characterized by a flattened ventral pons, cerebellar vermal hypoplasia, and vaulted pontine tegmentum, which forms a caplike or beaklike bulge projecting into the fourth ventricle.[122] Previous DTI studies identified ectopic transversely oriented nerve fibers in the cap, and absence of transverse fiber bundles in the ventral pons, characterizing PTCD as an embryonic axon guidance defect.[123] It was first described by Barth and colleagues.[2] The condition is believed to occur as a result of aberrant neuronal axonal guidance during embryologic development, but its genetic cause has not been identified.

DS is a CCDD affecting 1 in 1000 individuals and is considered the most common CCDD.[124] Affected individuals have restricted horizontal gaze, which is greatest with attempted abduction and globe retraction. Pathologic studies of patients with DS found absence of abducent motor neurons and nerve associated with aberrant innervations of the lateral rectus muscle by axons of the oculomotor nerve.[125,126] Up to 10% of cases of DS may be familial, and genetic studies of rare families segregating autosomal dominant DS led to the identification of CHN1 as a *DS* gene.[127] Neuroimaging findings of patients with DS show absence or hypoplasia of cranial nerve VI.[128] Absence of the abducent nerve bilaterally associated with underdevelopment of the vestibular apparatus in the temporal bone has been described in patients with mutations in *HOXA1* gene (HOXA1 spectrum disease).[129,130]

In MS, patients present with congenital facial weakness associated with restricted horizontal eye movements.[124] MS is usually sporadic, although *HOXA1* and *TUBB3* mutations have been described in atypical MS phenotypes. Brainstem hypoplasia associated with absence or hypoplasia of the facial or abducent nerves is the most common radiologic feature in MS.[131]

KS has been considered a human guidance disorder of cranial nerve guidance, although embryologically, the olfactory nerve is derived from the hindbrain. KS is genetically heterogeneous and can be inherited as an X-linked, autosomal dominant, and possibly autosomal recessive trait.[3] Six KS genes have been reported, accounting for approximately 30% of cases: *KAL1* (KS type 1), *FGFR1* (KS type 2), *PROKR2* (KS type 3), *PROK2* (KS type 4), *CHD7* (KS type 5), and *FGF8* (KS type 6). MR of patients with KS show absence or hypoplasia of the olfactory bulb or nerve associated with a shallow olfactory sulcus. However, more than 60% of males harboring *KAL1* mutations also have mirror movements and enlarged aberrant ipsilateral corticospinal tract.[132] Recently, Costa-Barbosa and colleagues[133] reported that certain clinical features are highly associated with the gene mutation in patient with

KS, including dental agenesis and digital bony abnormalities (for KS types 2 and 6) and hearing loss (for KS type 7).

SUMMARY

CMCNS are prevalent disorders, and recent data from the literature have shown that advances in MR techniques have been fostering neuroimaging as a guide to genetic analysis. It is expected that identification of a gene mutation based on the MR phenotype could help the neuroscientist to better understand these disorders. Although much progress has been made in neuroembryology, genetics, and imaging of CMCNS, further advances in these topics suggest that progress will continue.

REFERENCES

1. Barkovich AJ, Guerrini R, Kuzniecky RI, et al. A developmental and genetic classification for malformations of cortical development: update 2012. Brain 2012;135(Pt 5):1348–69.
2. Barth PG, Majoie CB, Caan MW, et al. Pontine tegmental cap dysplasia: a novel brain malformation with a defect in axonal guidance. Brain 2007; 130(Pt 9):2258–66.
3. Engle EC. Human genetic disorders of axon guidance. Cold Spring Harb Perspectives in Biology 2010;2(3):a001784.
4. Jansen A, Andermann E. Genetics of the polymicrogyria syndromes. Journal Medical Genetics 2005;42(5):369–78.
5. Leventer RJ, Jansen A, Pilz DT, et al. Clinical and imaging heterogeneity of polymicrogyria: a study of 328 patients. Brain 2010;133(Pt 5):1415–27.
6. Nugent AA, Kolpak AL, Engle EC. Human disorders of axon guidance. Current Opinion Neurobiology 2012;22(5):837–43.
7. Van Allen MI, Kalousek DK, Chernoff GF, et al. Evidence for multi-site closure of the neural tube in humans. American J Medical Genetics 1993; 47(5):723–43.
8. Sarnat HB, Flores-Sarnat L. Neuroembryology and brain malformations: an overview. Handb of Clinical Neurology 2013;111:117–28.
9. Kanekar S, Shively A, Kaneda H. Malformations of ventral induction. Seminars Ultrasound CT MR 2011;32(3):200–10.
10. Dubourg C, Bendavid C, Pasquier L, et al. Holoprosencephaly. Orphanet J Rare Diseases 2007;2:8.
11. Ribeiro LA, Quiezi RG, Nascimento A, et al. Holoprosencephaly and holoprosencephaly-like phenotype and GAS1 DNA sequence changes: Report of four Brazilian patients. Am J Med Genet A 2010; 152A(7):1688–94.
12. Barcovich AJ, Raybaud C. Pediatric neuroimaging. 5th edition. Philadelphia: Wolters Kluwer Health/ Lippincott Williams & Wilkins; 2012.
13. Solomon BD, Lacbawan F, Mercier S, et al. Mutations in ZIC2 in human holoprosencephaly: description of a novel ZIC2 specific phenotype and comprehensive analysis of 157 individuals. Journal Medical Genetics 2010;47(8):513–24.
14. Mercier S, Dubourg C, Garcelon N, et al. New findings for phenotype-genotype correlations in a large European series of holoprosencephaly cases. Journal Medical Genetics 2011;48(11):752–60.
15. Tatsi C, Sertedaki A, Voutetakis A, et al. Pituitary stalk interruption syndrome and isolated pituitary hypoplasia may be caused by mutations in holoprosencephaly-related genes. J Clinical Endocrinology Metabolism 2013;98(4):E779–84.
16. Glass HC, Shaw GM, Ma C, et al. Agenesis of the corpus callosum in California 1983-2003: a population-based study. American J Medical Genetics A 2008;146A(19):2495–500.
17. Wang LW, Huang CC, Yeh TF. Major brain lesions detected on sonographic screening of apparently normal term neonates. Neuroradiology 2004; 46(5):368–73.
18. Bodensteiner J, Schaefer GB, Breeding L, et al. Hypoplasia of the corpus callosum: a study of 445 consecutive MRI scans. Journal Child Neurology 1994;9(1):47–9.
19. Jeret JS, Serur D, Wisniewski K, et al. Frequency of agenesis of the corpus callosum in the developmentally disabled population as determined by computerized tomography. Pediatric Neuroscience 1985;12(2):101–3.
20. Edwards TJ, Sherr EH, Barkovich AJ, et al. Clinical, genetic and imaging findings identify new causes for corpus callosum development syndromes. Brain 2014;137(Pt 6):1579–613.
21. Schell-Apacik CC, Wagner K, Bihler M, et al. Agenesis and dysgenesis of the corpus callosum: clinical, genetic and neuroimaging findings in a series of 41 patients. American Journal Medical Genetics A 2008;146A(19):2501–11.
22. O'Driscoll MC, Black GC, Clayton-Smith J, et al. Identification of genomic loci contributing to agenesis of the corpus callosum. American Journal Medical Genetics A 2010;152A(9):2145–59.
23. Bedeschi MF, Bonaglia MC, Grasso R, et al. Agenesis of the corpus callosum: clinical and genetic study in 63 young patients. Pediatric Neurology 2006;34(3):186–93.
24. Barkovich AJ, Lyon G, Evrard P. Formation, maturation, and disorders of white matter. AJNR Am J Neuroradiol 1992;13(2):447–61.
25. Zanni G, Colafati GS, Barresi S, et al. Description of a novel TUBA1A mutation in Arg-390 associated with asymmetrical polymicrogyria and mid-hindbrain

dysgenesis. European J Paediatr Neurology 2013; 17(4):361–5.

26. Okumura A, Hayashi M, Tsurui H, et al. Lissencephaly with marked ventricular dilation, agenesis of corpus callosum, and cerebellar hypoplasia caused by TUBA1A mutation. Brain Dev 2013; 35(3):274–9.

27. Troester MM, Trachtenberg T, Narayanan V. A novel mutation of the ARX gene in a male with nonsyndromic mental retardation. J Child Neurology 2007;22(6):744–8.

28. Piccione M, Matina F, Fichera M, et al. A novel L1CAM mutation in a fetus detected by prenatal diagnosis. European Journal Pediatrics 2010; 169(4):415–9.

29. Fernandez RM, Nunez-Torres R, Garcia-Diaz L, et al. Association of X-linked hydrocephalus and Hirschsprung disease: report of a new patient with a mutation in the L1CAM gene. American Journal Medical Genetics A 2012;158A(4):816–20.

30. Slavotinek AM, Chao R, Vacik T, et al. VAX1 mutation associated with microphthalmia, corpus callosum agenesis, and orofacial clefting: the first description of a VAX1 phenotype in humans. Human Mutation 2012;33(2):364–8.

31. Uyanik G, Elcioglu N, Penzien J, et al. Novel truncating and missense mutations of the KCC3 gene associated with Andermann syndrome. Neurology 2006;66(7):1044–8.

32. Qazi QH, Reed TE. A problem in diagnosis of primary versus secondary microcephaly. Clinical Genetics 1973;4(1):46–52.

33. Dobyns WB. Primary microcephaly: new approaches for an old disorder. American J Medical Genetics 2002;112(4):315–7.

34. Rosenberg MJ, Agarwala R, Bouffard G, et al. Mutant deoxynucleotide carrier is associated with congenital microcephaly. Nature Genetics 2002; 32(1):175–9.

35. Passemard S, Titomanlio L, Elmaleh M, et al. Expanding the clinical and neuroradiologic phenotype of primary microcephaly due to ASPM mutations. Neurology 2009;73(12):962–9.

36. Rimol LM, Agartz I, Djurovic S, et al. Sex-dependent association of common variants of microcephaly genes with brain structure. Proc Natl Acad Sci U S A 2010;107(1):384–8.

37. Shen J, Gilmore EC, Marshall CA, et al. Mutations in PNKP cause microcephaly, seizures and defects in DNA repair. Nature Genetics 2010;42(3): 245–9.

38. Mochida GH, Walsh CA. Molecular genetics of human microcephaly. Current Opinion Neurology 2001;14(2):151–6.

39. Desir J, Cassart M, David P, et al. Primary microcephaly with ASPM mutation shows simplified cortical gyration with antero-posterior gradient

pre- and post-natally. American J Medical Genetics A 2008;146A(11):1439–43.

40. de Wit MC, de Coo IF, Halley DJ, et al. Movement disorder and neuronal migration disorder due to ARFGEF2 mutation. Neurogenetics 2009;10(4): 333–6.

41. Bilguvar K, Ozturk AK, Louvi A, et al. Whole-exome sequencing identifies recessive WDR62 mutations in severe brain malformations. Nature 2010; 467(7312):207–10.

42. Nicholas AK, Khurshid M, Desir J, et al. WDR62 is associated with the spindle pole and is mutated in human microcephaly. Nature Genetics 2010; 42(11):1010–4.

43. Bhat V, Girimaji SC, Mohan G, et al. Mutations in WDR62, encoding a centrosomal and nuclear protein, in Indian primary microcephaly families with cortical malformations. Clinical Genetics 2011; 80(6):532–40.

44. Najm J, Horn D, Wimplinger I, et al. Mutations of CASK cause an X-linked brain malformation phenotype with microcephaly and hypoplasia of the brainstem and cerebellum. Nature Genetics 2008;40(9):1065–7.

45. Takanashi J, Arai H, Nabatame S, et al. Neuroradiologic features of CASK mutations. AJNR Am J Neuroradiol 2010;31(9):1619–22.

46. Barth PG, Ryan MM, Webster RI, et al. Rhabdomyolysis in pontocerebellar hypoplasia type 2 (PCH-2). Neuromuscul Disorders 2008;18(1):52–8.

47. Namavar Y, Barth PG, Kasher PR, et al. Clinical, neuroradiological and genetic findings in pontocerebellar hypoplasia. Brain 2011;134(Pt 1):143–56.

48. Papetti L, Tarani L, Nicita F, et al. Macrocephaly-capillary malformation syndrome: description of a case and review of clinical diagnostic criteria. Brain Dev 2012;34(2):143–7.

49. Bhargava R, Au Yong KJ, Leonard N. Bannayan-Riley-Ruvalcaba syndrome: MRI neuroimaging features in a series of 7 patients. AJNR Am J Neuroradiol 2014;35(2):402–6.

50. Moon K, Ducruet AF, Crowley RW, et al. Complex dural arteriovenous fistula in Bannayan-Riley-Ruvalcaba syndrome. Journal Neurosurgery Pediatrics 2013;12(1):87–92.

51. Toelle S, Poretti A, Scheer I, et al. Bannayan-Riley-Ruvalcaba syndrome with progressive spinal epidural lipomatosis. Neuropediatrics 2012;43(4): 221–4.

52. DeLone DR, Brown WD, Gentry LR. Proteus syndrome: craniofacial and cerebral MRI. Neuroradiology 1999;41(11):840–3.

53. Vanderver A, Tonduti D, Kahn I, et al. Characteristic brain magnetic resonance imaging pattern in patients with macrocephaly and PTEN mutations. American J Medical Genetics A 2014;164A(3): 627–33.

54. Schaefer GB, Bodensteiner JB, Buehler BA, et al. The neuroimaging findings in Sotos syndrome. American J Medical Genetics 1997;68(4):462–5.

55. Riviere JB, Mirzaa GM, O'Roak BJ, et al. De novo germline and postzygotic mutations in AKT3, PIK3R2 and PIK3CA cause a spectrum of related megalencephaly syndromes. Nature Genetics 2012;44(8):934–40.

56. Mirzaa GM, Conway RL, Gripp KW, et al. Megalencephaly-capillary malformation (MCAP) and megalencephaly-polydactyly-polymicrogyria-hydrocephalus (MPPH) syndromes: two closely related disorders of brain overgrowth and abnormal brain and body morphogenesis. American J Medical Genetics A 2012;158A(2):269–91.

57. Baek ST, Gibbs EM, Gleeson JG, et al. Hemimegalencephaly, a paradigm for somatic postzygotic neurodevelopmental disorders. Current Opinion Neurology 2013;26(2):122–7.

58. Poduri A, Evrony GD, Cai X, et al. Somatic activation of AKT3 causes hemispheric developmental brain malformations. Neuron 2012;74(1):41–8.

59. Sheen VL, Topcu M, Berkovic S, et al. Autosomal recessive form of periventricular heterotopia. Neurology 2003;60(7):1108–12.

60. Neal J, Raju GP, Bodell A, et al. Periventricular heterotopia with complete agenesis of the corpus callosum: a case report. Journal Neurology 2006; 253(10):1358–9.

61. Sheen VL, Dixon PH, Fox JW, et al. Mutations in the X-linked filamin 1 gene cause periventricular nodular heterotopia in males as well as in females. Human Molecular Genetics 2001;10(17):1775–83.

62. Parrini E, Ramazzotti A, Dobyns WB, et al. Periventricular heterotopia: phenotypic heterogeneity and correlation with filamin A mutations. Brain 2006; 129(Pt 7):1892–906.

63. Dobyns WB, Truwit CL, Ross ME, et al. Differences in the gyral pattern distinguish chromosome 17-linked and X-linked lissencephaly. Neurology 1999;53(2):270–7.

64. Hong SE, Shugart YY, Huang DT, et al. Autosomal recessive lissencephaly with cerebellar hypoplasia is associated with human RELN mutations. Nature Genetics 2000;26(1):93–6.

65. Boycott KM, Flavelle S, Bureau A, et al. Homozygous deletion of the very low density lipoprotein receptor gene causes autosomal recessive cerebellar hypoplasia with cerebral gyral simplification. American J Human Genetics 2005;77(3):477–83.

66. Poirier K, Keays DA, Francis F, et al. Large spectrum of lissencephaly and pachygyria phenotypes resulting from de novo missense mutations in tubulin alpha 1A (TUBA1A). Human Mutation 2007;28(11):1055–64.

67. Kumar RA, Pilz DT, Babatz TD, et al. TUBA1A mutations cause wide spectrum lissencephaly (smooth brain) and suggest that multiple neuronal migration pathways converge on alpha tubulins. Human Molecular Genetics 2010;19(14):2817–27.

68. Dobyns WB, Curry CJ, Hoyme HE, et al. Clinical and molecular diagnosis of Miller-Dieker syndrome. American J Human Genetics 1991;48(3): 584–94.

69. Bonneau D, Toutain A, Laquerriere A, et al. X-linked lissencephaly with absent corpus callosum and ambiguous genitalia (XLAG): clinical, magnetic resonance imaging, and neuropathological findings. Annals Neurology 2002;51(3):340–9.

70. Beltran-Valero de Bernabe D, Currier S, Steinbrecher A, et al. Mutations in the O-mannosyltransferase gene POMT1 give rise to the severe neuronal migration disorder Walker-Warburg syndrome. American J Human Genetics 2002;71(5): 1033–43.

71. van Reeuwijk J, Maugenre S, van den Elzen C, et al. The expanding phenotype of POMT1 mutations: from Walker-Warburg syndrome to congenital muscular dystrophy, microcephaly, and mental retardation. Human Mutation 2006;27(5):453–9.

72. van Reeuwijk J, Janssen M, van den Elzen C, et al. POMT2 mutations cause alpha-dystroglycan hypoglycosylation and Walker-Warburg syndrome. Journal Medical Genetics 2005;42(12):907–12.

73. Mercuri E, D'Amico A, Tessa A, et al. POMT2 mutation in a patient with 'MEB-like' phenotype. Neuromuscul Disord 2006;16(7):446–8.

74. Manya H, Sakai K, Kobayashi K, et al. Loss-of-function of an N-acetylglucosaminyltransferase, POMGnT1, in muscle-eye-brain disease. Biochem Biophys Res Communications 2003;306(1):93–7.

75. de Bernabe DB, van Bokhoven H, van Beusekom E, et al. A homozygous nonsense mutation in the fukutin gene causes a Walker-Warburg syndrome phenotype. Journal Medical Genetics 2003;40(11): 845–8.

76. Manzini MC, Gleason D, Chang BS, et al. Ethnically diverse causes of Walker-Warburg syndrome (WWS): FCMD mutations are a more common cause of WWS outside of the Middle East. Human Mutation 2008;29(11):E231–41.

77. Yoshioka M. Phenotypic spectrum of Fukutinopathy: most severe phenotype of Fukutinopathy. Brain Dev 2009;31(6):419–22.

78. Yis U, Uyanik G, Heck PB, et al. Fukutin mutations in non-Japanese patients with congenital muscular dystrophy: less severe mutations predominate in patients with a non-Walker-Warburg phenotype. Neuromuscul Disord 2011;21(1):20–30.

79. Beltran-Valero de Bernabe D, Voit T, Longman C, et al. Mutations in the FKRP gene can cause muscle-eye-brain disease and Walker-Warburg syndrome. Journal Medical Genetics 2004; 41(5):e61.

80. van Reeuwijk J, Grewal PK, Salih MA, et al. Intragenic deletion in the LARGE gene causes Walker-Warburg syndrome. Human Genetics 2007; 121(6):685–90.

81. Piao X, Chang BS, Bodell A, et al. Genotype-phenotype analysis of human frontoparietal polymicrogyria syndromes. Annals Neurology 2005;58(5): 680–7.

82. Barak T, Kwan KY, Louvi A, et al. Recessive LAMC3 mutations cause malformations of occipital cortical development. Nature Genetics 2011;43(6):590–4.

83. Cantagrel V, Lefeber DJ, Ng BG, et al. SRD5A3 is required for converting polyprenol to dolichol and is mutated in a congenital glycosylation disorder. Cell 2010;142(2):203–17.

84. Barkovich AJ. Current concepts of polymicrogyria. Neuroradiology 2010;52(6):479–87.

85. Judkins AR, Martinez D, Ferreira P, et al. Polymicrogyria includes fusion of the molecular layer and decreased neuronal populations but normal cortical laminar organization. Journal Neuropathology Experimental Neurology 2011;70(6):438–43.

86. Luo R, Yang HM, Jin Z, et al. A novel GPR56 mutation causes bilateral frontoparietal polymicrogyria. Pediatric Neurology 2011;45(1):49–53.

87. Fujii Y, Ishikawa N, Kobayashi Y, et al. Compound heterozygosity in GPR56 with bilateral frontoparietal polymicrogyria. Brain Dev 2014;36(6):528–31.

88. Villard L, Nguyen K, Cardoso C, et al. A locus for bilateral perisylvian polymicrogyria maps to Xq28. American J Human Genetics 2002;70(4):1003–8.

89. Leventer RJ, Mills PL, Dobyns WB. X-linked malformations of cortical development. American J Medical Genetics 2000;97(3):213–20.

90. Guerreiro MM, Andermann E, Guerrini R, et al. Familial perisylvian polymicrogyria: a new familial syndrome of cortical maldevelopment. Annals Neurology 2000;48(1):39–48.

91. Herrera EP, Brandao-Almeida IL, Guimaraes CA, et al. Perisylvian syndrome: report of one Brazilian family with focus on the genetic mode of inheritance and clinical spectrum. Arq Neuropsiquiatr 2005;63(2B):459–63 [in Portuguese].

92. Castro A, Rodrigues N, Pereira M, et al. Bilateral polymicrogyria: always think in chromosome 22q11.2 deletion syndromes. BMJ Case Reports 2011;2011.

93. Chitayat D, Moore L, Del Bigio MR, et al. Familial Dandy-Walker malformation associated with macrocephaly, facial anomalies, developmental delay, and brain stem dysgenesis: prenatal diagnosis and postnatal outcome in brothers. A new syndrome? American J Medical Genetics 1994;52(4): 406–15.

94. Millen KJ, Gleeson JG. Cerebellar development and disease. Current Opinion Neurobiology 2008; 18(1):12–9.

95. Murray JC, Johnson JA, Bird TD. Dandy-Walker malformation: etiologic heterogeneity and empiric recurrence risks. Clinical Genetics 1985;28(4):272–83.

96. Osborns A, Salzman K, Barkovich AJ. Diagnostic imaging brain. 2nd edition. Salt Lake City: Amirsys; 2009.

97. Romanengo M, Tortori-Donati P, Di Rocco M. Rhombencephalosynapsis with facial anomalies and probable autosomal recessive inheritance: a case report. Clinical Genetics 1997;52(3):184–6.

98. Ramocki MB, Scaglia F, Stankiewicz P, et al. Recurrent partial rhombencephalosynapsis and holoprosencephaly in siblings with a mutation of ZIC2. American J Medical Genetics A 2011;155A(7): 1574–80.

99. Dill P, Poretti A, Boltshauser E, et al. Fetal magnetic resonance imaging in midline malformations of the central nervous system and review of the literature. Journal Neuroradiol 2009;36(3):138–46.

100. Yachnis AT. Rhombencephalosynapsis with massive hydrocephalus: case report and pathogenetic considerations. Acta Neuropathol 2002; 103(3):301–4.

101. Millonig JH, Millen KJ, Hatten ME. The mouse Dreher gene Lmx1a controls formation of the roof plate in the vertebrate CNS. Nature 2000;403(6771):764–9.

102. Romani M, Micalizzi A, Valente EM. Joubert syndrome: congenital cerebellar ataxia with the molar tooth. Lancet Neurology 2013;12(9):894–905.

103. Bachmann-Gagescu R, Ishak GE, Dempsey JC, et al. Genotype-phenotype correlation in CC2D2A-related Joubert syndrome reveals an association with ventriculomegaly and seizures. Journal Medical Genetics 2012;49(2):126–37.

104. Parisi MA. Clinical and molecular features of Joubert syndrome and related disorders. American Journal of Medical Genetics. C Seminars in Medical Genetics 2009;151C(4):326–40.

105. Parisi MA, Doherty D, Eckert ML, et al. AHI1 mutations cause both retinal dystrophy and renal cystic disease in Joubert syndrome. Journal Medical Genetics 2006;43(4):334–9.

106. Parisi MA, Bennett CL, Eckert ML, et al. The NPHP1 gene deletion associated with juvenile nephronophthisis is present in a subset of individuals with Joubert syndrome. American Journal Human Genetics 2004;75(1):82–91.

107. Castori M, Valente EM, Donati MA, et al. NPHP1 gene deletion is a rare cause of Joubert syndrome related disorders. Journal Medical Genetics 2005; 42(2):e9.

108. Graeber CP, Hunter DG, Engle EC. The genetic basis of incomitant strabismus: consolidation of the current knowledge of the genetic foundations of disease. Seminars Ophthalmology 2013;28(5-6):427–37.

109. Ferreira RM, Amaral LL, Goncalves MV, Lin K. Imaging findings in congenital cranial dysinnervation

disorders. Topics in Magnetic Resonance Imaging 2011;22(6):283–94.

110. Dretakis E. Familial idiopathic scoliosis associated with encephalopathy in three children of the same family. Acta Orthop Hell 1970;22:51–5.

111. Jen JC, Chan WM, Bosley TM, et al. Mutations in a human ROBO gene disrupt hindbrain axon pathway crossing and morphogenesis. Science 2004; 304(5676):1509–13.

112. Sicotte NL, Salamon G, Shattuck DW, et al. Diffusion tensor MRI shows abnormal brainstem crossing fibers associated with ROBO3 mutations. Neurology 2006;67(3):519–21.

113. Haller S, Wetzel SG, Lutschg J, Functional MR. DTI and neurophysiology in horizontal gaze palsy with progressive scoliosis. Neuroradiology 2008;50(5): 453–9.

114. Irahara K, Saito Y, Sugai K, et al. Pontine malformation, undecussated pyramidal tracts, and regional polymicrogyria: a new syndrome. Pediatric Neurology 2014;50(4):384–8.

115. Mackey DA, Chan WM, Chan C, et al. Congenital fibrosis of the vertically acting extraocular muscles maps to the FEOM3 locus. Human Genetics 2002; 110(5):510–2.

116. Tischfield MA, Baris HN, Wu C, et al. Human TUBB3 mutations perturb microtubule dynamics, kinesin interactions, and axon guidance. Cell 2010;140(1):74–87.

117. Jiang YQ, Oblinger MM. Differential regulation of beta III and other tubulin genes during peripheral and central neuron development. Journal Cell Science 1992;103(Pt 3):643–51.

118. Ying M, Han R, Hao P, et al. Inherited KIF21A and PAX6 gene mutations in a boy with congenital fibrosis of extraocular muscles and aniridia. BMC Medical Genetics 2013;14:63.

119. Merino P, Gomez de Liano P, Fukumitsu H, et al. Congenital fibrosis of the extraocular muscles: magnetic resonance imaging findings and surgical treatment. Strabismus 2013;21(3):183–9.

120. Demer JL, Clark RA, Tischfield MA, et al. Evidence of an asymmetrical endophenotype in congenital fibrosis of extraocular muscles type 3 resulting from TUBB3 mutations. Investigative Ophthalmology Visual Science 2010;51(9):4600–11.

121. Shaaban S, Ramos-Platt L, Gilles FH, et al. RYR1 mutations as a cause of ophthalmoplegia, facial weakness, and malignant hyperthermia. JAMA Ophthalmology 2013;131(12):1532–40.

122. Rudaks LI, Patel S, Barnett CP. Novel clinical features in pontine tegmental cap dysplasia. Pediatric Neurology 2012;46(6):393–6.

123. Jissendi-Tchofo P, Doherty D, McGillivray G, et al. Pontine tegmental cap dysplasia: MR imaging and diffusion tensor imaging features of impaired axonal navigation. AJNR Am J Neuroradiol 2009; 30(1):113–9.

124. Oystreck DT, Engle EC, Bosley TM. Recent progress in understanding congenital cranial dysinnervation disorders. J Neuroophthalmol 2011;31(1): 69–77.

125. Hotchkiss MG, Miller NR, Clark AW, et al. Bilateral Duane's retraction syndrome. A clinical-pathologic case report. Archives Ophthalmology 1980;98(5): 870–4.

126. Miller NR, Kiel SM, Green WR, et al. Unilateral Duane's retraction syndrome (type 1). Archives Ophthalmology 1982;100(9):1468–72.

127. Miyake N, Chilton J, Psatha M, et al. Human CHN1 mutations hyperactivate alpha2-chimaerin and cause Duane's retraction syndrome. Science 2008; 321(5890):839–43.

128. Yonghong J, Kanxing Z, Zhenchang W, et al. Detailed magnetic resonance imaging findings of the ocular motor nerves in Duane's retraction syndrome. Journal Pediatric Ophthalmology Strabismus 2009;46(5):278–85 [quiz: 286–7].

129. Bosley TM, Alorainy IA, Salih MA, et al. The clinical spectrum of homozygous HOXA1 mutations. American J Medical Genetics A 2008;146A(10): 1235–40.

130. Tischfield MA, Bosley TM, Salih MA, et al. Homozygous HOXA1 mutations disrupt human brainstem, inner ear, cardiovascular and cognitive development. Nature Genetics 2005;37(10): 1035–7.

131. Wu SQ, Man FY, Jiao YH, et al. Magnetic resonance imaging findings in sporadic Mobius syndrome. Chinese Medical Journal 2013;126(12): 2304–7.

132. Krams M, Quinton R, Ashburner J, et al. Kallmann's syndrome: mirror movements associated with bilateral corticospinal tract hypertrophy. Neurology 1999;52(4):816–22.

133. Costa-Barbosa FA, Balasubramanian R, Keefe KW, et al. Prioritizing genetic testing in patients with Kallmann syndrome using clinical phenotypes. Journal Clinical Endocrinology Metabolism 2013; 98(5):E943–53.

Genetic Markers and Their Influence on Cerebrovascular Malformations

Hortensia Alvarez, MD[a], Mauricio Castillo, MD[b],*

KEYWORDS

- Cerebral vascular malformation • Hereditary hemorrhagic telangiectasia • Cerebral aneurysm
- Congenital vascular disorder • Gene expression

KEY POINTS

- Cerebral vascular malformations include anomalies of the arterial wall (ie, cerebral aneurysm), anomalies of the capillary–venous interface (ie, arteriovenous malformation), and venous anomalies (ie, cavernous malformations).
- Familial disorders caused by mutations in single genes are associated with cerebral aneurysms (polycystic renal disease), arteriovenous malformations (hereditary disorders such as hemorrhagic hereditary telangiectasia), and cavernous malformations.
- Recent studies identified critical genes involved in the development of sporadic forms of the same vascular disorders, emphasizing the role played by genetic and epigenetic factors in their genesis and evolution.
- Identification of genetic markers and therapeutic tools and strategies directed to alter the molecular pathways of vascular disorders are in the scope of future research.

ANEURYSMS

The term *aneurysm* encompasses a variety of lesions affecting the arterial vascular wall through different mechanisms, leading some investigators to use the term, *aneurysmal vasculopathy*, which allows categorization of these lesions in different subgroups.[1,2] Aneurysms result from luminal, parietal, or abluminal injuries or from a combination of all of these.[3]

Endothelial or adventitial chronic focal dissections causing recurrent mural hematomas, intramural thrombosis, intrathrombotic channels, and inflammatory changes in the adventitia are seen in serpentine or partially thrombosed aneurysms (Fig. 1). Giant aneurysms (larger than 2.5 cm) without intralesional thrombosis should be considered a type of focal dissections associated with failed angiogenesis in their walls (Fig. 2).[4] Proteins involved in the biological functions of proliferation, development, and apoptosis are highly expressed in large and giant unruptured aneurysms but scarcely expressed in unruptured aneurysms, suggesting that certain proteins are associated with aneurysm growth but not with their ruptures. Giant, serpentine, fusiform, and partially thrombosed aneurysms are associated with mural inflammatory processes. High-resolution black-blood contrast-enhanced T1-weighted magnetic resonance (MR) sequences can be used to detect macrophage activity and inflammation in the arterial walls and show focal contrast enhancement of the walls of inflamed aneurysms (Fig. 3). Patients with familial or acquired disorders mediated by immunologic pathways, such as familial candidiasis,[5] or patients with the acquired

The authors have nothing to disclose.
[a] Interventional Neuroradiology, UNC at Chapel Hill, Chapel Hill, NC 27516, USA; [b] UNC at Chapel Hill, Chapel Hill, NC 27516, USA
* Corresponding author.
E-mail address: castillo@med.unc.edu

neuroimaging.theclinics.com

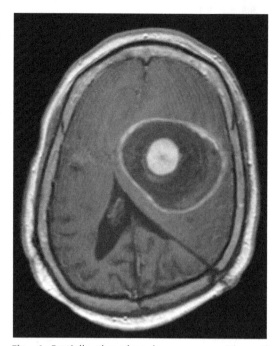

Fig. 1. Partially thrombosed aneurysm with wall enhancement. Axial T1 postcontrast image shows a left-sided giant aneurysm with contrast filling only its central aspect and the rest of it filled with clot. Note contrast enhancement of its wall, signifying adventitial inflammatory changes.

immunodeficiency syndrome,[6] may harbor multiple fusiform dysplastic aneurysms, but the responsible molecular mechanisms are unknown. Other inherited disorders, such as neurofibromatosis

type 1 (OMIM# 162200 autosomal dominant), and connective tissue diseases such as Ehlers-Danlos syndrome type IV (OMIM #130050, autosomal dominant) and Marfan syndrome (OMIM #154700, autosomal dominant) are associated with dysplastic vascular segments and fusiform or giant aneurysms. Noninflammatory conditions such as fibromuscular dysplasia[7,8] are also associated with intracranial aneurysms (IA), and although their cause is unknown, there have been reports of familial cases. Fusiform and large aneurysms may also be associated with cardiac myxoma in both the sporadic and familiar autosomal dominant forms.[9,10]

Most of the research on genetics of aneurysms is focused on the study of formation, growth, and rupture of saccular aneurysms or "berry aneurysms" (**Fig 4**). Saccular intracranial aneurysms are defined as vascular out pouches located mainly around the circle of Willis, usually measuring less than 25 mm (with most ruptured ones measuring 5–7 mm),[11] more frequent in women between 40 and 60 years, very infrequent in pediatric populations, and associated to risk factors such as high blood pressure, cigarette smoking, and alcohol consumption. They are considered the most frequent type of aneurysm, accounting for 80% to 90%[12] of all IA; however, the term *saccular aneurysm* is not used homogenously in the literature. In a recent meta-analysis,[13] the prevalence of saccular IA was estimated at 3.2% of patients without comorbidities, whereas the prevalence was 6.9% in patients with Autosomal dominant polycystic kidney disease

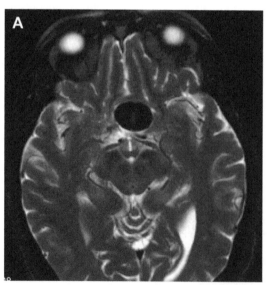

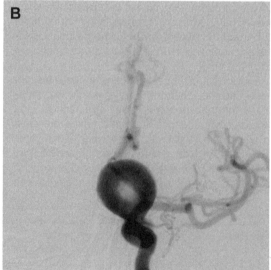

Fig. 2. Giant patent unruptured aneurysm. (*A*) Axial T2 image shows a left supraclinoid internal carotid artery giant aneurysm without any clot. (*B*) Frontal digital subtraction angiography view shows the aneurysm to be completely patent with earlier contrast filling peripherally rather than centrally.

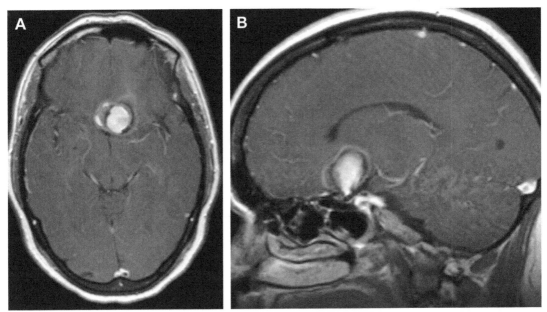

Fig. 3. Giant partially thrombosed aneurysm. (*A*) Axial T1 postcontrast image shows a left-sided supraclinoid internal carotid artery aneurysm with nonenhancing clot surrounding the contrast-filled lumen and wall enhancement caused by inflammation in the adventia. (*B*) Parasagittal postcontrast T1 image clearly shows wall contrast enhancement.

(ADPKD) and 3%–4% in patients with a positive family history of IA or subarachnoid hemorrhage. The same investigators point out that the high incidence of subarachnoid hemorrhage in Finland and Japan does not correlate with a higher incidence of IA but rather with a high rate of rupture. ADPKD is a genetic disorder caused by mutations in 2

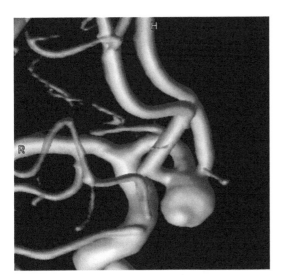

Fig. 4. Common saccular aneurysm. Oblique 3-dimensional view from digital subtraction angiography shows a common saccular aneurysm in the anterior communicating artery region. Note small protuberance at dome in this aneurysm which had ruptured.

genes, PDK1 and PDK2, accounting for 85% to 90% and 10% to 15% of cases, respectively, and characterized by multiple renal cysts leading to progressive renal failure and hypertension. Cerebral aneurysms in ADPKD are 5 times more frequent than those found in the general population, and the average age for their rupture is 41 years, a decade earlier than in the general population.[1] IA in ADPKD is probably not related to early onset of hypertension. Recessive or infantile forms of PKD are not associated with IA. Proteins involved in ADPKD are expressed in vascular smooth muscle and endothelium, suggesting that they have a direct role in the vascular manifestations of ADPKD.[1] ADPKD accounts for 9% of familial IA. The tuberous sclerosis complex (OMIM#191100) is an autosomal dominant disorder caused by mutations in 2 genes (TSC1 and TSC2). TSC2 is located immediately adjacent to PDK1, and large deletions could result in a contiguous gene syndrome.[14] IA associated with tuberous sclerosis complex is thought to be a part of a continuous gene syndrome (**Fig. 5**).

In the absence of any heritable disorder, the prevalence of IA in first-degree relatives of patients with IA is estimated at 6% to 20%.[15] The Familial Aneurysm study,[16] a multicentric study comparing the characteristics of familiar and nonfamilial IA in more than 3000 participants found that familial IA are more likely multiple, are more likely to be located in the middle cerebral artery, and present

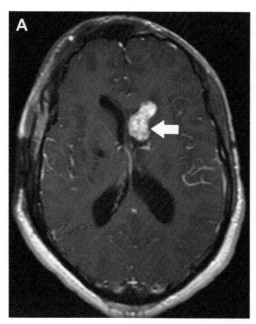

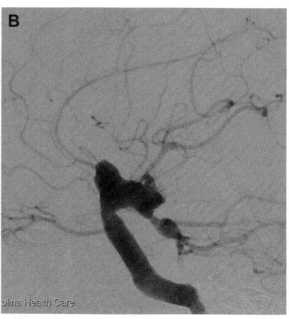

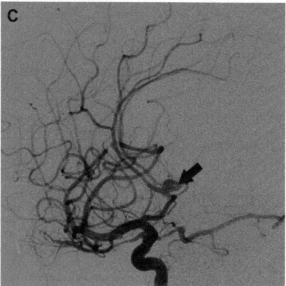

Fig. 5. Tuberous sclerosis and vascular anomalies. (*A*) Axial postcontrast T1 image shows a left-sided enhancing giant cell subependymal astrocytoma (*arrow*), mild hydrocephalus, and multiple skull fibrous plaques. (*B*) Oblique DSA view of left internal carotid artery injection shows dilated and dysplastic arteries. (*C*) Oblique DSA view of right internal carotid artery injection shows an anterior communicating artery aneurysm (*arrow*) in the same patient.

higher risk of rupture than sporadic IA.[17,18] Similar data are reported in several other population-based and non–population-based studies.

It seems that genetic factors likely influence the occurrence of IA in association with hemodynamic factors or modifiable risk factors such as hypertension, alcohol abuse, and cigarette smoking.[19] Candidate gene studies in sporadic IA have identified several potential risk loci with the affected proteins involved in the regulation of the extracerebral matrix, endothelium maintenance, and the inflammatory pathways through the regulation of macrophages, lymphocytes, and interleukins.[20] More recently, genomewide association studies (GWAS) using large cohorts of affected and nonaffected individuals are trying to identify variations in the entire genome (instead of in a candidate gene) that are common in individuals with a particular trait but not in the general population. Using this technology, several loci associated to IA were identified, and the loci 9p21.3, which is involved in multiple molecular pathways of cellular proliferation, seems to be the most consistent and significant one associated with IA. Genes on chromosomes 8, 4, 10, 13, and 18 expressed in smooth muscle and endothelial cells and collectively involved in regulating the cell cycle progression, cellular proliferation, and mechanisms of vasculogenesis and angiogenesis are also thought to be involved in the mechanism of IA formation and growth. A recent meta-analysis of all genetic studies in IA including candidate gene studies and GWAS in 116,000 individuals[19] found that multiple pathologic pathways involved in vascular endothelial maintenance and extracellular matrix integrity are present in the formation and rupture of IA, confirming that variants on chromosomes 4, 8, and 9 are strongly associated with IA. Interesting work is ongoing and focused on identifying molecular markers in peripheral blood to predict the risk of rupture, occurrence, and development of IA.[21]

The annual risk of rupture of IA is estimated at about 1%.[22] More than 30,000 subarachnoid hemorrhages (SAH) caused by ruptured IA are diagnosed every year in the United States. Mortality associated with IA rupture is estimated at 40% to 50% and with two-thirds of survivors having permanent neurologic deficits.[20] However, most of IA will not rupture. Identification of risk factors and mechanisms leading to aneurysms rupture is one of the goals of current research. The next generation of genetics tools and mega-analysis studies[20] with high power of predictions will likely help us understand the mechanisms of formation and rupture of IA and the links between genetic and environmental factors.

Guidelines from the American Heart Association published in 2012[22] consider it reasonable to offer noninvasive screening to patients with familial (at least 1 first-degree relative) SAH and/or a history of SAH to evaluate for de novo aneurysms or late regrowth of treated aneurysms, but the risks and benefits of this screening still require further study (class IIb; level of evidence B). Based on a cost-effectiveness study, Bor and colleagues[23] consider it acceptable to screen patients with 2 or more affected first-degree relatives. Screening should start at 20 years of age and be repeated every 7 years up to 80 years.

Digital subtraction angiography (DSA) is the gold standard to detect IA, but it carries a 0.5% risk of permanent neurologic sequelae. Noninvasive imaging techniques (computed tomography angiography/magnetic resonance [MR] imaging) should be considered the first option for screening of high-risk asymptomatic populations.

ARTERIOVENOUS MALFORMATIONS

Arteriovenous malformations (AVM) are anomalies of the arterial-venous capillary interface. They occur in 2 different forms: the nidal type, with a network of vessels connecting feeding arteries to draining veins, and the fistulae type, consisting of a connection between an artery and a vein without an interposed nidus. The size of an AVM is variable and extends from a microshunt measuring less than 1 cm to large lobar or multilobar shunts. AVM size and architectural type embody a genetically determined specific phenotypic expression, and, thus, a small microshunt does not become a large AVM and a nidus type AVM will not evolve into a fistula type. Single nucleotide polymorphism (SNP) on chromosome 9p21, previously reported to be associated with intracranial aneurysms and stroke, was recently found to be associated with sporadic brain AVM, in particular, with large nidus AVM, suggesting that this SNP could be a candidate marker for AVM dimension[24] and underlines the notion of the genetically predetermined specific features of AVM. The prevalence of AVM in the general population is 10 to 18:100,000 adults and 1.2 to 1.3 per 1000,000 new cases per person-year.[25] Studies on sporadic AVM identified several SNPs associated with an increased risk of AVM or their progression to rupture, but the molecular pathway leading to the initial formation of AVM is not yet known. Genomewide expression profiling of peripheral blood have recently been conducted to identify different expression profiles in ruptured and unruptured AVM.[26]

Most AVM are sporadic and exhibit differing sizes, types, and localizations. Only in few instances are cerebral or medullary AVM a part of a hereditary syndrome. Among those, HHT and AVM-capillary malformation are the most common hereditary disorders presenting with cerebral or medullary familiar AVM.

HHT, also known as Osler-Rendu-Weber syndrome, is an autosomal dominant condition with a highly variable expression among members of the same family, suggesting that the phenotype of this monogenetic disease could be influenced by other genes or by environmental or epigenetic factors. Three different genes are mutated in HHT: ENG, ACRVL1/ALK1, and SMAD 4, resulting in 3 phenotypes known as HHT1 (OMIM #187300), HHT2 (OMIM # 600376), and Juvenile Polyposis-HHT overlap syndrome (OMIM#175050). Cerebral and medullary AVM are more frequent in HHT1. In a large cross-sectional study including 171

HHT-affected patients with brain AVM, 69% had HHT1 mutation, 17% had HHT2, 2% had SMAD4, and in 13% no mutation was found.[25] The genes mutated in HHT encode proteins that mediate signaling by the transforming growth factor–ß superfamily, which is involved in the process of vascular remodeling and hemostasis.[27] The incidence of HHT in the general population is 1:5000 individuals with some regional variations caused by the founder's effect, which refers to first mutations occurring in common ancestors located in particular geographic regions. Conversely, brain AVM are associated with HHT in 2% of cases.[28,29]

In an interesting study by Park and colleagues[30] a de novo AVM was created and its development recorded in an HHT-mutated mouse model after inducing a wound in the animal's skin. The skin wound triggered an aberrant local angiogenic response of endothelial cells with creation of an arteriovenous shunt. The control mouse responded to the same injury by replicating normal vessels. In accordance with this observation is the second hit hypothesis, which considers that 2 different events are needed to develop a vascular lesion: a genetic silent defect and epigenetic trigger acting during a particular time window. It is also interesting to note that the levels of endoglin are reduced by 50% in the endothelium of AVM in HHT1 patients and that they are also reduced in regions with no AVM.

HHT clinical manifestations as defined by the HHT Foundation International are known as the *Curacao criteria*[27] and include recurrent epistaxis, mucocutaneous telangiectasia in distinctive sites (such as lips, oral cavity, and fingers) and arteriovenous malformations on liver, lung, gastrointestinal, or nervous system. Neurologic symptoms in HHT patients are related in two-thirds of patients to cerebral emboli or abscesses caused by paradoxic emboli from pulmonary arteriovenous fistula,[31] and one-third are caused by cerebral AVM.

Sporadic and HHT-related cerebral AVM are found to have different phenotypic expressions. Multiple cerebral AVM are present in 0.7% to 3% of sporadic AVM patients[31,32] (**Fig. 6**) reaching 39%[29] and 50%[32] in HHT patients. Micro-AVM (less than 1 cm) are present in 7% of patients with sporadic AVM but in 23.7% to 42.9% in HHT patients.[32,33] Furthermore, HHT-related AVM exhibit a lower annual risk of bleeding (0.4%–0.7%)[31] compared with the accepted annual risk of bleeding of sporadic AVM (2%–4%).[34,35] Finally, HHT-AVM in pediatric populations are frequently of the high-flow fistula AVM type.[34] Cerebral (supra- or infratentorial) and spinal cord[36,37] single-hole, fast-flow fistulae have been repeatedly reported in children with HHT.[36,37] Thus, HHT should be considered in children (and their family members) presenting with cerebral or medullary high-flow fistulae. Additionally, it has been suggested that these malformations should be included in the Curacao criteria.

Screening for asymptomatic AVM in HHT patients is controversial. International guidelines from the HHT International Foundation[38] recommend, despite a low level of evidence, to screen for cerebral AVM in adults with definite and possible HHT and in children at 6 months of age or at the moment of diagnosis. DSA is the gold standard to detect cerebral AVM but because it carries a 0.5% risk of permanent stroke MR imaging is judged a safer noninvasive modality. Owing to the lack of development of new cerebral AVM in adult HHT patients, follow-up MR imaging is not required after an initial negative result. However, a normal MR image during childhood should be

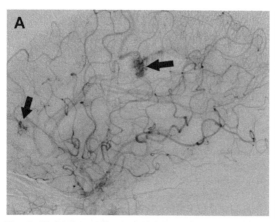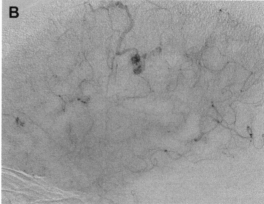

Fig. 6. Multiple small AVM in hemorrhagic hereditary telangiectasia. (*A*) Midarterial phase lateral DSA view shows 2 small frontal AVM (*arrows*). (*B*) Venous phase of DSA in the same patient shows the 2 small AVM and their venous drainage.

followed by an MR image in adult life. In the authors' institution, for purposes of AVM screening, a routine contrast-enhanced MR imaging study is performed but with the addition of susceptibility-weighted imaging and a time-of-flight magnetic resonance angiography using 3.0T units to obtain a higher spatial resolution.

CAPILLARY MALFORMATION-ARTERIOVENOUS MALFORMATION

Capillary malformation-arteriovenous malformation CM-AVM (OMIM#608354) is a recently described autosomal dominant condition associating multiple skin capillary malformations with fast-flow AVM caused by mutations in the RASA1 gene, which is involved in the modulation of a wide range of growth factor receptor signaling.[39] Fast-flow AVM have been described in the brain, face, and limbs in 18.5% of patients with RSA1 mutation but not in the lungs, liver, and gastrointestinal tract.[40] More recently, an association between RASA1 and spinal cord AVM[40] was reported in some patients. CMs, also known as port-wine stains, are present in 0.3% of newborns.[41] Most of these are isolated birthmarks and only a few are accompanied by cerebral or spinal vascular lesions such as CM-AVM or Sturge-Weber syndrome. CMs in CM-AVM syndrome are small, pale pink to red lesions, usually multiple and randomly located in the head, neck, trunk, and extremities. Most of them are present at birth, although new lesions can develop during childhood or young adulthood. RASA1 mutation was identified in CM-AVM patients but not in patients with isolated CM, isolated cerebral AVM, or patients with Sturge-Weber syndrome (SWS).[42] Cerebral and spinal AVM are describe as high-flow pial arteriovenous fistulas, draining into dilated venous pouches and are symptomatic in the first years of life. The molecular mechanism of the CM-AVM is not known. The highly variable intrafamilial and interfamilial phenotypic expressions suggest a somatic second hit mechanism in addition to the germline mutation.

STURGE-WEBER SYNDROME

SWS (OMIM # 185300) is a congenital, sporadic disorder in which patients harbor a facial port-wine stain, cortical dysplasias, ocular abnormalities, and choroid plexus hypertrophy. Intracerebral anomalies consist of lobar or multilobar cortical venular thrombosis with a secondary capillary venous proliferation and collateral venous circulation (Fig. 7).[43] The chronic venular ischemia leads to cerebral calcifications and focal atrophy (Fig. 8). The occipital lobes are the most commonly affected regions, but other regions including the cerebellar hemispheres or bilateral involvement can be seen. Progression of cortical and subcortical lesions is seen in patients during the first years of life.[44] Clinical manifestations related to cerebral anomalies include seizures, mental retardation, and hemiparesis. Seizures are present in 75% of SWS patients with unilateral brain involvement and in 95% of patients with bilateral brain lesions.[45] Ocular abnormalities include glaucoma, colobomas, and cataracts. Glaucoma occurs in one-third of patients and is caused by a retinal vascular venous malformation.[44] In a review of the literature, Schmidt and colleagues[46] found a total of 121 patients with retinal malformations; 52 lesions were associated with other cerebral or facial anomalies belonging to the spectrum of SWS. Thus, screening for cerebral abnormalities should be considered in patients with isolated retinal vascular malformations.

The facial port-wine stain is classically described as involving the region innervated by the first division of a trigeminal cranial nerve; however, it can extend to the mandibular region or be bilateral. SWS was considered by Lasjaunias and colleagues[43] as a metameric venous syndrome with cerebral and facial expressions caused by an early embryologic defect in a group of neural crest cells before their migration to their final territories (cerebral or facial). Recently, Shirley and colleagues[47] sequenced entire genomes of DNA samples of port-wine stain patients with and without SWS, brain tissue from SWS patients, and normal controls and they identified a somatic mutation in the GNAQ gene in SWS patients, in port-wine stain samples from syndromic and nonsyndromic patients but in none of the controls, suggesting that a single underlying mechanism is involved in the expression of SWS and nonsyndromic port-wine stains. Isolated port-wine stains may represent the late origin of somatic mutations involving a reduced number of cells, whereas the complete expression of the syndrome may represent an early mutation affecting a larger number of progenitor cells. Thus, an isolated port wine stain may represent an incomplete phenotypic expression of SWS.

On MR imaging, the classic finding of SWS is thick pial enhancement in the occipital, parietal, and cerebellar regions. One or both choroid plexuses may be enlarged. Susceptibility-weighted image may show prominent deep medullary veins generally converging in a choroid plexus glomus. The choroid layer of the eye may be thick and enhances more than usual and eventually the eye shrinks (phthisis bulbi). The skin corresponding

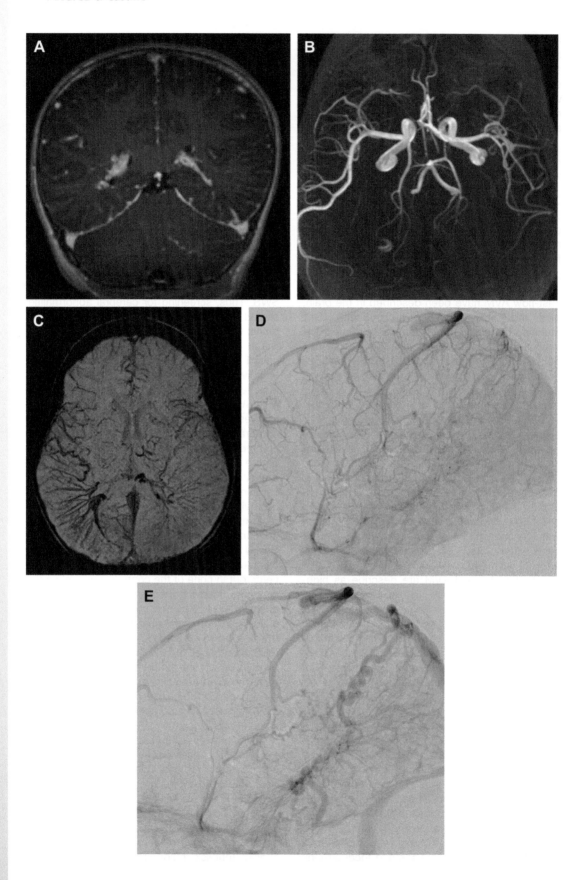

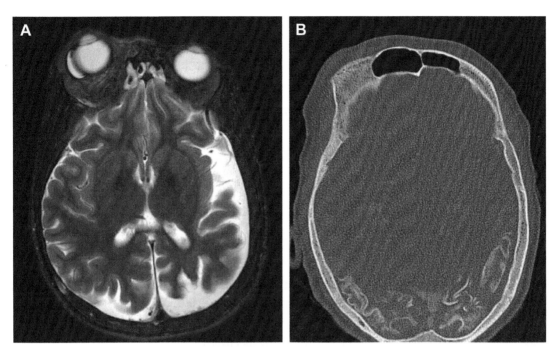

Fig. 8. Sturge-Weber syndrome, chronic changes. (*A*) Axial T2 image shows atrophy of the posterior cerebral hemispheres, left greater than right. Lateral to the right globe there is a glaucoma valve/reservoir. (*B*) Axial CT, bone windows, in same patient show posterior cortical calcifications. A right side glaucoma valve is present lateral to the globe.

to the port-wine stain may be thickened and the bones and muscles ipsilateral to it hypertrophied. Perfusion imaging shows increased blood flow and volume early in the course of the disease, but between 5 and 10 years of age the perfusion in those areas decreases, becomes low, and eventually leads to ischemia manifested as cortical calcifications on computed tomography (CT).

CEREBRAL CAVERNOUS MALFORMATION

Cerebral cavernous malformations (CCM) (OMIM# 116860), also known as cavernomas, cavernous angiomas, or cryptic vascular malformations, are vascular venous malformations. They comprise clusters of venous spaces lined by a single layer of endothelial cells embedded in a collagen matrix[48] with a variable layer of fibrous adventitia. They do not contain any brain cells and can occur in any region of the brain, including the ventricles, and spinal cord. Intralesional hemorrhages are

frequent as demonstrated by the different ages of blood seen by MR imaging. CCM can occur in familiar or sporadic forms accounting for 80% and 20% each, respectively. Mutations in 3 genes were identified in the familial forms: KRITI/CCM1, MGC4607CCM2, and PDCD10/CCM3 with CCM1 being the most frequent.[49] CCM1 is frequent in Hispanic Americans of Mexican descent attributed to the inheritance of the same mutation from a common ancestor (founder effect).[50]

Other vascular abnormalities are associated with CCM. In a prospective study[51] of 417 patients with familial CCM, cutaneous vascular malformations were found in 9%, an incidence significantly higher compared with incidence of CCM in the general population (0.3%), suggesting a link between the 2 conditions. Capillary malformations and hyperkeratotic cutaneous capillary venous malformations were the most common type of cutaneous vascular malformations and CCM1 the most commonly associated mutation.

Fig. 7. Sturge-Weber syndrome. (*A*) Coronal postcontrast T1 image shows bilateral cerebral pial enhancement and abnormal enhancing veins in white matter of the left cerebellar hemisphere. (*B*) Axial time-of-flight MR angiogram is normal. (*C*) Axial susceptibility-weighted image shows abnormal deep veins in most of the right cerebral hemisphere and, to a lesser degree, in the left one. (*D*) Lateral DSA view of a right-side injection shows absence of cortical veins and collateral venous circulation through deep veins. (*E*) Later venous phase in same patient shows collateral venous circulation caused by obliteration of superficial draining veins.

Developmental venous anomalies (DVA) are extreme anatomic variations of the cerebral venous drainage. They represent normal veins, draining normal nervous tissue with normal expression of structural and functional proteins and lack of angiogenetic activity. The incidence of DVA was found to be 2.6% in a series of 4069 brain autopsies.[52] DVA and CCM are seen together 14% to 30% of times. Petersen and colleagues,[53] in a retrospective study involving 112 patients and 2212 CCM, found DVA associated with CCM in 44% of sporadic forms and only in one patient with a familial form, suggesting that 2 different molecular mechanisms are involved. However, the link between these 2 abnormalities is not yet known. Because of the proximity between DVA and CCM in certain patients, it has been suggested that DVA could trigger the development of CCM by a focal release of angiogenetic signals, but that hypothesis has not been proven (Fig. 9). A recent report suggests that the 3 CCM genes are expressed in neurons rather than in blood vessels,[54] questioning the accepted view that endothelial instead of neuronal cells are the targets of the primary defect. As in other vascular anomalies, a 2-hit mechanism is probably responsible for them: first a germline mutation plus a

second somatic mutation explain the differences between familial and inter- and intrafamilial varieties of CCM.

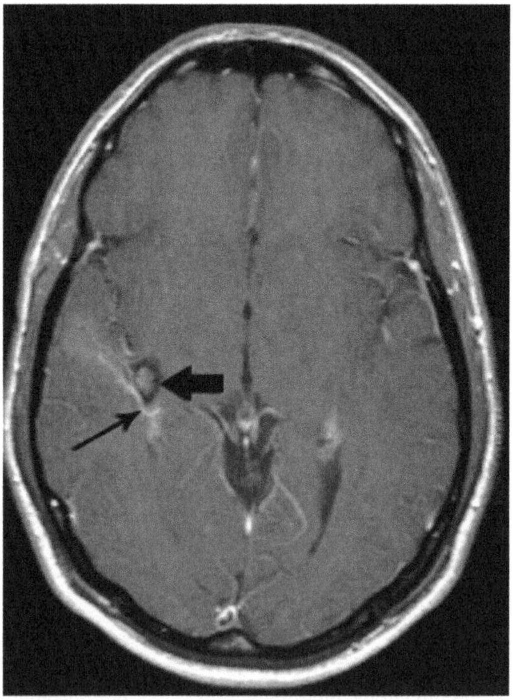

Sporadic CCMs tend to be single and associated with DVA, whereas familial CCMs are multiples and not associated with DVA (Fig. 10). De novo CCM is also more frequent in familial forms with an incidence of 0.2% to 0.4% of de novo CCM per patient year, and they are reported to develop at any time during the patients' lifespans.[55] De novo CCM have also been reported in patients treated with radiation. In a series of 171 patients treated with cranial irradiation for cerebral and head and neck tumors and leukemia or total body irradiation before hematopoietic stem cell transplantation, the authors observed a cumulative incidence of CCM of 2.24%, 3.86%, 4.95%, and 6.74% within 5, 10, 15, and 20 years, respectively, after the radiation therapy and an increased incidence in children irradiated within the first 10 years of life (4.42%, 7.04%, and 8.49% within 5, 10, and 15 years after radiation therapy, respectively).[56]

MR imaging is the gold standard to detect CCM lesions. T2-weighted gradient-echo and susceptibility-weighted imaging are the most sensitive sequences to detect CCM. The sensitivity of susceptibility-weighted images to identify multiples lesions in patients with familial CCM is higher

Fig. 9. Cavernous malformation and developmental venous anomaly. Axial postcontrast image shows a right temporal cavernous malformation (*thick arrow*) with an adjacent developmental venous anomaly (*thin arrow*).

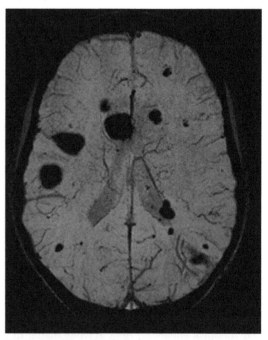

Fig. 10. Multiple familial cavernous malformations. Axial susceptibility-weighted image shows multiple dark spots corresponding to cavernous malformation in a young Mexican man.

than that of other sequences. de Souza and colleagues[57] found that this sequence showed 73% more lesions than T2-weighted gradient echo images. Associated DVA are also easily recognized with susceptibility-weighted or T1-weighted postcontrast images. CCM are not opacified during digital subtraction catheter angiography, making this technique less useful in their diagnosis. However, complex DVAs close to a CCM should be delineate before a surgical approach using digital subtraction angiography.

VENOUS MALFORMATIONS

Venous malformations (VM) are focal defects of the vascular venous morphogenesis and correspond to dilated venous spaces connected to the local venous circulation by tortuous channels resulting in a slow flow circulation. VM are lined by endothelial cells surrounded by loose and irregularly distributed smooth muscle cells. They affect the skin, mucosa, and deep structures such as muscles and bones. In the head and neck they are localized in the skin, soft tissues, tongue, oral cavity, pharyngeal or laryngeal regions, or conjunctivas causing maxillofacial deformities and functional (ie, respiratory) disturbances. VM undergo frequent thromboses and thrombolysis episodes leading to secondary calcifications by forming phleboliths, a pathognomonic feature of VM. Up to 93% of VM are sporadic, unifocal lesions.[58] Inherited forms comprise cutaneous-mucosal venous malformations (OMIM# 6000195) and glomulovenous malformations (GVM) (OMIM# 138000) representing 1% and 5%, respectively, of all venous malformations. GVM are autosomal dominant inherited lesions caused by a mutation in the glomulin gene, the function of which is not known. Unlike other VM in which the primary cell dysfunction is in the endothelial vascular cell, in GVM the primary defect is in smooth muscle cells.[59] GVM are more superficial than sporadic forms of VM involving the skin and mostly located in the extremities. GVM are considered a separate group of VM with genetic, clinical, and histologic differences.[60]

VCMC is caused by a germline mutation in TIE2 gene that encodes for endothelial cell tyrosine kinase receptor TIE2. They affect the maxillofacial and neck regions and involve the skin, mucosa, and deep structures, although they tend to be more superficial than the sporadic forms.[58] A somatic mutation in TIE2 was recently reported to cause 40% of the sporadic forms of VM.[61] This discovery could have an important impact in the research for therapeutic tools to treat VM, particularly targeting TIE2 signaling pathways.[61]

The process of thrombosis and thrombolysis that occurs inside of VM is known as localized intravascular coagulopathy,[58] and this phenomenon can be measured by quantification of D-dimer in peripheral blood. D-dimer is permanently elevated in patients with VM except in those with GVM lesions. D-dimer level is normal in patients with lymphatic malformations or fast-flow vascular lesions; thus, it is considered a biomarker for VM in patients without other comorbidities susceptible to produce modifications of D-dimer levels such as cancer, inflammatory disease, thrombophilia, ischemic heart disease, and pregnancy. It is recommended to measure the D-dimer levels in patients presenting with VM. Imaging of these lesions is best done with combination of CT and MR imaging. MR imaging offers the better soft tissue resolution and shows superficial enhancing masses, which at times may involve multiple compartments and may compromise the airway by direct extension or compression. Precontrast T1-weighted images and postcontrast fat-suppressed T1 images are best for outlining the malformation. CT may be helpful in characterizing bone involvement and detection of phleboliths. MR angiography, both static and contrast enhanced time resolved, show no significant arterial contributions in these lesions.

LYMPHATIC MALFORMATIONS

Lymphatic malformations (LM) are composed of cystic vascular channels lined by endothelial cells derived from the lymphatic cellular line and filled with lymph. About 60% of LM are located in the head and neck (Fig. 11).[62] Lymphatic vessels originate from the primitive lymph sacs located in the jugular region. Classical theories that attempt to explain their formation consider obstructions or sequestrations of lymph tissue as the origin of LM. Recent studies suggest that single lymphatic vessels may develop a tumorlike proliferative behavior triggered by trauma or infections.[62] Markers of lymphatic endothelial cells are detected in LM, and specific lymphangiogenic growth factors are expressed in normal lymphatic endothelium, and they correlate with LM genesis. There is no evidence of inheritance in LM.

Lymphedema consists of a separate disorder, usually affecting the lower extremities causing extensive swelling. Lymphedema may be acquired, secondary to surgery or infection, or primary. The latter is an autosomal dominant congenital condition usually presenting at birth (Milroy disease or type I lymphedema, OMIM#135100) or later in puberty (Meige disease or type I lymphedema, OMIM#135200).

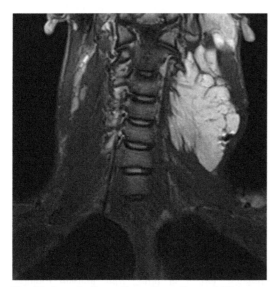

Fig. 11. Lymphatic malformation. Coronal T2 image shows a large lobulated hyperintense lymphatic malformation involving multiple anatomic compartments in the left neck.

LM are better imaged with MR imaging, which allows mapping for their common multicompartmental nature. Postcontrast fat-suppressed T1 images show absence of enhancement, which separates them from venous and other vascular lesions. LM are bright on T2 images and diffusion-weighted images and show no arterial flow on time-resolved contrast-enhanced MR angiography.

REFERENCES

1. Rossetti S, Chauveau D, Kubly V, et al. Association of mutation position in polycystic kidney disease 1 (PKD1) gene and development of a vascular phenotype. Lancet 2003;361:2196–201.
2. Krings T, Piske RL, Lasjaunias P. Intracranial arterial aneurysm vasculopathies: targeting the outher vessel wall. Neuroradiology 2005;47:931–7.
3. Krings T, Madell DM, Kiehl TR, et al. Intracranial aneurysms: from vessel wall pathology to therapeutic approach. Nat Rev Neurol 2011;7:547–59.
4. Nakajima N, Nagahiro S, Sano T, et al. Krüppel-like zinc-finger transcription factor 5 (KLF5) is highly expressed in large and giant unruptured cerebral aneurysms. World Neurosurg 2012;78:114–21.
5. Soltész B, Tóth B, Shabashova N, et al. New and recurrent gain-of-function STAT1 mutations in patients with chronic mucocutaneous candidiasis from Eastern and Central Europe. J Med Genet 2013;50:567–78.
6. Sedat J, Alvarez H, Rodesch G, et al. Multifocal cerebral fusiform aneurysms in children with immune

deficiencies report of four cases. Interv Neuroradiol 1999;5:151–6.
7. Cloft HJ, Kallmes DF, Kallmes MH, et al. Prevalence of cerebral aneurysms in patients with fibromuscular dysplasia: a reassessment. J Neurosurg 1998;88:436–40.
8. Begelman SM, Olin JW. Fibromuscular dysplasia. Curr Opin Rheumatol 2000;12:41–7.
9. Viganò S, Papini GD, Cotticelli B, et al. Prevalence of cerebral aneurysms in patients treated for left cardiac myxoma: a prospective study. Clin Radiol 2013;68(11):e624–8.
10. Ryou KS, Lee SH, Park SH, et al. Multiple fusiform myxomatous cerebral aneurysms in a patient with Carney complex. J Neurosurg 2008;109:318–20.
11. Juvela S. Prevalence of and risk factors for intracranial aneurysms. Lancet Neurol 2011;10:595–7.
12. Wiebers DO, Piepgras DG, Meyer FB. Pathogenesis, natural history, and treatment of unruptured intracranial aneurysms. Mayo Clin Proc 2004;79:1572–83.
13. Vlak MH, Algra A, Brandenburg R, et al. Prevalence of unruptured intracranial aneurysms, with emphasis on sex, age, comorbidity, country, and time period: a systematic review and meta-analysis. Lancet Neurol 2011;10(7):626–36.
14. Oyazato Y, Iijima K, Emi M, et al. Molecular analysis of TSC2/PKD1 contiguous gene deletion syndrome. Kobe J Med Sci 2011;57(1):E1–10.
15. Ronkainen A, Hernesniemi J, Puranen M. Familial intracranial aneurysms. Lancet 1997;349:380–4.
16. Mackey J, Brown RD Jr, Moomaw CJ, et al, FIA and ISUIA Investigators. Unruptured intracranial aneurysms in the familial intracranial aneurysm and international study of unruptured intracranial aneurysms cohorts: differences in multiplicity and location. J Neurosurg 2012;117(1):60–4.
17. Broderick JP, Brown RD Jr, Sauerbeck L, et al, FIA Study Investigators. Greater rupture risk for familial as compared to sporadic unruptured intracranial aneurysms. Stroke 2009;40(6):1952–7.
18. Brown RD Jr, Huston J, Hornung R, et al. Screening for brain aneurysm in the Familial Intracranial Aneurysm study: frequency and predictors of lesion detection. J Neurosurg 2008;108:1132–8.
19. Alg VS, Sofat R, Houlden H, et al. Genetic risk factors for intracranial aneurysms: a meta-analysis in more than 116,000 individuals. Neurology 2013;80(23):2154–65.
20. Hussain I, Duffis EJ, Gandhi CD, et al. Genome-wide association studies of intracranial aneurysms: an update. Stroke 2013;44(9):2670–5.
21. Sabatino G, Rigante L, Minella D, et al. Transcriptional profile characterization for the identification of peripheral blood biomarkers in patients with cerebral aneurysms. J Biol Regul Homeost Agents 2013;27(3):729–38.

22. Connolly ES Jr, Rabinstein AA, Carhuapoma JR, et al. Guidelines for the management of aneurysmal subarachnoid hemorrhage: a guideline for health-care professionals from the American Heart Association/American Stroke Association. Stroke 2012; 43(6):1711–37.

23. Bor AS, Koffijberg H, Wermer MJ. Optimal screening strategy for familial intracranial aneurysms: a cost-effectiveness analysis. Neurology 2010;74(21): 1671–9.

24. Sturiale CL, Gatto I, Puca A, et al. Association between the rs1333040 polymorphism on the chromosomal 9p21 locus and sporadic brain arteriovenous malformations. J Neurol Neurosurg Psychiatry 2013; 84(9):1059–62.

25. Nishida T, Faughnan ME, Krings T, et al. Brain arteriovenous malformations associated with hereditary hemorrhagic telangiectasia: gene-phenotype correlations. Am J Med Genet A 2012;158A(11):2829–34.

26. Kim H, Su H, Weinsheimer S, et al. Brain arteriovenous malformation pathogenesis: a response-to-injury paradigm. Acta Neurochir Suppl 2011;111:83–92.

27. Shovlin CL, Guttmacher AE, Buscarini E, et al. Diagnostic criteria for hereditary hemorrhagic telangiectasia (Rendu-Osler-Weber syndrome). Am J Med Genet 2000;91:66–7.

28. Lesca G, Genin E, Blachier C, et al. Hereditary hemorrhagic telangiectasia: evidence for regional founder effects of ACVRL1 mutations in French and Italian patients. Eur J Hum Genet 2008;16(6): 742–9.

29. Bharatha A, Faughnan ME, Kim H, et al. Brain arteriovenous malformation multiplicity predicts the diagnosis of hereditary hemorrhagic telangiectasia: quantitative assessment. Stroke 2012;43(1):72–8.

30. Park SO, Wankhede M, Lee YJ. Real-time imaging of de novo arteriovenous malformation in a mouse model of hereditary hemorrhagic telangiectasia. J Clin Invest 2009;119(11):3487–96.

31. Willemse RB, Mager JJ, Westermann C, et al. Bleeding risk of cerebrovascular malformations in hereditary hemorrhagic telangiectasia. J Neurosurg 2000;92(5):779–84.

32. Matsubara S, Mandzia JL, ter Brugge K, et al. Angiographic and clinical characteristics of patients with cerebral arteriovenous malformations associated with hereditary hemorrhagic telangiectasia. AJNR Am J Neuroradiol 2000;21(6):1016–20 [Erratum appears in AJNR Am J Neuroradiol 2001; 22(7):1446. Manzia JL [corrected to Mandzia JL]].

33. Krings T, Ozanne A, Chng SM, et al. Neurovascular phenotypes in hereditary haemorrhagic telangiectasia patients according to age. Review of 50 consecutive patients aged 1 day-60 years. Neuroradiology 2005;47(10):711–20.

34. Crawford PM, West CR, Chadwick DW, et al. Arteriovenous malformations of the brain: natural history in unoperated patients. J Neurol Neurosurg Psychiatry 1986;49(1):1–10.

35. Krings T, Chng SM, Ozanne A, et al. Hereditary hemorrhagic telangiectasia in children: endovascular treatment of neurovascular malformations: results in 31 patients. Neuroradiology 2005;47:946–54.

36. Calhoun AR, Bollo RJ, Garber ST, et al. Spinal arteriovenous fistulas in children with hereditary hemorrhagic telangiectasia. J Neurosurg Pediatr 2012;9(6):654–9.

37. Cullen S, Alvarez H, Rodesch G, et al. Spinal arteriovenous shunts presenting before 2 years of age: analysis of 13 cases. Childs Nerv Syst 2006;22(9):1103–10.

38. Faughnan ME, Palda VA, Garcia-Tsao G, et al. International guidelines for the diagnosis and management of hereditary haemorrhagic telangiectasia. J Med Genet 2011;48:73–87.

39. Eerola I, Boon LM, Mulliken JB, et al. Capillary malformation-arteriovenous malformation, a new clinical and genetic disorder caused by RASA1 mutations. Am J Hum Genet 2003;73(6):1240–9.

40. Thiex R, Mulliken JB, Revencu N, et al. A novel association between RASA1 mutations and spinal arteriovenous anomalies. AJNR Am J Neuroradiol 2010; 31(4):775–9.

41. Jacobs AH, Walton RG. The incidence of birthmarks in the neonate. Pediatrics 1976;58:218–22.

42. Revencu N, Boon LM, Mendola A, et al. RASA1 mutations and associated phenotypes in 68 families with capillary malformation-arteriovenous malformation. Hum Mutat 2013;34(12):1632–41.

43. Lasjaunias P, ter Brugge KG, Berenstein A. Cerebro-facial venous metameric syndromes (Sturge Weber syndrome). In: Lasjaunias P, ter Brugge KG, Berenstein A, editors. Surgical neuroangiography: vol. 3: Clinical and interventional aspects in children. Berlin: Springer; 2006. p. 45–7.

44. Pascual-Castroviejo I, Pascual-Pascual SI, Velazquez-Fragua R, et al. Sturge-Weber syndrome: study of 55 patients. Can J Neurol Sci 2008;35(3):301–7.

45. Comi AM. Presentation, diagnosis, pathophysiology, and treatment of the neurological features of Sturge-Weber syndrome. Neurologist 2011;17(4):179–84.

46. Schmidt D, Pache M, Schumacher M. The congenital unilateral retinocephalic vascular malformation syndrome (bonnet-dechaume-blanc syndrome or wyburn-mason syndrome): review of the literature. Surv Ophthalmol 2008;53(3):227–49.

47. Shirley MD, Tang H, Gallione CJ, et al. Sturge-Weber syndrome and port-wine stains caused by somatic mutation in GNAQ. N Engl J Med 2013;368(21):1971–9.

48. Clatterbuck RE, Eberhart CG, Crain BJ, et al. Ultrastructural and immunocytochemical evidence that an incompetent blood-brain barrier is related to the pathophysiology of cavernous malformations. J Neurol Neurosurg Psychiatry 2001;71(2):188–92.

49. Fischer A, Zalvide J, Faurobert E, et al. Cerebral cavernous malformations: from CCM genes to

endothelial cell homeostasis. Trends Mol Med 2013;
19(5):302–8.

50. Gunel M, Awad IA, Finberg K, et al. A founder mutation as a cause of cerebral cavernous malformation
in Hispanic Americans. N Engl J Med 1996;334(15):
946–51.

51. Sirvente J, Enjolras O, Wassef M, et al. Frequency
and phenotypes of cutaneous vascular malformations in a consecutive series of 417 patients with familial cerebral cavernous malformations. J Eur Acad
Dermatol Venereol 2009;23(9):1066–72.

52. Ruíz DS, Yilmaz H, Gailloud P. Cerebral developmental venous anomalies: current concepts. Ann
Neurol 2009;66(3):271–83.

53. Petersen TA, Morrison LA, Schrader RM, et al.
Familial versus sporadic cavernous malformations:
differences in developmental venous anomaly association and lesion phenotype. AJNR Am J Neuroradiol 2010;31(2):377–82.

54. Revencu N, Vikkula M. Cerebral cavernous malformation: new molecular and clinical insights. J Med
Genet 2006;43(9):716–21.

55. Brunereau L, Levy C, Laberge S, et al. De novo
lesions in familial form of cerebral cavernous malformations: clinical and MR features in 29 non-Hispanic
families. Surg Neurol 2000;53(5):475–82 [discus-
sion: 482–3].

56. Strenger V, Sovinz P, Lackner H, et al. Intracerebral
cavernous hemangioma after cranial irradiation in
childhood. Incidence and risk factors. Strahlenther
Onkol 2008;184(5):276–80.

57. de Souza JM, Domingues RC, Cruz LC Jr, et al.
Susceptibility-weighted imaging for the evaluation
of patients with familial cerebral cavernous malformations: a comparison with T2-weighted fast spin-
echo and gradient-echo sequences. AJNR Am J
Neuroradiol 2008;29(1):154–8.

58. Dompmartin A, Vikkula M, Boon LM. Venous malformation: update on aetiopathogenesis, diagnosis
and management. Phlebology 2010;25(5):224–35.

59. Brouillard P, Vikkula M. Genetic causes of vascular
malformations. Hum Mol Genet 2007;16(Spec No
2):R140–9.

60. Boon LM, Mulliken JB, Enjolras O. Glomuvenous
malformation (glomangioma) and venous malformation: distinct clinicopathologic and genetic entities.
Arch Dermatol 2004;140(8):971–6.

61. Limaye N, Wouters V, Uebelhoer M, et al. Somatic
mutations in angiopoietin receptor gene TEK cause
solitary and multiple sporadic venous malformations. Nat Genet 2009;41(1):118–24.

62. Wiegand S, Eivazi B, Barth PJ, et al. Pathogenesis of lymphangiomas. Virchows Arch 2008;
453(1):1–8.

Imaging Phenotypes in Multiple Sclerosis

Stefan Dirk Roosendaal, MD, PhD*, Frederik Barkhof, MD, PhD

KEYWORDS

- Multiple sclerosis • Genetics • MR imaging • Imaging

KEY POINTS

- Multiple sclerosis is a heterogeneous disease with complex interacting environmental and genetic causative factors.
- Several genes have been associated with multiple sclerosis susceptibility and found to be related to imaging patterns.
- Magnetic resonance imaging can especially contribute to the current research of genetic associations with disease prognosis and severity.

INTRODUCTION

Multiple sclerosis (MS) is a progressive disease of the central nervous system with a usual onset in young adulthood, often leading to severe disability. Patients can experience a wide range of symptoms, including motor and sensory problems, ataxia, fatigue, and cognitive impairment.[1] The disease course similarly varies to a large extent between patients. Nevertheless, a limited number of different clinical phenotypes can be distinguished.[2] Before definite diagnosis, patients who experience an acute clinical attack that is suspect for a demyelinating event can be labeled as clinically isolated syndrome (CIS). Many of these patients subsequently develop a phenotype called relapsing-remitting (RR) MS, in which exacerbations are followed by full or partial remissions. In about two-thirds of patients this disease type is succeeded by secondary progressive (SP) MS, characterized by a gradual worsening without recovery. A small proportion of patients (10%–15%) experience progressive decline from onset, defined as primary progressive (PP) MS. In addition to these disease courses, there are MS variants and diseases that mimic MS clinically and radiologically, such as neuromyelitis optica (NMO).[3]

There are multiple findings indicating that environmental factors have a causative role in MS that may interplay with genetic variables. The risk of MS is strongly influenced by region of residence in early life,[1] and the global prevalence of MS is related to distance from the equator, being highest in northern Europe and southern parts of Australia and New Zealand. Furthermore, women are more often affected than men and in recent years they may be increasingly affected.[4] Environmental factors suspected to be (partly) causative have been infections such as Epstein-Barr virus,[5] vitamin D deficiency,[6] smoking, and other toxins. However, from familial recurrence rates of 15% to 20% it can be assumed that part of the risk for the disease is influenced by genetic variables. Maybe even more interesting are effects that genes have on MS disease course and progression of disability, although twins concordant for the diagnosis of MS can have different disease courses. In this context, magnetic resonance (MR) imaging

Disclosures: S.D. Roosendaal has no conflicts of interest; F. Barkhof has no conflicts of interest; The MS Center Amsterdam is supported by a program grant from the Dutch MS Research Foundation (grant number 09-538d).
Department of Radiology & Nuclear Medicine, Neuroscience Campus Amsterdam, VU University Medical Center, PO Box 7057, Amsterdam, 1007 MB, The Netherlands
* Corresponding author. De Boelelaan 1117, Amsterdam 1081 HV, The Netherlands.
E-mail address: stefanmed@yahoo.com

parameters can be used as more accurate and pathologically representative outcome measures than any other clinical parameter.

This article summarizes genetic and imaging findings in MS, reviews correlations between genetics and MR imaging parameters, and discusses implications for current knowledge. It also proposes future perspective and research strategies.

GENETICS OF MULTIPLE SCLEROSIS

A large part of genetic research in MS has been focused on genetic susceptibility to MS. Many studies have found clues for a genetic role in susceptibility in the familial clustering of MS.[7,8] The risk of developing MS is highest for a monozygotic twin; approximately 20% when the other twin is already affected. The risk decreases with the number of shared genes to approximately 2.5% for siblings and 1.5% when one of the parents has MS.[7] Although a low risk, it is still greater than the prevalence of MS in the general population (0.1%–0.3%).

In the past decade, most associations found by linkage studies and candidate gene studies concentrated on the human leukocyte antigen (HLA) locus on chromosome 6. The strongest of associations have been found with the HLA-DRB1*1501 allele of the HLA-DRB1 gene,[9] which is part of a set of genes involved in self versus nonself immune recognition: the major histocompatibility complex (MHC) class II region. Other alleles in immunity-related genes found in these studies have weaker associations to MS susceptibility (odds ratios that are smaller than 2).[10]

The recent ability to use genome-wide association (GWA) studies by assessing single-nucleotide polymorphisms (SNPs) has allowed the detection of new genetic variations with even smaller effects on susceptibility,[11] although these studies require large groups of patients with MS.[12] The GWA studies have resulted in the notion that MS is a complex multigenetic disease, in which several genes are likely to interplay with each other and with environmental factors.

In addition to the aforementioned hypothesis-generating studies, in several studies specific genes have been subject of investigation; for example, those known to be related to neurodegeneration in general, such as brain-derived neurotrophic factor (BDNF) and apolipoprotein E (ApoE).

IMAGING OF MULTIPLE SCLEROSIS

Focal white matter lesions in the brain can be depicted with T2-weighted and fluid-attenuated inversion recovery (FLAIR) images,[13] representing a combination of inflammation, demyelination, axonal loss, and gliosis. Locations considered to be characteristic for MS are the periventricular and juxtacortical areas (Fig. 1), the posterior fossa, and the spinal cord. The appearance of new lesions is considered to be a measure of disease activity, and lesion enhancement on postgadolinium T1-weighted images represents blood-brain barrier leakage in the acute stage of a lesion. These MR imaging features of MS contribute to the most recent diagnostic criteria.[14,15]

Axonal degeneration in MS occurs both in acute and in chronic MS lesions,[16] and when focally extensive it is mirrored by persistent T1 hypointensity (also referred to as T1 black holes [T1BH]). However, widespread axonal loss can also be found outside focal lesions in the normal-appearing and diffusely abnormal white matter, where it can be detected by more advanced quantitative MR imaging techniques (Box 1), such as diffusion-weighted imaging (DWI)/diffusion tensor imaging (DTI), magnetic transfer imaging (MTR), and MR spectroscopy.[17,18]

In the last decade, it has come to light that gray matter pathology in MS are abundant and clinically meaningful.[19] Focal gray matter lesions are more difficult to identify with conventional MR imaging than white matter lesions, although their visualization can be improved by a more sensitive MR imaging technique called double-inversion recovery (DIR; see Fig. 1) and by using (ultra)high-field MR imaging. Loss of brain volume (BV) over time, or atrophy, can be reliably measured for both white matter and gray matter (Fig. 2), and assesses the end-stage of the disease process.[20]

Spinal cord abnormalities, either focal or diffuse, are found in most patients with MS and are strongly related to prognosis.[21,22] They can be accurately depicted with proton density–weighted and T2-weighted imaging. Similar to the brain, quantitative MR imaging measures of the spinal cord are more specific with respect to the underlying pathophysiologic process and correlate well with disability.[23] The extent of spinal cord abnormalities varies greatly between patients with MS and is not strongly related to the extent of brain abnormalities within patients.

MR imaging is able to characterize imaging phenotypes that are more directly influenced than clinical outcome measures by pathophysiologic mechanisms, and therefore can be more straightforwardly linked to genotypes. The use of MR imaging in MS genotype-phenotype studies does not only add an objective and repeatable measure of disease severity, it also allows selection of patient groups based on imaging patterns. The goal of using MR imaging as an intermediate

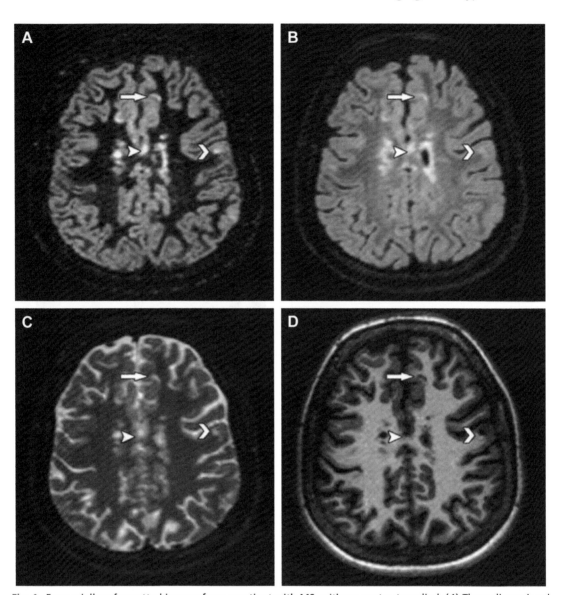

Fig. 1. Four axially reformatted images from a patient with MS, with no contrast applied. (A) Three-dimensional (3D) double-inversion recovery (3D-DIR), (B) 3D-FLAIR, (C) 3D-T2, and (D) 3D magnetization prepared rapid gradient echo. Images show several white and gray matter lesions. Straight arrows point to juxtacortical lesions. Delta arrows point to mixed white matter–gray matter lesions. Arrowheads point to cortical lesions clearly seen on 3D-DIR and to a lesser extent on the other images. (From Moraal B, Roosendaal SD, Pouwels PJ, et al. Multi-contrast, isotropic, single-slab 3D MR imaging in multiple sclerosis. Eur Radiol 2008;18:2311–20; with permission.)

phenotype in MS can be 2-fold: it may allow detection of new genetic polymorphisms that relate to MS and thereby induce new insights in disease mechanisms, and it can also provide new prognostic markers for disease severity.

ASSOCIATIONS OF MULTIPLE SCLEROSIS SUSCEPTIBILITY GENES WITH BRAIN MAGNETIC RESONANCE IMAGING

Several studies have investigated whether susceptibility genes can explain differences in disease

severity. For example, large variation can be found between patients with MS with regard to the number and volume of T2 lesions in the brain. An association between the allele with the strongest effect on MS susceptibility, HLA-DRB1*1501, and T2 lesion volume was found by Okuda and colleagues.[24] However, this association was not confirmed in other studies.[25–31] Likewise, although some studies have reported associations between susceptibility genes with T1BH,[25,26] in others no significant relations could be found.[32,33] The dissimilar results between the studies described

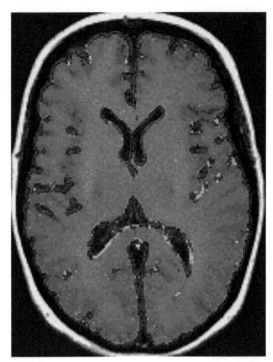

Box 1
MR imaging parameters

Conventional MR imaging

T2 lesions

- Non-specific mixture of pathologic processes including demyelination, gliosis, inflammation, axonal loss

T1 enhancing lesions

- Disruption of the blood-brain barrier by active inflammation

Persistent T1 hypointense lesions (black holes)

- Associated with severe tissue damage

Brain atrophy

- Significant volume loss occurs in MS, correlated with neurodegeneration

Spinal cord imaging

Nonconventional MR imaging

Diffusion-weighted imaging (DWI)/diffusion tensor imaging (DTI)

- Measures diffusional motion of water, relates to axonal loss and demyelination

Magnetic transfer imaging

- Estimate of tissue structure disruption, associated with axonal damage and demyelination

¹H (proton) MR spectroscopy

- Metabolites (eg, *N*-acetylaspartate and glutamate) can be quantified both in lesions and normal-appearing brain matter

Functional MR imaging

- Can be measured during task or rest
- Changes may represent functional reorganization

Voxel-based techniques

Fig. 2. Measurement of whole-brain atrophy by sequential MR imaging. Scans from an individual with RR MS were obtained 1 year apart. The scans were coregistered by use of the structural image evaluation using normalization of atrophy (SIENA) method. The colored voxels identify where changes in BV have occurred (blue represents contraction and red represents expansion). Overall, a 1.45% decrease in BV occurred over the year. (*From* Barkhof F, Calabresi PA, Miller DH, et al. Imaging outcomes for neuroprotection and repair in multiple sclerosis trials. Nat Rev Neurol 2009;5:256–66; with permission.)

above could in part be caused by the heterogeneity of the patient groups, often consisting of several disease types.

In patients with CIS, associations between HLA status and number and volume of gadolinium-enhancing lesions were found.[34] However, in a longitudinal study by the same group with 179 patients with CIS and 16 susceptibility SNPs, including HLA-DRB1, no relations with T2 lesion load (T2LL) or BV were found.[33]

In most of the studies using BV as an outcome measure, no associations with known susceptibility genes have been found (**Table 1**). Among the SNPs investigated have been HLA genes, KIF1B

(a gene involved in axonal transport),[35] and interleukin receptor genes.[33,36]

In addition to the large range of number and volume of lesions in patients with MS, anatomic location of lesions within the brain varies widely among patients. This variety in involvement of the cerebrum, brainstem, and cerebellum may partly be explained by genetic differences. This possibility was investigated by examining the effect of 69 candidate SNPs on a lesion probability map of 208 patients with MS, showing increased probability for lesions in certain brain areas for 5 SNPs and decreased probability for lesions in 6 SNPs.[29] The most statistically robust finding was the increased probability of having a lesion in the cerebral white matter against the frontal and occipital horn of the left lateral ventricle, for the heterozygous genotype of rs2227139, located within the MHC class II region. In another study

Table 1
Relations between MS susceptibility genes and brain MR imaging

Study, Year	Patients (CIS/RR/SP/PP)	HC	MR Imaging	Most Important Findings
Baranzini et al,[30] 2009	987 (100/659/137/72)[a]	883	T2LL, BV	GWA; T2LL and BV associated with multiple (non-HLA) SNPs, not with HLA-DRB1*1501
Gourraud et al,[38] 2013	484 (76/343/45/20)	—	LPM	GWA; 31 SNPs associated with lesion pattern
Healy et al,[87] 2010	532 (17/351/123/37)[b]	776	T2LL, BV	HLA B44 associated with higher BV and lower T2LL
Hooper-van Veen et al,[36] 2003	492 (-/221/172/99)[c]	228	T1BH, T2LL, BV	No associations interleukin-1 polymorphism with MR imaging
Hooper-van Veen et al,[88] 2006	489 (-/220/175/440)[d]	180	T1BH, T2LL, BV	Change in T1BH associated with CD28, IFNGR2, IL1B-511
Horakova et al,[34] 2011	205 (CIS only)	—	T2LL, T1Gad, BV	HLA-DRB1*1501 associated with higher T1Gad, not with BV
Jensen et al,[89] 2010	1006 (RR and SP[e])	—	BV (ICR)	No associations 7 susceptibility SNPs with BV
Kalincik et al,[33] 2013	179 (CIS only)	—	T2LL, BV	No associations 16 susceptibility SNPs with T2LL and BV
Karrenbauer et al,[32] 2013	100 (-/79/19/2)	—	T2LL, T1BH, lesion location	No associations HLA-DRB1*15 or *04 with MR imaging
Okuda et al,[24] 2009	505 (88/352/46/14)	—	T2LL, T1Gad, MRS	Higher T2LL and lower NAA in NAWM in HLA-DRB1*1501 + patients
Qiu et al,[70] 2011	252 (-/119/117/16)	—	T2SC	No associations HLA-DRB1 alleles and number/location SC lesions
Sepulcre et al,[37] 2008	50 (15/28/3/4)	—	T2LL, BV, LPM	No association HLA-DR2 status with lesion distribution and BV
Schreiber et al,[28] 2002	71 (21/40/10)	—	T2LL	No associations HLA with T2LL
Sombekke et al,[27] 2009	150 (-/88/32/30)	—	T2LL, T2SC	HLA-DRB1*1501 not associated with T2LL
Sombekke et al,[29] 2011	208 (-/126/42/40)	—	T2LL, LPM	MHC II region SNP associated with lesion distribution
Van der Walt et al,[90] 2011	978 (-/639/339/-)[f]	—	BV (ICR)	No associations HLA-DRB1 alleles with BV
Zivadinov et al,[25,91] 2003; 2009	100 (-/71/16/13)	122	T2LL, T1BH, BV	B7 associated with higher T2LL and T1BH; DRB1*12 with higher T1BH and lower BV
Zivadinov et al,[26] 2007	41 (-/27/7/7)	—	T2LL, T1BH, BV	Multiple HLA alleles associated with MR imaging (eg, HLA-DRB1*1501 associated with lower BV and higher T1BH)

Abbreviations: CIS, clinically isolated syndrome; HC, healthy controls; LPM, lesion probability mapping; NAA, *N*-acetylaspartate; SC, spinal cord; T1Gad, T1 gadolinium-enhancing lesions.
[a] MR imaging analysis limited to RR and SP.
[b] MR imaging available in 375 patients.
[c] MR imaging available in 96 patients.
[d] MR imaging available in 94 patients.
[e] Precise distribution not mentioned.
[f] MR imaging available in 745 patients.

comparing T1BH and T2 lesion probability maps between 50 patients with MS with negative and positive HLA-DR2 status (determined by the presence of the HLA-DRB1*1501 allele, present in 30% of patients),[37] no significant differences in lesion distribution were found, and neither did gray or white matter atrophy differ. A GWA study[38] found several SNPs associated with one of the lesion distribution patterns found in a group of 284 patients with MS. The genes involved have immunity-related but also neural functions. Also, a different lesion pattern in this study was found between patients with versus without the HLA-DR1*1501 allele.

Cortical lesions were recently found to be abundant in MS, in post-mortem studies[39] as well as in vivo with MR imaging,[40] and to be correlated with disability including cognitive impairment.[41] No studies assessing potential genetic associations with the prevalence of cortical lesions have yet been conducted. In one case report[42] 4 sisters with RR MS were described, each of them having a disproportionally high number of cortical lesions, suggesting a genetic predisposition.

GENETIC ASSOCIATIONS WITH NEURODEGENERATION IN MULTIPLE SCLEROSIS

Pathologic and radiological studies have revealed that neurodegeneration is an important feature of MS. This insight is stressed by patients treated with antiinflammatory drugs having fewer exacerbations but nevertheless experiencing gradual ongoing functional loss.[43] MR imaging parameters that may represent neurodegeneration are BV measurements, spectroscopic assessment of N-acetylaspartate (NAA) levels, and T1BH. In this context, longitudinal studies may more accurately create contrasting patient groups for neurodegeneration.

Several genes that have been associated with either neurodegeneration or a neuroprotection in animal analogs of MS or in other diseases have been studied and are reviewed here.

Brain-derived Neurotrophic Factor

BDNF is a growth factor produced in the brain and that is heavily involved in synaptic plasticity and neuronal growth. A well-studied BDNF polymorphism in which the amino acid valine is substituted for methionine at codon 66 (Val66Met) leads to reduced secretion. Although the effect of this polymorphism on cognition in healthy subjects is inconsistent, it has been associated with many neurodegenerative disorders.[44] Release of BDNF by immune cells has been shown in active MS

lesions,[45] which hypothetically may have an impact on neuronal preservation. Studies on the BDNF polymorphisms on MR imaging measures in MS have shown inconsistent results (Table 2), although most of the relations found affected gray matter volume (GMV) and only 1 of the studies[46] found a relation with lesion volume. Presence of the BDNF Met66 allele in patients with MS has been associated with lower GMV compared with the homozygous BDNF Val66 allele in patients with MS,[47] and was associated with low GMV values in another study.[48] In contrast, higher GMV was related to presence of BDNF Met66 in a study consisting of 209 patients with MS,[46] with post-hoc analysis using voxel-based morphometry (VBM) specifically showing higher GMV in the cingulate.[49] Lower GMV was found in patients homozygous for BDNF Val66 compared with controls but not in patients with BDNF Met66 in a study by Dinacci and colleagues.[50] In a study in which polymorphisms at another BDNF location (rs2030324) were evaluated, associations with left thalamus volume were found.[51]

Apolipoprotein E

Genetic variation in ApoE, an important lipid carrier protein in the central nervous system mainly produced by astrocytes, has been strongly associated with susceptibility to Alzheimer disease.[52] A contribution of ApoE polymorphisms to MS susceptibility has been suspected, because of genetic linkage and its possible role in neuronal repair and plasticity. However, in large meta-analyses including thousands of patients with MS and controls, an effect of ApoE variation in MS susceptibility has not been proved.[53,54]

Although most of the imaging studies assessing the influence of ApoE on MS severity could not show significant associations,[28,55–60] some studies have reported more brain damage in carriers of the ε4 allele (Table 3).[61–64] In a study consisting of 99 patients with RR MS,[63] MR imaging was performed at 2 points in time with a minimum interval of 2 years. Patients with the ε4 allele (either ε3/ε4 or ε4/ε4) showed a significantly larger annual BV decrease and a more increased black hole ratio (T1 black hole volume divided by T2 lesion volume) compared with patients without the ε4 allele. In another study by the same group, significantly lower NAA levels were shown in patients with ε4 compared with patients without ε4, using MR spectroscopy (MRS).[62] Also, a larger decrease of NAA levels in patients with ε4 was noticed during an interval of 3 years. Although ApoE polymorphisms are not likely to be related to MS susceptibility, they might have a modest role in modifying

Table 2
Relations between brain-derived neurotrophic factor polymorphisms and MR imaging

Study, Year	Patients (CIS/RR/SP/PP)	HC	MR Imaging	Most Important Findings
Cerasa et al,[48] 2010	29 (RR only)	61	T2LL, BV, fMR imaging	Lower GMV in Met+ patients, no differences in T2LL; no MS-specific action on fMR imaging
Dinacci et al,[50] 2011	45 (-/32/10/3)	34	T1BH, T2LL, BV	Lower GMV in Met− patients compared with healthy controls; no differences for all MR imaging parameters between Met+ and Met− patients
Fera et al,[73] 2013	26 (RR only)	25	T2LL, BV, VBM fMR imaging	Effect of Met+ on functional connectivity differs between patients and controls; BV or T2LL not different between Met+ and Met− patients
Liguori et al,[47] 2007	50 (RR only)	50	T2LL, BV	Lower GMV in Met+ patients compared with Met− patients; no differences in T2LL
Ramasamy et al,[49] 2011	188 (-/142/46/-)	—	T1BH, T2LL, VBM	Higher cingulate-GMV in Met+ patients compared with Met− patients; no differences in T1BH or T2LL
Weinstock-Guttman et al,[51] 2011	209 (-/167/40/2)	—	T1BH, T2LL, BV (Freesurfer), DWI, MTR	No significant relations rs2030324 polymorphism of BDNF with MR imaging; borderline association with thalamic volume
Zivadinov et al,[46] 2007	209 (-167/40/2)	—	T1BH, T1Gad, T2LL, BV, DWI, MTR	Met+ in patients associated with higher GMV and lower T2LL

Abbreviations: BDNF, brain-derived neurotrophic factor; DWI, diffusion-weighted imaging; fMR, functional MR; GMV, gray matter volume; Met+, carrier of the BDNF methionine 66 (Met66) allele; Met−, homozygous for valine at BDNF codon 66; VBM, voxel-based morphometry.

disease severity, possibly through an effect on axonal damage.

Glutamate

Glutamate is the major excitatory neurotransmitter in the central nervous system. Dysregulation of glutamate homeostasis leads to excitotoxicity and has been associated with neurodegeneration in neurologic disorders, including MS.[65,66] SNPs in 34 genes known to be involved in the glutamatergic pathway were analyzed using a new multivariate statistical model, using (longitudinal) BV measures and T1/T2 ratio in 326 patients with RR and SP MS.[67] Five SNPs in the *N*-methyl-D-aspartate (NMDA) receptor-2A subunit (GRIN2A) domain were associated with total BV, as well as with gray and white matter volume. NMDA is one of the ionotropic channels activated by glutamate. GRIN2A polymorphisms have been associated with variation of the medial temporal lobe in healthy controls.[68] In a study using gray matter glutamate concentration measured by MRS as a phenotype, associations with a gene involved in the function of postsynaptic neurotransmitter receptors was found with both a pathway and a GWA approach.[69] It was then related to neurodegeneration using atrophy and a decrease in NAA concentration over 1-year follow-up.

GENETICS OF SPINAL CORD LESIONS IN MULTIPLE SCLEROSIS

In a study in which 150 patients with MS were assessed for brain and spinal cord lesions, carriership of HLA-DRB1*1501 was associated with the extent of focal lesions in the spinal cord.[27] This association was not confirmed in a more recent study with 252 patients with MS, of whom 83% had spinal cord lesions,[70] although DRB1*1501 was associated with the presence of diffuse spinal cord lesions. Moreover, correlations were found between minor alleles DRB1*1104 and DRB1*0701

Table 3
Relations between ApoE alleles and MR imaging

Study, Year	Patients (CIS/RR/SP/PP)	HC	MR Imaging	Most Important Findings
De Stefano et al,[61] 2004	76 (RR only)	22	T2LL, BV	Lower BV in ε4+ patients
Enzinger et al,[62] 2003	72, FU in 44 (RR only)	—	MRS	Lower baseline and larger decrease NAA in ε4+ patients
Enzinger et al,[63] 2004	99 (RR only)	—	T1BH, T1Gad, T2LL, BV	Larger increase in T1BH and atrophy in ε4+ patients
Fazekas et al,[64] 2000	83 (-/76/5/2)	—	T1BH, T2LL	More T1BH in ε4+ patients
Ghaffar et al,[55] 2011	90 (-/66/18/6)	—	T1BH, T2LL, BV, DTI	No MR imaging differences between ε4+ and ε4− patients
Lanzillo et al,[60] 2006	52 (RR only)	—	T1Gad, T2LL, BV	No relations ApoE polymorphisms and MR imaging
Portaccio et al,[56] 2009	50 (RR only)	—	T2LV, BV	No differences between ε4+ and ε4− patients
Schreiber et al,[28] 2002	71 (-21/40/10)	—	T2LV	No relation ApoE polymorphisms with T2LV
Van der Walt et al,[57] 2009	1006 (-/663/343/-)[a]	—	BV (ICD)	No relation ApoE polymorphisms with atrophy
Zakrzewska-Pniewska et al,[58] 2004	117 (-/85/31/1)	100	T2LL, BV (visual rating)	No relations ApoE polymorphisms with MR imaging
Zwemmer et al,[59] 2004	408 (-/159/159/90)[b]	144	T1BH, T2LL, BV	No MR imaging differences between ε4+ and ε4− patients

Abbreviations: ε4+, homozygous or heterozygous carrier of ε4 allele; ε4−, noncarrier of ε4 allele; ApoE, apolipoprotein E; ICD, intercaudate distance; MRS, MR spectroscopy.
[a] MR imaging available in 792 patients.
[b] MR imaging available in 174 patients.

and higher number of focal lesions. More research is warranted in this area, especially because spinal cord pathology in MS are strongly associated with clinical disability.[71,72] By including quantitative MR imaging measures, such as spinal cord atrophy, sensitivity may be increased.

ADVANCED MAGNETIC RESONANCE IMAGING MEASURES

Limited experience exists regarding the relationship of genetic findings and advanced MR techniques. Functional MR imaging has been used in several BDNF polymorphism studies. Opposite effects of the Val66Met polymorphism on memory activation were found in patients with MS and controls.[73] In another study using a working memory task, increased activation was found in healthy BDNF Met66 carriers, but not in patients with MS.[48]

MRS is a sophisticated tool that can be used for the assessment of specific hypotheses. So far it has only been used in a small number of studies to investigate glutamate excitotoxicity[69] and axonal damage (NAA).[24,62] DTI is another

technique that may assess subtle damage in MS. It is increasingly available as an MR imaging outcome measure, but so far has scarcely been used for genetic correlation.[55]

The effect of genes on differences in the distribution of brain damage in patients with MS is relevant and can be investigated using lesion probability mapping (LPM; **Fig. 3**) for lesions, and VBM or cortical thickness measurements (eg, using Freesurfer[74]) for atrophy. These methods have been used in analyses involving HLA genes,[37] BDNF polymorphisms,[49] and genetic variants of a cannabinoid receptor.[75] In addition, they may be of advantage in GWA studies.[29,37,38] Statistical power may be increased by simultaneously performing analyses using hypothesis-driven regions of interest.

GENETICS OF MULTIPLE SCLEROSIS–RELATED DISEASES AND MIMICS

There are several diseases that are closely related to MS pathologically, clinically, and/or radiologically. Studying the imaging phenotypes of these

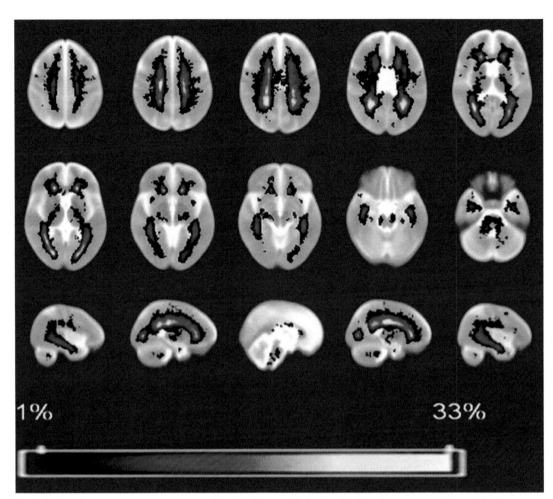

1%

33%

Fig. 3. Lesion-frequency map in a group of 208 patients with MS, indicating for every voxel the lesion frequency throughout the patient sample, and showing a range from 1% (2 patients having a lesion in that voxel) to the maximum of 33% (69 patients). (*From* Sombekke MH, Vellinga MM, Uitdehaag BM, et al. Genetic correlations of brain lesion distribution in multiple sclerosis: an exploratory study. AJNR Am J Neuroradiol 2011;32:695–703; with permission. Copyright © 2011 by American Society of Neuroradiology.)

diseases may be of interest and might also provide clues about certain genetic aspects that are shared with MS.

Cerebral autosomal dominant arteriopathy with subcortical infarcts and leukoencephalopathy (CADASIL) often presents in young adulthood and may mimic MS clinically and radiographically.[76] Involvement of the temporal pole and external capsule by T2-hyperintense lesions suggests CADASIL more than MS. Several mutations of the NOTCH3 gene are known to cause CADASIL. In a missense NOTCH3 mutation, C212Y, an inherited pattern of spinal cord lesions may be seen in combination with CADASIL.[77] No associations between MS and the NOTCH3 gene have been found,[78] although there is a case report of a 26-year-old patient with Balo concentric sclerosis with a transition mutation of the NOTCH3

gene (1750C>T). Balo concentric sclerosis is a rare disease associated with MS and NMO. On MR imaging, typical lesions consisting of multiple concentric rings can be found, and are thought to represent the host response to injury (Fig. 4).

NMO (or Devic disease) was originally considered a variant of MS. Patients with NMO experience severe episodes of optic neuritis and transverse myelitis, and have spinal lesions extending multiple segments as the dominant abnormalities on MR imaging. The recent discovery of antibodies directed against the predominant water channel in the central nervous system (aquaporin-4) clearly defines NMO as a separate disease, although this antigen is not found in all patients with NMO.[79] With respect to genetic associations, NMO is, in contrast with MS, not linked with a positive HLA-DRB1*1501 status.[80] The high frequency of familial NMO may

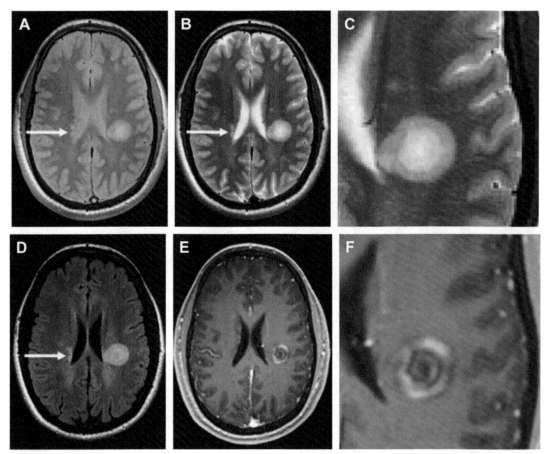

Fig. 4. Balo concentric sclerosis. Note the alternating bands of signal intensity on proton-density–weighted (*A*), T2-weighted (*B, C*) and FLAIR (*D*) images. The pattern of multiple concentric rings is best seen on contrast-enhanced T1-weighted scans (*E, F*). Parts *C* and *F* are magnifications. Other nonenhancing areas of signal hyperintensity partly adjacent to the right lateral ventricle (*white arrow*) are also seen, suggesting foci of earlier demyelination. (*From* Seewann A, Enzinger C, Filippi M, et al. MRI characteristics of atypical idiopathic inflammatory demyelinating lesions of the brain: a review of reported findings. J Neurol 2008;255:1–10; with permission.)

suggest a partly genetic cause, even though an association with a genetic variation of aquaporin-4 was not found.[81] In Asian people, a form of MS called opticospinal MS exists, which resembles a relapsing form of NMO. HLA-DPB1*0501 is associated with opticospinal MS but also with more classic MS in Japanese patients.[82]

Leber hereditary optic neuropathy (LHON) is a maternally inherited disease causing optic nerve degeneration by loss of retinal ganglion cells, resulting in bilateral vision loss. Three mitochondrial DNA point mutations are known (m.11778G>A, m.14484T>C and m.3460G>A), with incomplete penetrance and male dominance. The prevalence in Europe is estimated to be 1 in 45,000.[83] The combination of LHON and a clinical phenotype of MS is referred to as Harding disease or LHON-MS. It differs from LHON in having a long interval between the other eye being affected and from

MS in having painless neuritis and poor visual prognosis. In a recent review, all of the 56 reported cases had MS-compatible abnormalities on MR imaging.[84] It was suggested in the same review that having the LHON mitochondrial DNA mutation may direct an inflammatory reaction at the already vulnerable optic nerves in those individuals susceptible to developing MS.

FUTURE PERSPECTIVES

Because MS is a multigenetic and heterogeneous disease, correlations found in MS are often not strong for individual genes, both when searching for genes associated with susceptibility and for genes related to disease severity or prognosis. In order to further increase knowledge about MS, future research studies can adapt for this difficulty in several ways (**Box 2**).

MR imaging parameters as intermediate outcome measures are more precise than clinical outcome measures and should increasingly be used. When hypotheses concerning specific pathophysiologic mechanisms are examined, MR imaging may be helpful; for example, by allowing researchers to select patients with various amounts of axonal damage (T1BH) or cortical glutamate levels (MRS). Furthermore, certain imaging patterns are clinically relevant and therefore already deserve more attention in genetic research. For instance, why is the spinal cord heavily involved in some patients, whereas in others it is not? Another example is cortical pathology in MS, which can be detected in vivo and have been related to cognitive disability. MR imaging allows clinicians to select patient groups for these and other imaging patterns. It may be opportunistic to select extremes for an MR imaging trait while keeping other potentially confounding variables comparable, to increase statistical power and specificity.

Quantitative MR imaging techniques, such as (longitudinal) atrophy measurement, DTI, MTR, and MRS, provide more information than conventional MR imaging measures by allowing detection of abnormalities outside focal lesions in the normal-appearing white matter, and should therefore increasingly be used in MS genotype-phenotype studies. Mapping analysis techniques such as VBM and LPM can help to link spatial MS pathology patterns to genetic polymorphisms on a group level. Functional MR imaging may help to identify potential genetic variability in adaptive neuronal plasticity.

It seems that genes associated with MS susceptibility are not strongly involved in disease severity and prognosis, and that other genes may be partly responsible. The search for polymorphisms involved in disease severity will be even more rewarding, because they are immediately clinically relevant by allowing better patient selection for early and more aggressive therapy. One inventive method to test specific hypotheses with regard to the genetics of MS severity and different MR imaging patterns is the pathway-based approach, allowing much less stringent statistical correcting than GWA studies, and therefore smaller patient groups. An example is the investigation of the glutamate pathway, using MR spectroscopy for in vivo measurement of brain glutamate levels.[69] Furthermore, although only a few studies have addressed influences of epigenetics or messenger RNA expression on disease severity in MS,[31,85,86] these are promising strategies.

The increased and more sophisticated use of MR imaging as outcome measures, selection of well-defined MS patient groups, and pathway-based analyses may benefit genetic research in MS, thereby leading to a better understanding of, and prognostic ability for, this complex disease.

REFERENCES

1. Compston A, Coles A. Multiple sclerosis. Lancet 2008;372:1502–17.
2. Lublin FD, Reingold SC. Defining the clinical course of multiple sclerosis: results of an international survey. National Multiple Sclerosis Society (USA) Advisory Committee on Clinical Trials of New Agents in Multiple Sclerosis. Neurology 1996;46:907–11.
3. Miller DH, Weinshenker BG, Filippi M, et al. Differential diagnosis of suspected multiple sclerosis: a consensus approach. Mult Scler 2008;14:1157–74.
4. Koch-Henriksen N, Sørensen PS. The changing demographic pattern of multiple sclerosis epidemiology. Lancet Neurol 2010;9:520–32.
5. Almohmeed YH, Avenell A, Aucott L, et al. Systematic review and meta-analysis of the sero-epidemiological association between Epstein Barr virus and multiple sclerosis. PLoS One 2013;8: e61110.
6. Ascherio A, Munger KL, White R, et al. Vitamin D as an early predictor of multiple sclerosis activity and progression. JAMA Neurol 2014;71:306–14.
7. O'Gorman C, Lin R, Stankovich J, et al. Modelling genetic susceptibility to multiple sclerosis with family data. Neuroepidemiology 2013;40:1–12.
8. Hansen T, Skytthe A, Stenager E, et al. Concordance for multiple sclerosis in Danish twins: an update of a nationwide study. Mult Scler 2005;11:504–10.

9. Hafler DA, Compston A, Sawcer S, et al. Risk alleles for multiple sclerosis identified by a genomewide study. N Engl J Med 2007;357:851–62.

10. Muñoz-Culla M, Irizar H, Otaegui D. The genetics of multiple sclerosis: review of current and emerging candidates. Appl Clin Genet 2013;6:63–73.

11. Sawcer S, Hellenthal G, Pirinen M, et al. Genetic risk and a primary role for cell-mediated immune mechanisms in multiple sclerosis. Nature 2011; 476:214–9.

12. Manolio TA. Genomewide association studies and assessment of the risk of disease. N Engl J Med 2010;363:166–76.

13. Filippi M, Rocca MA. MR imaging of multiple sclerosis. Radiology 2011;259:659–81.

14. Polman CH, Reingold SC, Banwell B, et al. Diagnostic criteria for multiple sclerosis: 2010 revisions to the McDonald criteria. Ann Neurol 2011;69:292–302.

15. Montalban X, Tintoré M, Swanton J, et al. MRI criteria for MS in patients with clinically isolated syndromes. Neurology 2010;74:427–34.

16. Trapp BD, Peterson J, Ransohoff RM, et al. Axonal transection in the lesions of multiple sclerosis. N Engl J Med 1998;338:278–85.

17. Moll NM, Rietsch AM, Thomas S, et al. Multiple sclerosis normal-appearing white matter: pathology-imaging correlations. Ann Neurol 2011;70:764–73.

18. Seewann A, Vrenken H, van der Valk P, et al. Diffusely abnormal white matter in chronic multiple sclerosis: imaging and histopathologic analysis. Arch Neurol 2009;66:601–9.

19. Geurts JJ, Calabrese M, Fisher E, et al. Measurement and clinical effect of grey matter pathology in multiple sclerosis. Lancet Neurol 2012;11:1082–92.

20. Barkhof F, Calabresi PA, Miller DH, et al. Imaging outcomes for neuroprotection and repair in multiple sclerosis trials. Nat Rev Neurol 2009;5:256–66.

21. Lycklama G, Thompson A, Filippi M, et al. Spinal-cord MRI in multiple sclerosis. Lancet Neurol 2003; 2:555–62.

22. Sombekke MH, Wattjes MP, Balk LJ, et al. Spinal cord lesions in patients with clinically isolated syndrome: a powerful tool in diagnosis and prognosis. Neurology 2013;80:69–75.

23. Rocca MA, Horsfield MA, Sala S, et al. A multicenter assessment of cervical cord atrophy among MS clinical phenotypes. Neurology 2011; 76:2096–102.

24. Okuda DT, Srinivasan R, Oksenberg JR, et al. Genotype-phenotype correlations in multiple sclerosis: HLA genes influence disease severity inferred by 1HMR spectroscopy and MRI measures. Brain 2009;132:250–9.

25. Zivadinov R, Uxa L, Zacchi T, et al. HLA genotypes and disease severity assessed by magnetic resonance imaging findings in patients with multiple sclerosis. J Neurol 2003;250:1099–106.

26. Zivadinov R, Uxa L, Bratina A, et al. HLA-DRB1*1501, -DQB1*0301, -DQB1*0302, -DQB1*0602, and -DQB1*0603 alleles are associated with more severe disease outcome on MRI in patients with multiple sclerosis. Int Rev Neurobiol 2007;79:521–35.

27. Sombekke MH, Lukas C, Crusius JB, et al. HLA-DRB1*1501 and spinal cord magnetic resonance imaging lesions in multiple sclerosis. Arch Neurol 2009;66:1531–6.

28. Schreiber K, Oturai A, Ryder L, et al. Disease severity in Danish multiple sclerosis patients evaluated by MRI and three genetic markers (HLA-DRB1*1501, CCR5 deletion mutation, apolipoprotein E). Mult Scler 2002;8:295–8.

29. Sombekke MH, Vellinga MM, Uitdehaag BM, et al. Genetic correlations of brain lesion distribution in multiple sclerosis: an exploratory study. AJNR Am J Neuroradiol 2011;32:695–703.

30. Baranzini SE, Wang J, Gibson RA, et al. Genome-wide association analysis of susceptibility and clinical phenotype in multiple sclerosis. Hum Mol Genet 2009;18:767–78.

31. Inkster B, Strijbis EM, Vounou M, et al. Histone deacetylase gene variants predict brain volume changes in multiple sclerosis. Neurobiol Aging 2013;34:238–47.

32. Karrenbauer VD, Prejs R, Masterman T, et al. Impact of cerebrospinal-fluid oligoclonal immunoglobulin bands and HLA-DRB1 risk alleles on brain magnetic-resonance-imaging lesion load in Swedish multiple sclerosis patients. J Neuroimmunol 2013; 254:170–3.

33. Kalincik T, Guttmann CR, Krasensky J, et al. Multiple sclerosis susceptibility loci do not alter clinical and MRI outcomes in clinically isolated syndrome. Genes Immun 2013;14:244–8.

34. Horakova D, Zivadinov R, Weinstock-Guttman B, et al. HLA DRB1*1501 is only modestly associated with lesion burden at the first demyelinating event. J Neuroimmunol 2011;236:76–80.

35. Sombekke MH, Jafari N, Bendfeldt K, et al. No influence of KIF1B on neurodegenerative markers in multiple sclerosis. Neurology 2011;76:1843–5.

36. Hooper-van Veen T, Schrijver HM, Zwiers A, et al. The interleukin-1 gene family in multiple sclerosis susceptibility and disease course. Mult Scler 2003; 9:535–9.

37. Sepulcre J, Masdeu JC, Palacios R, et al. HLA-DR2 and white matter lesion distribution in MS. J Neuroimaging 2008;18:328–31.

38. Gourraud PA, Sdika M, Khankhanian P, et al. A genome-wide association study of brain lesion distribution in multiple sclerosis. Brain 2013;136: 1012–24.

39. Kutzelnigg A, Lucchinetti CF, Stadelmann C, et al. Cortical demyelination and diffuse white matter injury in multiple sclerosis. Brain 2005;128:2705–12.

40. Geurts JJ, Pouwels PJ, Uitdehaag BM, et al. Intracortical lesions in multiple sclerosis: improved detection with 3D double inversion-recovery MR imaging. Radiology 2005;236:254–60.

41. Roosendaal SD, Moraal B, Pouwels PJ, et al. Accumulation of cortical lesions in MS: relation with cognitive impairment. Mult Scler 2009;15:708–14.

42. Calabrese M, Seppi D, Cocco E, et al. Cortical pathology in RRMS: taking a cue from four sisters. Mult Scler Int 2012;2012:760254.

43. Vigeveno RM, Wiebenga OT, Wattjes MP, et al. Shifting imaging targets in multiple sclerosis: from inflammation to neurodegeneration. J Magn Reson Imaging 2012;36:1–19.

44. Zuccato C, Cattaneo E. Brain-derived neurotrophic factor in neurodegenerative diseases. Nat Rev Neurol 2009;5:311–22.

45. Stadelmann C, Kerschensteiner M, Misgeld T, et al. BDNF and gp145trkB in multiple sclerosis brain lesions: neuroprotective interactions between immune and neuronal cells? Brain 2002;125:75–85.

46. Zivadinov R, Weinstock-Guttman B, Benedict R, et al. Preservation of gray matter volume in multiple sclerosis patients with the Met allele of the rs6265 (Val66Met) SNP of brain-derived neurotrophic factor. Hum Mol Genet 2007;16:2659–68.

47. Liguori M, Fera F, Gioia MC, et al. Investigating the role of brain-derived neurotrophic factor in relapsing-remitting multiple sclerosis. Genes Brain Behav 2007;6:177–83.

48. Cerasa A, Tongiorgi E, Fera F, et al. The effects of BDNF Val66Met polymorphism on brain function in controls and patients with multiple sclerosis: an imaging genetic study. Behav Brain Res 2010;207: 377–86.

49. Ramasamy DP, Ramanathan M, Cox JL, et al. Effect of Met66 allele of the BDNF rs6265 SNP on regional gray matter volumes in patients with multiple sclerosis: a voxel-based morphometry study. Pathophysiology 2011;18:53–60.

50. Dinacci D, Tessitore A, Russo A, et al. BDNF Val66-Met polymorphism and brain volumes in multiple sclerosis. Neurol Sci 2011;32:117–23.

51. Weinstock-Guttman B, Benedict RH, Tamaño-Blanco M, et al. The rs2030324 SNP of brain-derived neurotrophic factor (BDNF) is associated with visual cognitive processing in multiple sclerosis. Pathophysiology 2011;18:43–52.

52. Verghese PB, Castellano JM, Holtzman DM. Apolipoprotein E in Alzheimer's disease and other neurological disorders. Lancet Neurol 2011;10:241–52.

53. Burwick RM, Ramsay PP, Haines JL, et al. APOE epsilon variation in multiple sclerosis susceptibility and disease severity: some answers. Neurology 2006;66:1373–83.

54. Lill CM, Liu T, Schjeide BM, et al. Closing the case of APOE in multiple sclerosis: no association with disease risk in over 29 000 subjects. J Med Genet 2012;49:558–62.

55. Ghaffar O, Lobaugh NJ, Szilagyi GM, et al. Imaging genetics in multiple sclerosis: a volumetric and diffusion tensor MRI study of APOE ε4. Neuroimage 2011;58:724–31.

56. Portaccio E, Goretti B, Zipoli V, et al. APOE-epsilon4 is not associated with cognitive impairment in relapsing-remitting multiple sclerosis. Mult Scler 2009;15:1489–94.

57. Van der Walt A, Stankovich J, Bahlo M, et al. Apolipoprotein genotype does not influence MS severity, cognition, or brain atrophy. Neurology 2009;73: 1018–25.

58. Zakrzewska-Pniewska B, Styczynska M, Podlecka A, et al. Association of apolipoprotein E and myeloperoxidase genotypes to clinical course of familial and sporadic multiple sclerosis. Mult Scler 2004;10: 266–71.

59. Zwemmer JN, Van Veen T, Van Winsen L, et al. No major association of ApoE genotype with disease characteristics and MRI findings in multiple sclerosis. Mult Scler 2004;10:272–7.

60. Lanzillo R, Prinster A, Scarano V, et al. Neuropsychological assessment, quantitative MRI and ApoE gene polymorphisms in a series of MS patients treated with IFN beta-1b. J Neurol Sci 2006;245:141–5.

61. De Stefano N, Bartolozzi ML, Nacmias B, et al. Influence of apolipoprotein E epsilon4 genotype on brain tissue integrity in relapsing-remitting multiple sclerosis. Arch Neurol 2004;61:536–40.

62. Enzinger C, Ropele S, Strasser-Fuchs S, et al. Lower levels of N-acetylaspartate in multiple sclerosis patients with the apolipoprotein E epsilon4 allele. Arch Neurol 2003;60:65–70.

63. Enzinger C, Ropele S, Smith S, et al. Accelerated evolution of brain atrophy and "black holes" in MS patients with APOE-epsilon 4. Ann Neurol 2004;55: 563–9.

64. Fazekas F, Strasser-Fuchs S, Schmidt H, et al. Apolipoprotein E genotype related differences in brain lesions of multiple sclerosis. J Neurol Neurosurg Psychiatry 2000;69:25–8.

65. Werner P, Pitt D, Raine CS. Multiple sclerosis: altered glutamate homeostasis in lesions correlates with oligodendrocyte and axonal damage. Ann Neurol 2001;50:169–80.

66. Srinivasan R, Sailasuta N, Hurd R, et al. Evidence of elevated glutamate in multiple sclerosis using magnetic resonance spectroscopy at 3 T. Brain 2005;128:1016–25.

67. Strijbis EM, Inkster B, Vounou M, et al. Glutamate gene polymorphisms predict brain volumes in multiple sclerosis. Mult Scler 2013;19:281–8.

68. Inoue H, Yamasue H, Tochigi M, et al. Functional (GT) n polymorphisms in promoter region of N-methyl-D-aspartate receptor 2A subunit (GRIN2A) gene affect

hippocampal and amygdala volumes. Genes Brain Behav 2010;9:269–75.

69. Baranzini SE, Srinivasan R, Khankhanian P, et al. Genetic variation influences glutamate concentrations in brains of patients with multiple sclerosis. Brain 2010;133:2603–11.

70. Qiu W, Raven S, James I, et al. Spinal cord involvement in multiple sclerosis: a correlative MRI and high-resolution HLA-DRB1 genotyping study. J Neurol Sci 2011;300:114–9.

71. Lycklama à Nijeholt GJ, Barkhof F, Scheltens P, et al. MR of the spinal cord in multiple sclerosis: relation to clinical subtype and disability. AJNR Am J Neuroradiol 1997;18:1041–8.

72. Lukas C, Sombekke MH, Bellenberg B, et al. Relevance of spinal cord abnormalities to clinical disability in multiple sclerosis: MR imaging findings in a large cohort of patients. Radiology 2013;269: 542–52.

73. Fera F, Passamonti L, Cerasa A, et al. The BDNF Val66Met polymorphism has opposite effects on memory circuits of multiple sclerosis patients and controls. PLoS One 2013;8:e61063.

74. Fischl B, Dale AM. Measuring the thickness of the human cerebral cortex from magnetic resonance images. Proc Natl Acad Sci U S A 2000;97:11050–5.

75. Rossi S, Bozzali M, Bari M, et al. Association between a genetic variant of type-1 cannabinoid receptor and inflammatory neurodegeneration in multiple sclerosis. PLoS One 2013;8:e82848.

76. Federico A, Di Donato I, Bianchi S, et al. Hereditary cerebral small vessel diseases: a review. J Neurol Sci 2012;322:25–30.

77. Bentley P, Wang T, Malik O, et al. CADASIL with cord involvement associated with a novel and atypical NOTCH3 mutation. J Neurol Neurosurg Psychiatry 2011;82:855–60.

78. Broadley SA, Sawcer SJ, Chataway SJ, et al. No association between multiple sclerosis and the Notch3 gene responsible for cerebral autosomal dominant arteriopathy with subcortical infarcts and leukoencephalopathy (CADASIL). J Neurol Neurosurg Psychiatry 2001;71:97–9.

79. Jacob A, McKeon A, Nakashima I, et al. Current concept of neuromyelitis optica (NMO) and NMO spectrum disorders. J Neurol Neurosurg Psychiatry 2013;84:922–30.

80. Matiello M, Schaefer-Klein J, Brum DG, et al. HLA-DRB1*1501 tagging rs3135388 polymorphism is not associated with neuromyelitis optica. Mult Scler 2010;16:981–4.

81. Matiello M, Schaefer-Klein JL, Hebrink DD, et al. Genetic analysis of aquaporin-4 in neuromyelitis optica. Neurology 2011;77:1149–55.

82. Fukazawa T, Kikuchi S, Miyagishi R, et al. HLA-dPB1*0501 is not uniquely associated with opticospinal multiple sclerosis in Japanese patients. Important role of DPB1*0301. Mult Scler 2006;12: 19–23.

83. Mascialino B, Leinonen M, Meier T. Meta-analysis of the prevalence of Leber hereditary optic neuropathy mtDNA mutations in Europe. Eur J Ophthalmol 2012; 22:461–5.

84. Pfeffer G, Burke A, Yu-Wai-Man P, et al. Clinical features of MS associated with Leber hereditary optic neuropathy mtDNA mutations. Neurology 2013;81:2073–81.

85. Sellebjerg F, Hedegaard CJ, Krakauer M, et al. Glatiramer acetate antibodies, gene expression and disease activity in multiple sclerosis. Mult Scler 2012;18:305–13.

86. Van der Voort LF, Vennegoor A, Visser A, et al. Spontaneous MxA mRNA level predicts relapses in patients with recently diagnosed MS. Neurology 2010;75:1228–33.

87. Healy BC, Liguori M, Tran D, et al. HLA B*44: protective effects in MS susceptibility and MRI outcome measures. Neurology 2010;75:634–40.

88. Hooper-van Veen T, Berkhof J, Polman CH, et al. Analysing the effect of candidate genes on complex traits: an application in multiple sclerosis. Immunogenetics 2006;58:347–54.

89. Jensen CJ, Stankovich J, Van der Walt A, et al. Multiple sclerosis susceptibility-associated SNPs do not influence disease severity measures in a cohort of Australian MS patients. PLoS One 2010;5:e10003.

90. Van der Walt A, Stankovich J, Bahlo M, et al. Heterogeneity at the HLA-DRB1 allelic variation locus does not influence multiple sclerosis disease severity, brain atrophy or cognition. Mult Scler 2011;17:344–52.

91. Zivadinov R, Weinstock-Guttman B, Zorzon M, et al. Gene-environment interactions between HLA B7/A2, EBV antibodies are associated with MRI injury in multiple sclerosis. J Neuroimmunol 2009;209:123–30.

Molecular Genetics of Glioblastomas
Defining Subtypes and Understanding the Biology

 CrossMark

Ilana Zalcberg Renault, MD, PhD[a],*, Denise Golgher, PhD[b]

KEYWORDS

- Gliomas • Glioblastoma multiforme • Molecular genetics • Mutations

KEY POINTS

- Genomic studies have uncovered the molecular heterogeneity under the World Health Organization classification of glioblastoma multiforme (GBM).
- The cells that give rise to gliomas and the process of gliomagenesis are important to discriminate different subtypes (neural tumors correlate better with mature neurons, proneural tumors with oligodendrocytes, and classic and mesenchymal tumors with astrocytes).
- Microarray-based gene-expression studies have identified molecular subtypes and genes associated with stages and clinical evolution of the disease. Although there is still no consensus on how many subtypes, these studies agree on at least 3: neural, proneural, and mesenchymal.
- Several studies delineating a complex landscape of genetic alterations present in GBM may lead to target-specific treatments, better understanding of the biology of the disease, and better design and conduction of clinical trials.

INTRODUCTION

Among the cancers that affect the central nervous system, gliomas are those with the highest incidence. Their classification is based on morphology and the similarity between neoplastic cells and their normal glia counterparts: gliomas are tumors that have originated from the different cells of the glia, astrocytomas are histologically similar to astrocytes, oligodendrogliomas are similar to oligodendrocytes, and, in the case of mixed oligodendrogliomas, neoplastic cells similar to astrocytes and oligondendrocytes are present. Based on optical microscopy and immunohistochemistry, this classification also separates gliomas into 3 stages: stage II, stage III (anaplastic), and stage IV, which is the glioblastoma multiforme (GBM), the most malignant form of astrocytoma.[1] In clinical practice, the current parameters used for prognosis and treatment protocol are size and stage of the tumor.

Nonetheless, this classification is considered insufficient and controversial. The responses observed among patients diagnosed with tumors within the same class are too variable. There is a high degree of subjectivity when different observers analyze the morphologic distinction between an oligodendroglioma and an astrocytoma, for example. Considering that oligondendrogliomas are chemosensitive and the survival rate of patients with oligondendrogliomas is much higher than for a patient with astrocytoma, more precision

The authors have nothing to disclose.
[a] DASA, Rua João Borges 120/502, Gavea, Rio de Janeiro CEP 22451-100, Brazil; [b] Symbiosis-Biotechnology Consultancy, Rio de Janeiro, Brazil
* Corresponding author.
E-mail addresses: Zalcberg@inca.gov.br; ilanazalcberg@yahoo.com.br

in the diagnostic is markedly relevant for the medical care. By applying the knowledge of molecular genetics, it is possible to generate more information that can help in clinical practice: deletions of the 1p and 19q regions of the short arm of chromosome 1 and long arm of chromosome 19, respectively, are more frequent in tumors that are predominantly oligodendrocytic. The loss of heterozygosity (LOH) of 1p is correlated with chemosensitivity and of 1p/19q with a prolonged therapeutic response and survival rate in the patient.

GBM correspond to 54% of all brain gliomas. In the United States in 2012, statistics indicated an incidence of 3.19 per 100,000 inhabitants, with a higher incidence in men (men 1.6 times higher than women), and a survival rate after 5 years of less than 5%.[2] GBM are divided into primary (approximately 90%–95% and more frequent in older patients), and secondary (approximately 5%–10%, usually diagnosed in younger patients).[3,4] Differently from secondary gliomas, primary GBM show no evidence of a progression from lower-stage gliomas (grades II or III).

Despite comprehensive therapy, which includes surgery, radiotherapy and chemotherapy, the prognosis of patients with GBM is very poor. Diagnosed individuals present an average of 12 to 18 months of life, the prognosis being worse for patients older than 60 years and better for younger individuals.[5,6] Because of its aggressiveness, difficult treatment, and poor 5-year survival rate, gliomas have serious effects not only for the patient and immediate family but for the health system in general.[7] Nowadays little can be offered to patients to improve their prognosis. However, many studies are being conducted to enable better understanding of the molecular biology and genetics of GBM in the hope that, as has happened with other types of cancers such as breast, melanoma, leukemia, and lung, a better molecular characterization may lead to the development of target-specific drugs and innovative approaches in the diagnosis, prognosis, and treatment of gliomas.[8]

Cancer is a complex disease of the genome in which genes that regulate physiologic processes responsible for cellular differentiation, proliferation, and death are affected. When these genes are altered, still in the germinal cells or, more frequently, in somatic cells, and are not repaired, the mutations (the term here used to refer to any chromosomal alteration such as point mutation, deletion, insertion, amplification, and so forth), in most cases more than 1, are passed to daughter cells, which may confer characteristics that give the mutated cell advantages over normal cells.[4,9–11] Not only chromosomal alterations but also alterations in methylation patterns and other forms of transcriptional regulations contribute to the complexity of cancer.[4,9,10]

The mutations identified in cancer can be divided into 2 types, drivers and passengers. The former occurs in genes that belong to biological pathways essential for the survival of the malignant cell, and are frequently associated with an advantage in survival. The latter results from the genetic instability and does not have a pathologic role.[9,11,12]

Driver mutations seem to be tissue specific; in other words, only a minority of the driver mutations associated with GBM is also identified in breast or colorectal tumors.[13]

The comprehension of the biological pathway altered by a mutation is important for the genetic analysis of a tumor; mutations in different genes of the same biological pathway, present in one sample or in different samples, generally result in the same phenotype (exclusivity principle). For example, the analysis of GBM samples has indicated that the gene with the highest frequency of mutation is *TP53* (35.8% of the samples had an altered *TP53*). However, if the biological pathways are considered, pathways of apoptosis and guanosine triphosphatases have mutations in 79.2% of the analyzed samples.[10] The principle of exclusivity usually holds; it is rare to observe alterations in multiple genes the same biological pathway. For example, it is unlikely to find the same tumor bearing a mutation in *KRAS* with a mutation in *BRAF*, which is downstream of the same pathway.[11]

This review aims to provide an overview of the molecular genetics of glioblastomas, probably the most extensively studied type of cancer to this date. Therefore, the amount of information published and/or available is overwhelming.[14] Although it is by no means possible to give a thorough and complete picture on this topic, the reader is referred to other excellent reviews published, which will be able to complement the descriptions herein of an already very complex picture of the genomic alterations identified in these tumors.[4,6,15–17]

MOLECULAR CHARACTERIZATION OF GLIOBLASTOMA MULTIFORME: GENETIC ALTERATIONS

In 2008, 2 seminal studies were published delineating a complex landscape of genetic alterations present in GBM.[3,18] The *Tumor Cancer Genome Atlas* (TCGA) analyzed fewer genes in more samples than the group of Vogelstein, which analyzed more genes in fewer samples.[3]

Both studies pointed to the importance of 3 major biological pathways, responsible for cell survival, DNA repair, progression of G1/S, blockade of G2/M, cell migration, apoptosis, and progression of cell cycle: pathways of (1) RTK (tyrosine kinase receptors) signaling, and pathways of the tumor suppressor genes (2) *TP53* and (3) *RB*. The articles agreed on most of the genes altered and, in accordance with the principle of exclusivity, in general the alterations identified were in genes of different biological pathways. The TCGA study identified simultaneous alterations in 3 pathways in 74% of the samples of the study performed by the TCGA network.

Both studies identified samples with a hypermutated phenotype after treatment with the alkylating agent temozolomide (TMZ).[3,18] The TCGA network identified 7 samples with this profile. Of these, 6 had mutations in at least one DNA-repair gene of the MMR (mismatch repair) family that seem to have an influence in the methylation pattern of *MGMT*. The hypermethylation of the promoter of the gene *MGMT* results in the lack of expression of the protein O^6-methylguanine-DNA methyltransferase, which repairs DNA. The methylation of *MGMT* interferes with the susceptibility of cells to treatment with TMZ.[19] Results indicate that the administration of TMZ in combination with radiotherapy can increase the survival of patients diagnosed with GBM. Therefore, these observations can have a direct impact on the clinical practice and protocols administered today. In addition, mutations on MMR and the methylation pattern of *MGMT* can have an important role in the frequency of mutations observed in samples from treated patients.[18]

The most frequent alterations identified were: gene amplifications on *EGFR*, *CDK4*, *PDGFRA*, *MDM2*, *MDM4*, *MET CDK6*, *MYCN*, *CCND2*, *P1K3CA* and *AKT3*; homozygotic deletions in the genes *CDKN2A/B*, *PTEN*, *CDKN2C*, *RB1*, *PARK2*, and *NF1*; and higher-frequency mutations in the genes *TP53*, *PTEN*, *NF1*, *EGFR*, *ERBB2*, *RB1*, *P1K3R1*, and *P1K3CA*. Considering only alterations in copy number, 66%, 70%, and 59% of the 206 samples analyzed presented somatic alterations in the main pathways of *RB*, *TP53* and RTK, respectively. If sequencing results were included, this frequency would increase to 87%, 78%, and 88% in the respective pathways.[18]

In the genes identified as frequently mutated, Parsons and colleagues[3] indicated candidates that had more chances of being responsible for the process of tumor formation, in other words, driver mutations: *CDKN2A*, *TP53*, *EGFR*, *PTEN*, *NF1*, *CDK4*, *RB1*, *1DH1*, *P1K3CA*, and *P1K3R1*. It is worth pointing out that both studies identified mutations in the gene *NF1*, possibly a relevant

tumor suppressor gene in GBM; 23% and 15% of the samples in the TCGA network study and of Parsons and colleagues,[3] respectively, had some type of alteration in this gene.

Mutations in the *IDH1* gene were identified in almost all secondary GBM and correlated with a better prognosis, indicating their relevance in the refinement of the classification of these tumors. In primary GBM, these mutations were rarely detected.[3] A mutation in IDH1 correlates with a hypermethylation status of the DNA, denominated Glioma CpG Island Methylator Phenotype (G-CIMP).[20] Mutations in *IDH2* have also been identified in GBM samples, but are less recurrent than in *IDH1*.[21] *IDH1* and *IDH2* are NADP$^+$-dependent enzymes that catalyze the oxidative decarboxylation of isocitrate to α-ketoglutarate,[17] an important biological compound in the biochemical pathway of carbohydrates, lipids, and amino acids.[4] The identification of mutations on *IDH1* and *IDH2* were important not only because of their predominance but as possible biomarkers of progressive gliomas. They highlight an important characteristic of GBM, of a disease of altered cellular metabolism and correlated epigenetics.[17]

A previous report demonstrated the amplification of tyrosine kinase receptor genes in the GBM samples from TCGA.[22] Approximately 50% of the 206 samples had amplification in at least 1 of the 51 RTKs analyzed.[22] The most frequent was on the *EGFR* gene (41%), followed by *PDGFRA* (10%), which was frequently coamplified with *KIT* (7%) and *KDR* (4%). *MET* was the third most frequent (2%). The amplification of *EGFR* was associated with a worse prognosis.[4]

Lack of heterozygosity of chromosome 10 is also a frequent alteration in GBMs.[23,24]

Genomic alterations such as the ones described here produce altered patterns of gene expression. Several articles have been published reporting analysis of patterns of expression (transcriptomes) in gliomas.[25–30]

MOLECULAR CHARACTERIZATION OF GLIOBLASTOMA MULTIFORME: TRANSCRIPTOMES

Transcriptome analysis is performed using expression microarrays. Independently of the technology of choice, these experiments generate a huge amount of data that has to be treated by specific bioinformatics software and interpreted by specialists. The bioinformatics tools applied and the interpretation will depend, obviously, on the question being asked.

Whereas some studies aimed at the identification of biomarkers that could define molecular subtypes of GBM and correlate these subtypes with certain characteristics, others did the opposite, first selecting the desired characteristics (such as favorable or nonfavorable prognostic) and then searching for biomarkers within the group. Pope and colleagues,[31] for example, divided GBM samples according to their enhancement in the magnetic resonance image, dividing the samples into two groups: one group with incomplete enhancement and another group with complete enhancement. The pattern of expression was analyzed in both groups, indicating that the group with incomplete enhancement corresponded to secondary GBM and the group with complete enhancement with primary GBM.[31]

Phillips and colleagues[27], Verhaak and colleagues,[30] and earlier studies,[25,26] analyzed the transcriptome of several high-grade gliomas with the goal of defining genomic profiles that could classify GBM into subtypes.

Phillips and colleagues[27] grouped 76 astrocytomas according to the pattern of gene expression of 108 genes, and correlated the groups with survival. Three clusters with distinctive genomic profiles were identified: proneural, proliferative, and mesenchymal. The 3 profiles were validated with more samples and their prognostic value demonstrated. The proneural subtype (which may correspond to stages III or IV of the World Health Organization [WHO] classification), was the one with a better prognosis and was found in younger patients (<40 years); the proliferative and mesenchymal were found mostly in older patients (>50 years) and were associated with a worse prognosis. In posttreatment recurrent samples, the tumors of the proneural subtype changed to an expression pattern of the mesenchymal subtype.[27]

The work by Verhaak and colleagues[30] identified 4 different clusters and defined 4 subtypes based on the clustering of expression patterns: proneural, neural, classic, and mesenchymal. A correlation between response to more aggressive chemotherapy and a reduction in mortality rates was observed for the classic and mesenchymal subtypes, but not for the proneural. In this study, the proneural subtype was also associated with younger patients, with mutations in *IDH1* and *TP53*. In contrast to the study published by Phillips and colleagues,[27] no changes in genomic signatures were observed in recurrent posttreatment samples.

These transcriptome studies used different methodologies and different samples,[27,30] which could explain, in part, the differences observed. Some common and important observations should be pointed out: (1) microarray-based gene-expression studies were able to identify molecular subtypes and genes associated with stages and clinical evolution of the disease; (2) cells that originate the gliomas and the process of gliomagenesis are important in discriminating different subtypes (neural tumors correlate better with mature neurons, proneural with oligodendrocytes, and classic and mesenchymal with astrocytes)[6]; (3) the definition of subtypes can help in the development of target-specific drugs and more precise therapies, also laying the basis for design and conduction of clinical trials.

What is made clear by all of these studies is that the molecular heterogeneity identified in tumors denominated glioblastomas indicates a degree of complexity that does not correspond to the simple WHO classification for these tumors. There is still no consensus in the literature regarding the number of subtypes that will correspond better to the clinical development of the disease.

At least 2 of the subtypes, clustered according to the expression patterns identified by Phillips and colleagues[27] and Verhaak and colleagues,[30] the proneural and the mesenchymal, seem to correspond well to several experiments.[15,32] The proneural genomic signature, characterized by biomarkers associated with neurogenesis, has a more favorable prognostic, and is more frequent in younger patients and secondary GBM. The mesenchymal genomic signature has a less favorable prognostic, is more frequent in older patients, and is rich in biomarkers of tissues of mesenchymal origin. Several researchers believe that these patterns indicate an epithelial-mesenchymal transition in GBM with a worsening of the prognosis, similar to what happens in several other cancers.[32–34]

Huse and colleagues,[15] in their review with the very appropriate title "Molecular Subclassification of Diffuse Gliomas: Seeing Order in the Chaos," provided a comprehensive summary of the molecular alterations, genomic signatures, and WHO classification.

MOLECULAR CHARACTERIZATION OF GLIOBLASTOMA MULTIFORME: CLINICAL APPLICATIONS AND TECHNOLOGICAL TRENDS

Despite the overwhelming amount of information available about gliomas, little has been applied to medical practice. The LOH of 1p19q is used as a marker of oligodendrogliomas and the pattern of methylation of *MGMT* as an indicator of susceptibility to TMZ. Nevertheless, at the speed by which new data is being generated, it is very likely that innovative technologies will soon be able to benefit patients.

Colman and colleagues[32] analyzed data from samples of 4 different American institutions and identified 38 genes that had expression levels altered in patients who were considered long-term survivors (survival rates above average). Elevated expression levels of 31 genes were associated with a worse prognosis, whereas the elevated expression of 7 was associated with prolonged survival. From this genetic panel, the group standardized a test based on 9 biomarkers, which can be used as a predictive prognostic test for paraffin-embedded GBM samples. Genes with elevated expression and indicating a worse prognosis were associated with a mesenchymal origin and angiogenesis, whereas genes correlated with a more favorable prognosis were associated with a neural origin (proneural subtype).[32] This 9-gene test is available commercially.[35]

Amplifications, especially *EGFR* amplifications, are a hallmark of GBM, but even though mutant *EGFRs* could, in theory, constitute a target for therapy, the tyrosine kinase inhibitors erlotinib and gefitinib have brought little benefit in clinical trials. One of the hypotheses is that there is a mismatch between the sites of the mutations in the protein and the drugs that target it.[17] There is no doubt that the more information we have on altered genes, mutation sites, and 3-dimensional conformation of the resulting mutants, the more we will be able to develop target-specific drugs. Vogelstein and Kinzler,[36] in their historical perspective of cancer genes and the pathways they control, pointed out that "one important lesson from the use of these agents is that mutations are more reliable indicators of a good target than is abnormal expression."

More recently, a specific antigen was identified in a small percentage of GBM (3.1%).[37] This antigen is the product of a translocation and juxtaposition of the genes *FGFR* and *TACC* that codes for an oncoprotein. The industry, in need for innovative approaches for the treatment of gliomas, has already licensed the rights to commercialize the antigen for the development of target-specific therapies.[38] This example illustrates how next-generation sequencing will contribute to the identification of targets that can generate better therapies, even for a small percentage of patients.

To learn more about the technological trends in the treatment of gliomas, the authors analyzed the clinical trials from 1997 to 2013.[39] **Fig. 1** shows how the number of clinical trials in gliomas has been increasing, as have the amount of clinical trials using combinations of drugs and biomarkers.

Analysis of the ongoing clinical trials in 2013 (recruiting) indicated that the main areas of investigation were: immunotherapy (vaccines with tumor lysate or tumor antigens, dendritic cells, immunotherapy with specific T cells, peptides); recombinant viruses; drug combinations (inhibitors of tyrosine kinases [ITK] + antiangiogenics, ITK + biologicals); imaging (surgery and guided biopsy); other biologicals (bacterial toxins + cytokines, antibodies, mesenchymal stem cells). Clinical trials and other technological trends have been reviewed in detail elsewhere.[16,40] The Musella Foundation, a nonprofit organization dedicated to brain cancers, has a very useful Web site[41] with up-to-date information on clinical trials, treatments, specific reports, and information.

The diagnosis of GBM is a devastating one. Because of its location and invasive nature, even when the tumor is small and surgery is possible, a complete removal of malignant cells is impossible. Great effort is being made in trying to generate better imaging of malignant cells so

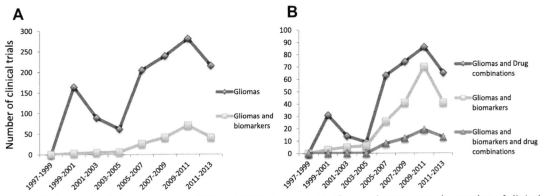

Fig. 1. Clinical trials of glioma between 1997 and 2013. Each point in the graph represents the number of clinical trials in a period of 3 years for searches with different keywords. (*A*) Number of clinical trials using the keywords "gliomas" or "gliomas and biomarkers." (*B*) Number of clinical trials using the keywords "gliomas and drug combination," "gliomas and biomarkers," and "gliomas and biomarkers and drug combination." (*Data from* Clinical-Trials.gov. Available at: http://clinicaltrials.gov/. Accessed April 23, 2014.)

that as much as possible might be surgically removed. It is known that GBM have infiltration of immune cells and the number of CD8$^+$ tumor-infiltrating lymphocytes correlates with a better prognosis.[42,43] The past decade has been a very successful one for the immunotherapy of cancer.[44] Therefore, it is not unrealistic to invest some hope in immunotherapy for the treatment of GBM, because T cells might help in killing the tumor cells that remain in the brain after surgery and the ones resistant to chemotherapy or radiotherapy.[45] Preclinical animal models certainly indicate that there is experimental reason for this hope.[40,46]

Ongoing clinical trials certainly indicate that many in the industry are speculating on immunotherapy. Obviously no one believes that immunotherapy alone will be a cure, but it is reasonable to assume that in combination with better surgery and imaging, innovative therapies (especially targeted ones) in the near future may offer a better prospect than the death sentence patients have today.

WHAT THE REFERRING PHYSICIAN NEEDS TO KNOW

- Some genetic tests are available for prognosis of glioblastomas.
- It is possible to analyze *MGMT* methylation patterns, lack of methylation being an indicator of less resistance to TMZ treatment.
- LOH of 1p/19q is a good indicator of oligodendrogliomas, which have a better prognosis than astrocytomas.
- Some integrated treatment centers for brain tumors around the world do not necessarily adopt TMZ as a first-line treatment, and depending on the profile of the tumor may choose a combination therapy (including antiangiogenesis).
- New data are being generated quickly; innovations in treatments will probably occur soon.

SUMMARY

The genomic analysis of GBM has uncovered a complex landscape of molecular alterations existing in tumors that are classified under the same anatomopathologic category according to the WHO classification system. The available information on these tumors is overwhelming and is way beyond the comprehension we have of the disease today. Although some of this knowledge has been successfully applied to medical practice, there is still a long way to go before it is translated into more benefits for the patient.

Researchers are paving the way to be able to develop new drugs and bring innovation to daily practice, in the form of better diagnostics, targeted drugs, and a more personalized treatment. Based on the heterogeneity of these tumors, their location, and invasive nature, this is a daunting task.

The ongoing clinical trials and the scientific effort being made indicate that in the near future novel treatment protocols based on chemotherapy, biologicals, and immunotherapy will become available, which will be able to improve the prognosis of GBM.

REFERENCES

1. Tumor grades and types. Available at: http://www.cancer.gov/cancertopics/wyntk/brain/page3#c2. Accessed April 20, 2014.
2. Dolecek TA, Propp JM, Stroup NE, et al. CBTRUS statistical report: primary brain and central nervous system tumors diagnosed in the United States in 2005-2009. Neuro Oncol 2012;14(5):v1–49.
3. Parsons DW, Jones S, Zhang X, et al. An integrated genomic analysis of human glioblastoma multiforme. Science 2008;321(5897):1807–12.
4. Dunn GP, Rinne ML, Wykosky J, et al. Emerging insights into the molecular and cellular basis of glioblastoma. Genes Dev 2012;26:756–84.
5. Gladson CL, Prayson RA, Liu WM. The pathobiology of glioma tumors. Annu Rev Pathol 2010;5:33–50.
6. Huse JT, Holland E, DeAngelis LM. Glioblastoma: molecular analysis and clinical implications. Annu Rev Med 2013;64:59–70.
7. Frosina G. DNA repair and resistance of gliomas to chemotherapy and radiotherapy. Mol Cancer Res 2009;7(7):989–99.
8. Impact of cancer genomics on precision medicine for the treatment of cancer. Available at: http://cancergenome.nih.gov/cancergenomics/impact. Accessed April 17, 2014.
9. Beerenwinkel N, Antal T, Dingli D, et al. Genetic progression and the waiting time to cancer. PLoS Comput Biol 2007;3(11):2239–46.
10. Gerstung M, Nicholas E, Jimmy L, et al. The temporal order of genetic and pathway alterations in tumorigenesis. PLoS One 2011;6(11):e27136.
11. Boca SM, Kinzler KW, Velculescu VE, et al. Patient-oriented gene set analysis for cancer mutation data. Genome Biol 2010;11(11):1–10.
12. Salk JJ, Horwitz MS. Passenger mutations as a marker of clonal cell lineages in emerging neoplasia. Semin Cancer Biol 2010;20(5):294–303.
13. Wong KM, Hudson TJ, McPherson JD. Unraveling the genetics of cancer: genome sequencing and beyond. Annu Rev Genomics Hum Genet 2011;12:407–30.

14. Glioblastoma multiforme. Available at: http://cancer genome.nih.gov/cancersselected/glioblastomamulti forme. Accessed April 21, 2014.

15. Huse JT, Phillips HS, Brennan CW. Molecular sub-classification of diffuse gliomas: seeing order in the chaos. Glia 2011;59(8):1190–9.

16. Ohka F, Natsume A, Wakabayashi T. Current trends in targeted therapies for glioblastoma multiforme. Neurol Res Int 2012;2012:878425. Article ID 878425.

17. Cloughesy TF, Cavenee WK, Mischel PS. Glioblastoma: from molecular pathology to targeted treatment. Annu Rev Pathol 2014;9:1–25.

18. TCGA Network. Comprehensive genomic characterization defines human glioblastoma genes and core pathways. Nature 2008;455(7216):1061–8.

19. Stupp R, Hegi ME, van den Bent MJ, et al. Changing paradigms–an update on the multidisciplinary management of malignant glioma. Oncologist 2006; 11(2):165–80.

20. Noushmehr H, Weisenberger DJ, Diefes K, et al. Identification of a CpG island methylator phenotype that defines a distinct subgroup of glioma. Cancer Cell 2010;17(5):510–22.

21. Yan H, Parsons DW, Jin G, et al. IDH1 and IDH2 mutations in gliomas. N Engl J Med 2009;360(8): 765–73.

22. Snuderl M, Fazlollahi L, Le LP, et al. Mosaic amplification of multiple receptor tyrosine kinase genes in glioblastoma. Cancer Cell 2011;20(6):810–7.

23. Fujisawa H, Reis RM, Nakamura M, et al. Loss of heterozygosity on chromosome 10 is more extensive in primary (de novo) than in secondary glioblastomas. Lab Invest 2000;80(1):65–72.

24. Yoshimoto K, Mizoguchi M, Hata N, et al. Molecular biomarkers of glioblastoma: current targets and clinical implications. Curr Biomark Find 2012;2: 63–76.

25. Freije WA, Castro-Vargas FE, Fang Z, et al. Gene expression profiling of gliomas strongly predicts survival. Cancer Res 2004;64:6503–10.

26. Nigro JM, Misra A, Zhang L, et al. Integrated array-comparative genomic hybridization and expression array profiles identify clinically relevant molecular subtypes of glioblastoma. Cancer Res 2005;65(5): 1678–86.

27. Phillips HS, Kharbanda S, Chen R, et al. Molecular subclasses of high-grade glioma predict prognosis, delineate a pattern of disease progression, and resemble stages in neurogenesis. Cancer Cell 2006;9(3):157–73.

28. Li A, Walling J, Ahn S, et al. Unsupervised analysis of transcriptomic profiles reveals six glioma subtypes. Cancer Res 2009;69:2091–9.

29. Gravendeel LA, Kouwenhoven MC, Gevaert O, et al. Intrinsic gene expression profiles of gliomas are a better predictor of survival than histology. Cancer Res 2009;69(23):9065–72.

30. Verhaak RG, Hoadley KA, Purdom E, et al. Integrated genomic analysis identifies clinically relevant subtypes of glioblastoma characterized by abnormalities in PDGFRA, IDH1, EGFR, and NF1. Cancer Cell 2010;17(1):98–110.

31. Pope WB, Chen JH, Dong J, et al. Relationship between gene expression and enhancement in glioblastoma multiforme: exploratory DNA microarray analysis. Radiology 2008;249(1):268–77.

32. Colman H, Zhang L, Sulman EP, et al. A multigene predictor of outcome in glioblastoma. Neuro Oncol 2010;12(1):49–57.

33. Kim Y, Koul D, Kim SH, et al. Identification of prognostic gene signatures of glioblastoma: a study based on TCGA data analysis. Neuro Oncol 2013; 15(7):829–39.

34. Zarkoob H, Taube JH, Singh SK, et al. Investigating the link between molecular subtypes of glioblastoma, epithelial-mesenchymal transition, and CD133 cell surface protein. PLoS One 2013;8(5):e64169.

35. Available at: http://www.castlebiosciences.com/. Accessed April 23, 2014.

36. Vogelstein B, Kinzler KW. Cancer genes and the pathways they control. Nat Med 2014;10(8):789–99.

37. Singh D, Chan JM, Zoppoli P, et al. Transforming fusions of FGFR and TACC genes in human glioblastoma. Science 2012;337(6099):1231–5.

38. Genetic engineering and biotechnology news. July 2013.

39. Available at: http://clinicaltrials.gov/. Accessed April 23, 2014.

40. Castro MG, Candolfi M, Kroeger K, et al. Gene therapy and targeted toxins for glioma. Curr Gene Ther 2011;11(3):155–80.

41. Available at: http://virtualtrials.com/. Accessed April 23, 2014.

42. Lohr J, Ratliff T, Huppertz A, et al. Effector T-cell infiltration positively impacts survival of glioblastoma patients and is impaired by tumor-derived TGF-β. Clin Cancer Res 2011;17:4296–308.

43. Han S, Zhang C, Li Q, et al. Tumour-infiltrating CD4+ and Cd8+ lymphocytes as predictors of clinical outcome in glioma. Br J Cancer 2014;110(10):2560–8.

44. Couzin-Frankel J. Cancer immunotherapy. Science 2013;342:1432–3.

45. Wainwright DA, Chang AL, Dey M, et al. Durable CTLA-4 and PD-L1 in mice with brain tumors. Clin Cancer Res 2014. [Epub ahead of print].

46. Mineharu Y, Muhammad AK, Yagiz K, et al. Gene therapy-mediated reprogramming tumor infiltrating T cells using IL-2 and inhibiting NF-KB signaling improves the efficacy immuno-therapy in a brain cancer model. Neurotherapeutics 2012;9:827–43.

Genomics of Brain Tumor Imaging

Whitney B. Pope, MD, PhD

KEYWORDS

- Imaging genomics • Radiogenomics • Glioblastoma • Microarray • Glioma • Bioinformatics

KEY POINTS

- Imaging genomics seeks to develop a method that leverages and integrates large datasets to identify predictive and prognostic biomarkers and new therapeutic targets in patients with glioblastoma.
- A substantial methodological framework including new data analysis methods has been developed to meet the challenge of working with big data.
- Malignant imaging phenotypes determined by MRI have genetic correlates; therefore, imaging may provide a means of panoramic and noninvasive surveillance of oncogenic pathway activation as patients are treated for GBM.

INTRODUCTION

Imaging genomics, radiogenomics, and radiomics are different names for essentially the same thing, a field of study focused on understanding the relationship between medical imaging data and molecular features of disease.[1–4] It is the integration of big data, quantitative imaging features taken from large numbers of images (typically MRI and computed tomography [CT]) and "-omic" data, which represent gene, protein or metabolite expression, as well as gene copy number, DNA methylation, and other important molecular markers. In oncology, this approach is being used to combine cancer phenotypes that can be globally assessed by imaging, with relevant molecular data, in order to develop prognostic and predictive biomarkers (Fig. 1). Improved diagnostic tests, better clinical decision making, new therapeutic targets, and improved understanding of tumor biology are all potential deliverables. Another promise of this approach is the ability to tailor therapy to enhance treatment effectiveness at the individual patient level. This article focuses on the application of imaging genomics to glioblastoma, one of the first pathologies for which this concept was applied.

BACKGROUND

Microarray Technology

Genomic information is a measure of gene expression based on mRNA isolated from tissue of interest. Microarrays, which contain thousands of complementary oligonucleotide or cDNA sequences (referred to as probes) are affixed in designated positions to a glass slide, so that mRNA-derived nucleic acids can be specifically detected via hybridization. The plates are washed, and the signal from these hybridized probes is detected and recorded. In this way the expression of thousands of genes can be quantified in a single experiment (Fig. 2).[5] Microarray technology and analysis have generated great interest among investigators of brain cancer for over a decade.[6]

Microarray Technology—Limitations

Oftentimes tissue for microarray analysis will be derived from surgical resections without precise tissue sample localization. This introduces sampling error in tumors such as glioblastoma (GBM) that are spatially heterogeneous in gene expression and imaging features. Additionally, tissue may not be composed of 100% tumor cells but may be of variable tumor cell concentration. This

The author has nothing to disclose.
Department of Radiological Sciences, David Geffen School of Medicine at UCLA, 757 Westwood Plaza, 1621E, Los Angeles, CA 90095, USA
E-mail address: wpope@mednet.ucla.edu

Neuroimag Clin N Am 25 (2015) 105–119
http://dx.doi.org/10.1016/j.nic.2014.09.006
1052-5149/15/$ – see front matter © 2015 Elsevier Inc. All rights reserved.

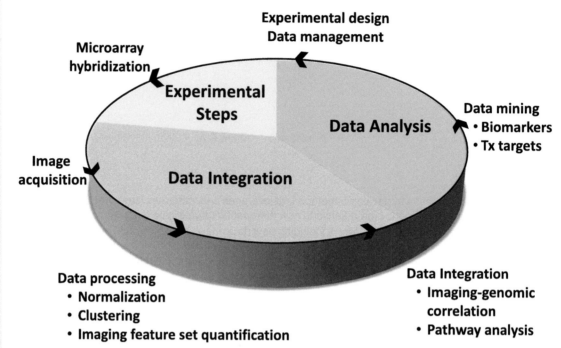

Fig. 1. Cycle of data acquisition, integration, analysis, and hypothesis generation/testing for imaging-genomics. Tx, treatment.

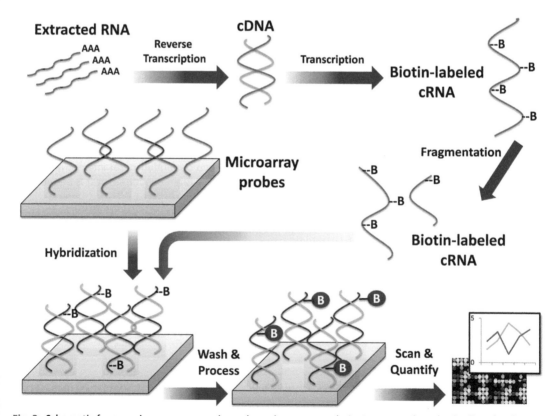

Fig. 2. Schematic for assessing gene expression using microarray analysis. Automated methods allow for the measurement of expression of thousands of genes in a single experiment. B, biotin.

will be reflected in the average tissue expression of tumor-associated genes and can lead to spurious conclusions about gene expression levels when unaccounted for.

Another limitation of microarray analysis is that multiple probes recognizing the same gene may be present. These probes can have varying sensitivity and specificity for the target gene, and some probes may more accurately reflect the dynamic range of gene expression than others. This variability can be a source of error or potentially lead to varying conclusions about gene expression from the same dataset. If multiple microarray platforms are used, then data will need to be normalized across platforms.[5,7] Another caveat is that gene expression levels do not always reflect protein concentrations, and proteins are typically the effector molecules of interest.[8,9]

Caveats in Interpreting Genomic Data

Once genomic data is acquired, association with imaging features must be performed. This presents some difficulties due to multiple-hypothesis testing leading to type 1 error (false positives). Clearly when there are thousands of genes that are being tested for a relationship to multiple imaging features, numerous correlations in expression (at the $P<.05$ level) occur by chance. Conversely, if one were to use a Bonferroni correction for multiple hypothesis testing, the requisite P values to demonstrate a statistically significant link would be so small that few associations would be found, even when those associations exist (that is, type 2 error or false negative).[10] To overcome these issues, various techniques have been employed. For instance, Tusher and colleagues[11] described a method called Significance Analysis of Microarrays (SAM) that "assigns a score to each gene on the basis of change in gene expression relative to the standard deviation of repeated measurements." A false discovery rate is determined by using permutations of the repeated measures in order to develop an estimate of the percentage of genes that will show such a change by chance. Using this method, the authors were able to reduce the false discovery rate from 60% to 84% to a more reasonable 12% in their analysis.

Another method to account for multiple hypothesis testing is gene set enrichment analysis (GSEA).[12] GSEA involves ranking genes from 2 sample groups by their differential expression, scoring enrichment by the Kolmogorov-Smirnov statistic using a predetermined set of genes common to a particular biological function, chromosomal location, or regulation. The significance of the scoring is assigned based on an empirical permutation method that corrects for multiple hypothesis testing.

In addition to identifying associations between single genes and imaging features, it also is possible to group genes by pathways based on prior knowledge. There are several proprietary as well as freely available computer programs that cluster genes based on potentially congruous function or patterns of activation. Commonly used methods include The Database for Annotation, Visualization and Integrated Discovery (DAVID), the Kyoto Encyclopedia of Genes and Genomes (KEGG), and the Ingenuity Pathway Analysis (IPA).[13] If genes that are known to be regulated as a functional unit are all correlated with a particular image feature, then the level of confidence that this represents a nonrandom association increases.

Gene expression levels of identified targets can be independently confirmed with reverse transcription polymerase chain reaction (RT-PCR),[5] but it is important to keep in mind that correlative microarray data analysis is, by necessity, somewhat of a fishing expedition (ie, a method that sweeps up a broad swath of potential associations for the purpose of directing further investigation). In this way, it can serve as a hypothesis-generating, rather than a hypothesis-testing, approach.[14]

Genes are typically organized via a hierarchical clustering analysis (to construct a dendrogram), arranged according to the degree of correlation between expression levels, and displayed as heat maps (**Fig. 3**).[15] This is among the many ways to organize gene expression information. Such hierarchical clustering analysis is the most common method used, albeit with several known limitations. For instance, varying ways of clustering yield (sometimes substantially) different results. Leaving out samples (for quality control or other reasons) can drastically affect the progression of the analysis, resulting in potentially different dendrograms. Any mistakes made early in the process are propagated throughout the analysis without the ability to be rectified.[7]

Imaging-Genomics—Advantages

Whereas microarray data usually represent a snapshot in time (ie, state of tumor at time of biopsy/resection), imaging surrogates of molecular features can potentially be followed for the lifetime of a patient. In addition, imaging has the advantage of providing a global assessment of the tumor, whereas microarray data represent gene expression from only a small fragment of tissue, and, as mentioned, are subject to sampling error.

A

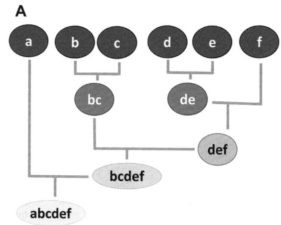

B

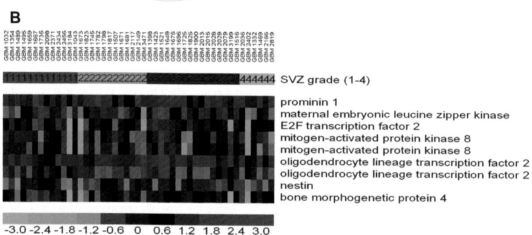

-3.0 -2.4 -1.8 -1.2 -0.6 0   0.6 1.2 1.8 2.4 3.0

Fig. 3. (*A*) Schematic of hierarchical clustering demonstrating iterative approach where the 2 genes with the most similar variation across tumor samples are grouped together and then treated as a single unit in subsequent iterations of the algorithm. (*B*) Heat map showing relative expression of a selection of genes (*right column*) across glioblastoma samples (*top row*) grouped according to SVZ grade. Color according to bar at bottom corresponding to relative gene expression levels. ([*B*] *From* Kappadakunnel M, Eskin A, Dong J, et al. Stem cell associated gene expression in glioblastoma multiforme: relationship to survival and the subventricular zone. J Neurooncol 2010;96(3):359–67.)

History of Cancer Genome Atlas and the Visually Accessible Rembrandt Images Feature Set

The National Institutes of Health (NIH)-sponsored Cancer Genome Atlas (TCGA) is an open-access repository of genomic and clinical data for more than 20 tumor types, including GBM.[16] The TCGA is linked to The Cancer Imaging Archive (TCIA),[17] which contains presurgical MRI scans of GBM cases that are associated with the patient's genomic and clinical data. In addition, a multi-institutional group of neuroradiologists has developed a standardized feature set (**Fig. 4**) consisting of 24 observations[18] (expanded from a published report of potentially prognostic imaging features in malignant glioma).[19] This visually accessible rembrandt images (VASARI) feature set has been used to score over 100 tumors, and the results have been made freely accessible as part of the TCGA/TCIA initiative. The advantage of this approach is that it allows for the investigation of large data sets that are rarely available at the single institution level, resulting in the generation of more statistically robust findings. Another advantage is that open access to the source data allows analyses to be independently validated by other interested researchers. One of the limitations of the TCGA data is that the specific tumor location and accompanying imaging features are not reported, as many tissue samples are from standard surgical resections rather than stereotactic biopsies.

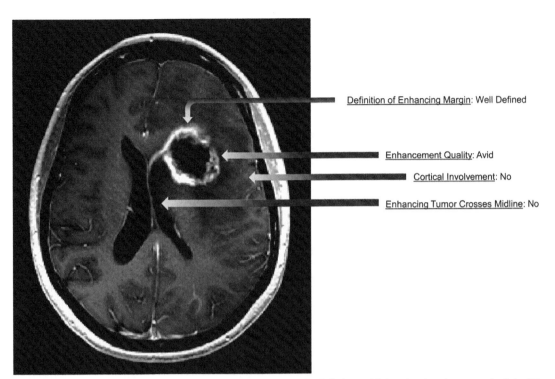

Definition of Enhancing Margin: Well Defined

Enhancement Quality: Avid

Cortical Involvement: No

Enhancing Tumor Crosses Midline: No

Fig. 4. T1 postcontrast axial image of a patient with GBM in the left frontal lobe. Scoring for several of the VA-SARI features is demonstrated.

Molecular Classification of Glioblastoma

In 2010, Verhaak and colleagues[20] published a seminal analysis of the TCGA database that divided GBM into 4 distinct molecular subtypes based on PDGFRA, IDH1, EGFR, and NF1 expression. EGFR was associated with classical GBM, NF-1 with mesenchymal, and PDGFRA/IDH1 with the proneural group. They also defined a neural group. The nomenclature used by Verhaak and colleagues was developed earlier by Phillips and colleagues[21] and was originally published in 2006. These authors divided malignant glioma into 3 subclasses based on similar gene expression profiles of tumors within a class and on inter-class survival differences. The groups were named proneural, proliferative, and mesenchymal. Proneural tumors had the best prognosis and were abundant in grade 3 tumors. Proneural tumors also were associated with increased gene expression of *OLIG-2* and *BCAN*. The authors additionally noted that tumors tended to shift to the mesenchymal class at recurrence. Thus molecular subclasses of GBM capture some of the molecular heterogeneity of GBM and appear to add value to histopathologic analysis for prognosis, and also identify potential driver pathways that are, or could be, therapeutic targets.

There are at least 2 additional molecular determinants in GBM that affect prognosis and potentially have imaging correlates. The first is the methylation, and therefore inactivation, of the O^6-methylguanine-DNA methyltransferase (MGMT) promoter.[22] MGMT is a key DNA repair enzyme that specifically removes promutagenic alkyl groups from the O^6 position of guanine in DNA, thereby diminishing toxicity of akylating agents used for chemotherapy. MGMT promoter methylated tumors carry a better prognosis than unmethylated tumors and are thought to be more sensitive to temozolomide therapy (TMZ, the chemotherapy agent used for standard treatment of malignant gliomas).[23,24]

Recently (2008), a cancer genome sequencing project discovered an association between mutations in the isocitrate dehydrogenase-1 (IDH-1) gene and GBM.[25] This mutation was subsequently shown to result in the production of the putative onco-metabolite 2-hydroxyglutarate (2-HG) and appears to be a driver of gliomagenesis, occurring before the p53 mutation.[26] The IDH-1 mutation is associated with DNA hypermethylation; it is linked to the CpG island methylator phenotype (G-CIMP), which includes methylation of the MGMT promoter. The IDH-1 mutation also acts to inhibit the differentiation of progenitor cells, is common in lower grade gliomas and secondary GBM, and is thought to be rare in primary GBM. The IDH-1 mutation, like MGMT promoter methylation with which it is associated, is linked to longer survival in glioma patients.[27]

Molecular Heterogeneity of Gliobastoma

Heterogeneity of GBM is an obstacle to successful treatment, and may indicate that effective therapy requires a combination approach to target multiple abnormal molecular pathways that drive malignant phenotypes.[28] Heterogeneity of GBM includes variations in imaging features and tissue histology and is found at the level of a single cell. Recently in a report published in *Science*, Patel and colleagues[29] performed a transcriptome analysis of single cells disassociated from GBM tumor samples. They demonstrated that gene expression was broadly spread between cells from the same tumor, indicating substantial intratumoral heterogeneity. They identified 4 genomic metasignatures that were enriched in genes for cell cycle, hypoxia, immune system, and oligodendrocyte function. Interestingly, molecularly defined subsets of GBM (proneural, proliferative, mesenchymal) were represented by single cells from the same tumor. The use of imaging to provide a multiple time point and panoramic view of this spatial and temporal heterogeneity in GBM is an important rationale underlying the potential of imaging–genomic analysis.

Imaging–Genomic Analyses for Glioma

One of the first papers to try to correlate imaging with "-omics" data, in this case proteomics, was authored by Hobbs and colleagues[30] in 2003. Using mass spectrometry as an alternate to 2-dimensional polyacrylamide gel electrophoresis (2D-PAGE), the authors examined the relationship between expression of approximately 100 proteins and peptides and contrast enhancement in 4 patients with GBM, generating protein profiles for comparison. Specifically, they compared protein levels in contrast-enhanced and nonenhanced regions of tumor derived from surgical resection specimens. They found that protein expression was different between enhancing and nonenhancing components of the same tumor. Protein expression varied in enhancing tumor even within areas of similar histology. Nonenhancing tumor appeared to be more similar between patients compared with enhancing tumor. Thus the authors demonstrated the molecular heterogeneity of GBM, and how that heterogeneity is most abundant in contrast-enhancing regions. Additionally, given similar histology, they demonstrated that

this heterogeneity is not captured by features visible in tissue sections by light microscopic evaluation. The authors hypothesized that underlying gene expression profiles correlate with imaging features of these tumors. It is exactly this hypothesis that has driven much of imaging–genomic analysis since. Although a remarkable paper, the authors were limited by the technology available at the time. For instance, only peptide/protein profiles generated by mass spectra were used for analysis; individual proteins were not identified. The study also was limited by the scope; only 4 patients, 1 imaging feature, and 100 peptides/proteins were considered. Microarrays and advanced proteomic techniques, which provide for the genome-wide compilation of expression data, were not available at that time. However, even using the limited means available, the authors were able to provide a proof-of-principle of the potential value in combining imaging and expression data to increase understanding of tumor biology.

The following year, a report was published that confirmed the hypothesis of Hobbs and colleagues, namely that there is a relationship between imaging features and gene expression levels. Raza and colleagues[31] examined the correlation between the amount of necrosis and gene expression in patients with GBM. Again limited by the technology available, the authors were able to examine the expression of 588 genes in 15 GBMs, finding that 9 genes positively correlated and 17 genes negatively correlated with necrosis grade. Importantly, these findings were corroborated with immunohistochemical analysis of tissue sections from these tumors, confirming the relationship between the microarray data and protein expression levels.

Necrosis is a hallmark of GBM and, previous to this work, had already been shown to be tightly associated with shortened patient survival.[32] Underscoring the prognostic impact of imaging features, Pope and colleagues demonstrated that histopathologically defined grade 3 tumors have survival times comparable to GBM if they show imaging evidence of necrosis.[19] Hypoxia, underlying the development of necrosis, is also thought to drive the malignant potential of GBM, resulting in increased invasion, and also, through the upregulation of VEGF, increased angiogenesis.[33] Imaging is the only method to obtain a global view of necrosis levels in these tumors. Thus the work of Raza and colleagues represents an important advance, because it is the first to specifically evaluate the relationship between gene expression and necrosis levels determined by MRI. Several subsequent studies have also investigated this association. And perhaps in the near future imaging with specific hypoxia markers (such as 18F-fluoromisonidazole, 18F-FMISO PET)[34] will provide additional understanding of the molecular mechanisms that drive hypoxia in malignant gliomas.

Several papers further characterized the regional variation of gene expression present in glioblastoma. For instance, Mariani and colleagues[35,36] used a 5700-gene cDNA array to examine gene expression in core versus peripheral invasive cells isolated from GBM tumor patients. A significant difference in gene expression between these 2 groups of cells was demonstrated. Van Meter and colleagues[37] used MRI-guided biopsies to compare intratumoral regional differences in gene expression, expanding the analysis to 22,283 probes by using more modern microarray technology. They established a consensus list of 643 genes that were expressed at a 2-fold difference in periphery versus core tissue samples from 6 GBMs. Importantly, results were validated with PCR and Western blotting analyses, and demonstrated, for instance, that VEGF expression was elevated in tumor core compared with the periphery. Barajas and colleagues[38] also analyzed differences in gene expression between the enhancing tumor core and peripheral nonenhancing GBM with similar results; the contrast-enhancing regions had more complex vascular hyperplasia as well as increased hypoxia and tumor cell density. Additionally, 846 genes were expressed differentially at the 2-fold level between the enhancing core and the tumor periphery. There is substantial overlap with the findings of Van Meter and colleagues[37] For instance, both groups showed up-regulation of VEGF and various collagen genes in the enhancing tumor core. However, there were also some differences in relative gene expression, which may be due to regional heterogeneity of GBM and the relatively small tumor sample size in the 2 studies. In general, the Van Meter paper emphasized increased expression of genes associated with cell migration, angiogenesis, cell survival, and integrin signaling in the enhancing core, whereas Barajas and colleagues[38] report increased expression of genes associated with mitosis, angiogenesis, and apoptosis. It is important to note that part of this discrepancy may be due to differences in gene classification schemes used in the 2 papers.

In 2007, Pope and colleagues published the first genome-wide analysis of the relationship between specific imaging traits and gene expression in malignant gliomas (grade 3 and 4 tumors), using microarrays to assess the expression of approximately 14,500 genes in 71 malignant tumors.[39] The analysis focused on the relationship between VEGF expression and edema, as VEGF is known to be a potent permeability factor and is the target of the antiangiogenic humanized monoclonal antibody bevacizumab.[40] VEGF gene expression levels were tightly correlated with tumor grade, being expressed approximately 4-fold higher in GBM than in grade 3 tumors. RT-PCR was used to confirm VEGF expression levels and showed good correspondence with the microarray data. As expected, VEGF expression was also correlated with several other known proangiogenic genes. Tumors with little or abundant edema had higher levels of VEGF than tumors with no edema. For tumors with no edema—but not tumors with little or abundant edema—VEGF stratified survival. This demonstrates how gene expression can provide prognostic information in subsets of tumors that are defined by imaging traits.

This study also addressed the question of whether VEGF is the sole driver of edema in malignant gliomas. To investigate this issue, gene expression was acquired from tumors that had both low VEGF expression levels and substantial edema. Using this method, neuronal pentraxin 2 (NPTX2) was identified as a gene whose expression levels correlated with edema, were prognostic for survival (independent of edema) and were independent of VEGF expression. Expression of NPTX2 was tightly correlated with the water channel aquaporin 3 (AQP3), in addition to several other genes including hepatocyte growth factor (HGH). Neuronal pentraxins are homologous to the acute phase-associated C-reactive protein.[41] Aquaporins are a family of membrane proteins that facilitate the movement of water molecules across cell membranes, and at least 1 member of the aquaporin family, aquaporin-4, has been shown to promote brain edema in ischemic stroke models.[42] Lastly HGF is a proangiogenic cytokine that acts on endothelial cells and has a variety of protumor effects in GBM.[43] The relationship between these proteins and the production of edema certainly requires further study, but this correlation of gene expression suggests the possibility of a proedema gene module that is VEGF-independent, and therefore could represent a complementary target to VEGF inhibition. Understanding the regulation of VEGF in GBM may be crucial, as VEGF is driven by hypoxia, and adaptation to hypoxia is a key phenotypic property of GBM.[44] The findings of this imaging–genomic analysis illustrate how this methodology can uncover potential gene modules that mediate tumor phenotypes and malignant cascades in GBM and other tumors. Additionally, these data may help to explain treatment failure (ie, why some tumors do not have reduction in edema following anti-*VEGF* therapy). Of note, these observations would not have been possible without the use of genomic–imaging analysis, because imaging is the only way to get a global perspective of edema for these tumors.

Pope and colleagues also assessed differences in gene expression in GBM based on the presence or absence of nonenhancing tumor (nCET).[45] This was based on previous work that had shown that nCET was associated with longer survival.[19] Fifty-two GBMs were split into 2 groups, those that contained regions of nCET, and those that did not. Microarray analysis showed that high expression levels of proangiogenic genes were associated with the lack of nCET, whereas the presence of nCET was associated with high expression levels of the stem cell and oligodendrocyte lineage marker *OLIG-2*[46] as well as genes previously shown to be associated with secondary GBM (GBM arising from lower-grade gliomas).[47] Later work demonstrated the association of nCET with the isocitrate dehydrogenase-1 (IDH-1) mutation.[48] The IDH-1 mutation is thought to be a marker of secondary, as opposed to de novo, GBM and drives the methylated, proneural GBM phenotype.[49] Synthesizing this information, it appears that 2 classes of GBM emerge. One includes tumors that are IDH-1 positive, MGMT promoter methylated, secondary GBMs that occur in younger patients, have nCET, are of the proneural molecular class, and carry a better prognosis. The other group is comprised of de novo GBMs that are highly necrotic, IDH-1 and nCET negative, have increased expression of proangiogenic factors, are not proneural, and have shorter survival (**Table 1**). Although clearly simplistic, this model shows how the integration of molecular, genomic, epigenetic, imaging, and clinical data can be used to generate a broad understanding of the heterogeneity of tumor biology in GBM and how this impacts prognosis. It also supports the argument that image–gene expression correlates do correspond with the understanding of tumor biology. There has been some concern that such associations might be random, given the high dimensionality of the gene expression data and lack of multiple hypothesis testing or other appropriate safeguards against type 1 error, but this does not seem to be the case.

A slightly different approach to imaging–genomic correlation was used by Diehn and colleagues.[50] Genes were initially grouped into clusters based on an unsupervised hierarchical analysis. Seven clusters of interest were identified based on gene functioning of the group members: EGFR overexpression (which should correspond to the classical subtype of GBM as defined by

Table 1
Potential associations of imaging, clinical, molecular and histopathologic features in glioblastoma

Type "A," Typical	Type "B," Atypical
Imaging	
nCET-negative	nCET-positive
More edema/necrosis	Less edema/necrosis
High ADC values	Low ADC values
Clinical	
1° GBM	2° GBM
Shorter survival	Longer survival
Older age	Younger age
Molecular	
Not proneural, IDH-1 WT	Proneural, IDH-1 mutant
Pathology	
No oligo component	Oligo component
Treatment	
High *VEGF* expression	Low *VEGF* expression
Anti-*VEGF* therapy effective	Anti-*VEGF* treatment less effective?

Abbreviations: ADC, apparent diffusion coefficient; IDH-1, isocitrate-dehydrogenase-1; nCET, non-contrast enhancing tumor (part or all); VEGF, vascular endothelial growth factor; WT, wild type.

Verhaak), hypoxia, extracellular matrix (ECM), immune system, proliferation, glial, and neuronal. The authors then demonstrated a statistically significant association (based on a random permutation analysis to control for multiple hypothesis testing) of these clusters with several binary imaging traits assessed in 22 GBMs. They found, for example, that tumors with a high contrast-to-necrosis ratio were associated with the EGFR overexpression gene cluster. The authors also identified an infiltrative imaging phenotype that was correlated with gene expression and shorter survival. The infiltrative phenotype appears to include tumors with nCET. Surprisingly, many genes associated with the proneural class of GBM, nCET, and independently prognostic of longer survival (OLIG-2, BCAN, ASCL-1)[21] were among the genes associated with higher expression in the infiltrative (worse prognosis) imaging phenotype. Additional prospective validation of the infiltrative phenotype and its relationship to nonenhancing tumor may be required to resolve this potential paradox.

The question of whether there is a relationship between subventricular zone (SVZ) involvement and gene expression was specifically analyzed in a paper by Kappadakunnel and colleagues[51] reporting an imaging–genomic study of 46 GBMs. Stem cell genes were not up-regulated in tumors that contacted the SVZ. However, overexpression of stem cells genes was associated with shorter survival. Instead of stem cell-related genes, tumors that contacted the SVZ showed up-regulation of immune system-related genes, in particular those of the human leukocyte antigen (HLA) group. The interest of this paper is that is seeks to address the question of how GBMs are generated. Is there a particular place in the brain where they form? Does that depend on stem cells or another cell type? Do stem cells migrate away from the SVZ and then form tumors? Do different locations tend to generate different kinds of tumors? The answer to this last question may be "yes" given more recent work by the authors' group using a radiographic atlas of the location of 507 de novo GBMs, which showed a predilection of particular GBM phenotypes for specific locations (eg, MGMT methylated tumors with the IDH-1 mutation tended to occur in the left frontal lobe, whereas amplified and variant EGFR-expressing tumors occurred most frequently in the left temporal lobe).[52]

The TCGA database, in addition to containing imaging and gene expression data, also contains expression values for microRNA (miRNA) for a subset of tumors. These small RNAs act to negatively regulate gene expression by binding specific sites in the 3′UTR of the target gene.[53] In the first imaging–genomic paper using the TCGA data set, Zinn and colleagues[54] analyzed 78 GBMs that had both gene and miRNA expression data available, providing information on 13,628 genes and 555 miRNAs. Using a discovery and validation set, the authors compared tumors with high versus low volumes of peritumoral fluid attenuation inversion recovery (FLAIR) signal abnormality (related to either edema, invasion, or both, Fig. 5). They found 53 genes and 5 miRNAs that were differentially expressed at the 1.5-fold level between the 2 groups of tumors. The most up-regulated gene was periostin (POSTN). Interestingly, the most downregulated miRNA was miR-219, which is predicted to bind (and thus negatively regulate) POSTN. Additionally, POSTN was associated with mesenchymal GBMs (which have a poorer prognosis), and POSTN levels, themselves, were associated with shorter survival. These findings are of great interest, because they suggest a regulatory link between gene and miRNA expression that impacts imaging features and survival. Identifying these regulatory pathways may help to develop targeted therapies. Further, targeting miRNA, while not well

developed at this time, is an intriguing possibility, as miRNA is a key regulator of oncogenic processes including invasion,[55] stemness,[56] apoptosis,[57] and proliferation.[58]

The authors also demonstrated the association of several collagen and collagen-binding genes (by ingenuity pathway analysis) with POSTN and the high-volume FLAIR imaging phenotype. It is known that tumor cells potentiate invasion by secreting factors such as metalloproteinases that degrade the existing ECM. This is followed by deposition of new tumor-derived ECM components requiring up-regulation of the associated genes.[59] Interestingly several collagen and collagen-binding genes such as COL6A3 and decorin (DCN) that were overexpressed in high FLAIR volume tumors have also been found to be up-regulated in association with high apparent diffusion coefficient (ADC) tumors.[60] In the latter study, tumoral ADC values were derived from the enhancing portion of tumors (rather than the region of peritumoral FLAIR signal abnormality), suggesting that this association with ECM genes can be captured within the enhancing core of the tumor itself. DCN may be of particular interest, since 4 papers[37,50,54,60] have independently associated overexpression of this gene with particular imaging phenotypes that correlate with poor survival. However, there are some data suggesting that DCN inhibits angiogenesis and invasion and thus may be an adaptive response to these tumor-driven processes.[61] Regardless, DCN may still retain value as a sensitive marker of a proinvasive phenotype.

Zinn and colleagues[62] also used the same TCGA data set to generate a prognostic model of GBM patient survival based on the volume of enhancing tumor (including the necrotic core), patient age, and Karnofsky performance status (KPS). Large-volume tumor, age of at least 60 years, and KPS less than 100 were all associated with poorer survival. Patients with 1 or none of these features (VAK-A) were compared against the remainders (VAK-B). As expected, the VAK-A cohort was found to have longer survival. The authors also identified a gene and miRNA expression profile that was differentially expressed between the 2 groups, and found that transcription factor analysis predicted an association between VAK-A and p53 activation, whereas VAK-B was predicted to be associated with p53 inhibition. Lastly further stratification of survival based on the Kaplan-Meier method was achieved by assessing MGMT promoter methylation status. Thus MGMT methylated VAK-A patients had 32-month median survival compared with only 12 months for VAK-B unmethylated patients. This work is another example of how imaging, molecular, and clinical data can

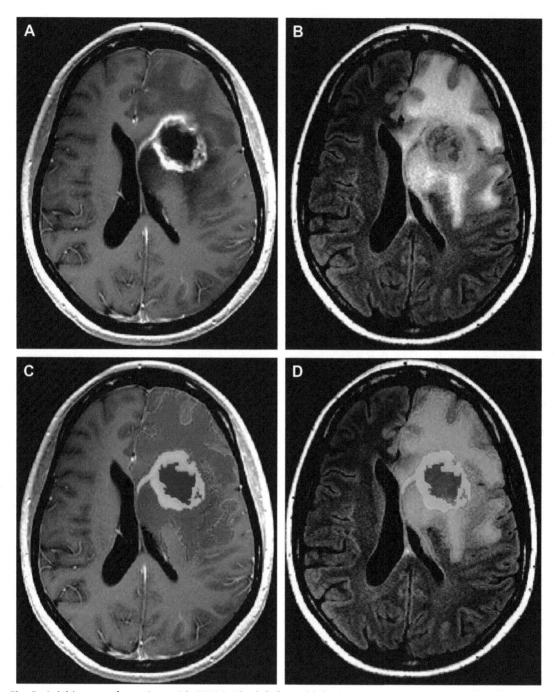

Fig. 5. Axial images of a patient with GBM in the left frontal lobe (same patient as in see Fig. 4). (*A*) T1 post-contrast, (*B*) FLAIR, (*C*) T1 postcontrast overlaid with segmented volumes, (*D*) FLAIR overlaid with segmented volumes. Red, necrotic tumor core; Green, enhancing tumor rim; Blue, peritumoral areas of T2/FLAIR signal abnormality comprising edema and/or nonenhancing tumor.

be integrated to generated highly prognostic models of patient survival. However, it is important to note that this determination is of somewhat limited clinical utility, since at this point prognosis has little impact on clinical decision making due to lack of treatment options for GBM patients.

In a pair of papers,[63,64] Jain and colleagues assessed the relationship between gene expression profiles and physiologic imaging, specifically tumor perfusion. Prior to these reports, most genomic–imaging analyses sought to identify links between anatomic imaging data and gene expression. However, recent advances have allowed the incorporation of physiologic imaging data acquisition including diffusion and perfusion protocols into routine clinical scanning. These physiologic imaging data are now available for a subset of patients in a TCGA database. Perfusion imaging is of particular interest, because perfusion is linked to angiogenesis and also can be altered by antiangiogenic treatments being investigated for antiglioma therapy.[65] In the first paper, 18 GBMs had CT to generate perfusion measurements of enhancing tumor. Out of 92 angiogenesis-related genes, 7 correlated with the permeability surface area product (PS, a measure related to vascular leakiness), and 5 genes correlated with tumoral cerebral blood volume (CBV) in a consistent manner. Correlated genes included hypoxia-inducible factor 1A (HIF1A), which is known to be induced by hypoxia and is a major driver of angiogenesis. One limitation of this paper is the use of CT, as most GBM patients are evaluated with MRI in the clinical setting. However, the work does confirm an expected relationship between molecular markers of angiogenesis and an increase in tumor perfusion parameters. In a subsequent work, Jain and colleagues[63] looked at MRI-derived perfusion metrics in a group of 57 patients with GBM and the relationship to the Verhaak and Phillips molecular classification of GBM. Somewhat disappointingly, the authors did not report association of perfusion data with particular gene expression levels, which might have provided some confirmation of the CT perfusion–genomic analysis of the earlier paper. The authors reported a lack of significant difference in CBV among the molecular classes of GBM, which is surprising, given the relative overexpression of proangiogenic molecules in some of the subclasses compared with others.

Although CBV appears to be unrelated to molecular classes of GBM, proneural tumors have been found to have significantly lower levels of contrast enhancement, while mesenchymal tumors lacked nCET.[66] These data support Pope and colleagues' previous findings that the presence of nCET is associated with genes that are overexpressed in the proneural class of GBM.[45] In another study, Pope and colleagues also found imaging features associated with mesenchymal GBMs.[67] Thus there is mounting evidence that, while some perfusion metrics such as CBV may be similar between molecular classes of GBM, there are interclass differences in imaging features that can be derived from standard MRI sequences.[48]

The issue of genes associated with an invasive imaging phenotype has recently been revisited in a study of 104 GBMs from the TCGA database.[68]

For this article, the invasive phenotype was defined as deep white matter tract involvement (enhancement of T2/FLAIR signal abnormality in the internal capsule, corpus callosum or brainstem) and tumor contiguous with the ependyma. Thus the definition is distinct from that used by Diehn and colleagues[50] in 2008. Nevertheless, similar to Diehn and colleagues, the authors report that the invasive phenotype was associated with shorter survival. They also used ingenuity pathway analysis to characterize gene clusters or canonical pathways associated with the 100 most over- and underexpressed genes between the 2 groups. They found associations with mitochondrial dysfunction and VEGF signaling, among other pathways. Lastly, the authors also report that transcription factor analysis of gene expression indicates that the transcription regulator and well-characterized oncogene Myc were likely activated in the invasive group. Thus the authors were able to leverage the information of gene cluster analysis to develop hypotheses related to oncogenic and metabolic pathways, which may be associated with a more aggressive and invasive GBM phenotype.

Following up prior work from 2008,[50] Jamshidi and colleagues[69] analyzed the relationship of 6 imaging features to genomic profiles in 23 patients with GBM. As in their prior work, imaging features included necrosis ratio, high versus low contrast, SVZ involvement, mass effect, an edematous versus infiltrative pattern, and a low versus high contrast-to-necrosis ratio. In addition to association with gene clusters, the authors also analyzed the relationship to copy-number variations (CNVs), the major difference with the prior study. A total of 376 genes had concordant correlative changes in mRNA and CNV. Genes increased with SVZ involvement were UBQLN1, APBA1, HJURP, LMO3, RAP2A, BFSP1, TYMS, and FAM83D. SVZ involvement also was associated with diminished expression of glioma stem cell-associated genes. Two prior papers[51,68] also assessed gene expression associated with SVZ involvement. Unfortunately there is no overlap between the SVZ-associated gene sets among these studies. Although Jamshidi and colleagues[69] do not speculate as to the cause of this discrepant finding, potentially it is related to the limitation of the small sample size used in their paper (n = 23), especially given the heterogeneity of GBM. Thus, as for many of these preliminary findings, further prospective investigation using new data sets will be required to resolve these apparent discrepancies.

Gevaert and colleagues[70] applied a sophisticated informatics methodology in constructing radiogenomic maps that are prognostic of patient survival. They generated 79 computational imaging features (eg, sharpness of lesion boundaries and boundary shapes) in 55 patients with GBM from the TCGA database. They then integrated gene expression, DNA methylation, and copy dumber data, creating 100 coexpressed gene expression modules, and selected the 35 modules that were prognostic of survival. The modules were than associated with imaging features to create a prognostic imaging–genomic dataset for regions of interest (ROIs) within necrotic, enhancing and edematous tumoral regions. Two potential advances of this approach over prior work are the initial screen for potential driver mutations and the use of a sophisticated, quantified, computational imaging feature set. The underlying logic for the identification of potential driver mutations is that it is unlikely that a significant proportion of samples will have changes in gene expression that are associated with multiple genomic events by chance. Instead, these nonrandom changes may indicate genes that drive gliomagenesis and progression. Similar to previous studies, the authors reported a significant correlation between various imaging features and molecular subtypes of GBM. The authors were also able to link 30 out of 54 imaging feature with biological processes. An example was an association between edema intensity and the Kyoto Encyclopedia of Genes and Genomes (KEGG) database cell cycle pathway.

FUTURE DIRECTIONS

Channeling big data such as imaging–genomics into clinically actionable information in an individual patient-tailored way remains a substantial challenge. To quote Rafii and colleagues[71] "the gap between our basic knowledge and clinical application is still wide. Closing the gap will require translational personalized trials, which may initiate a radical change in our routine clinical practice in oncology." Integration of gene expression and proteomic data may further this endeavor. For instance, Daemen and colleagues[72] have shown how this combination approach improves modeling of response to cetuximab in patients with rectal cancer. Further emphasis needs to be placed on these kinds of predictive, rather than prognostic, biomarkers. This is because, at least for GBM, prognostic models rarely convey actionable information for a particular patient.

There are several avenues to improve imaging–genomic analyses. In particular, sources of variation need to be considered. One obvious example remains the lack of standardized imaging terms.

For instance, there are significant differences in similarly named imaging phenotypes (for example what constitutes an invasive phenotype).[50,68] Variability in segmentation and ROI selection is another issue, which may be addressed by ever-improving automated methods of extracting imaging feature sets.[73] The use of stereotactic biopsies, rather than random sampling of the tumor, will help generate microarray analysis that is able to link gene expression data with specific imaging traits within a single tumor.[38] Physiologic imaging with perfusion, diffusion MRI, and PET scans provides a wealth of information that is only just beginning to be incorporated into these analyses.[74] Another significant variable is the wide array of software and protocols used to determine gene clusters and pathways. Because these genetic pathways are highly redundant, genes may get assigned to 1 pathway by 1 program and another pathway by another.[75] Also there is the question of how meaningful is the identification of overexpressed genes and pathways. Few genes and fewer cellular pathways cannot be plausibly linked in some way to cancer, given the vast impact oncogenesis has on virtually all aspects of cell functioning and metabolism. The specificity of these associations remains to be elucidated in many cases. Lastly, another current limitation in genomic–imaging analyses is that, even with multi-institutional participation in TCGA and other publically available datasets, small sample size remains problematic, especially when dealing with validation of potential associations in independent cohorts. Thus larger datasets need to be assembled.

To conclude, imaging–genomic analysis is a field in its infancy; its full potential is yet to be determined. Medical treatments will likely be optimized by improved integration of multiple, high-dimensional information streams, which currently tend to be unwieldy and not rigorously validated. Thus further development of not only imaging–genomic correlations, but also the underlying bioinformatics infrastructure this methodology requires, is important as we strive towards the goal of optimally personalized medicine.

ACKNOWLEDGMENT

The author would like to acknowledge Ms Diana Fang for help in figure preparation.

REFERENCES

1. Aerts HJ, Velazquez ER, Leijenaar RT, et al. Decoding tumour phenotype by noninvasive imaging using a quantitative radiomics approach. Nat Commun 2014;5:4006.

2. Kim N, Choi J, Yi J, et al. An engineering view on megatrends in radiology: digitization to quantitative tools of medicine. Korean J Radiol 2013;14(2):139–53.

3. Zinn PO, Colen RR. Imaging genomic mapping in glioblastoma. Neurosurgery 2013;60(Suppl 1): 126–30.

4. Kuo MD, Jamshidi N. Behind the numbers: decoding molecular phenotypes with radiogenomics—guiding principles and technical considerations. Radiology 2014;270(2):320–5.

5. De Cecco L, Dugo M, Canevari S, et al. Measuring microRNA expression levels in oncology: from samples to data analysis. Crit Rev Oncog 2013;18(4): 273–87.

6. Mischel PS, Cloughesy TF, Nelson SF. DNA-microarray analysis of brain cancer: molecular classification for therapy. Nat Rev Neurosci 2004;5(10):782–92.

7. Butte A. The use and analysis of microarray data. Nat Rev Drug Discov 2002;1(12):951–60.

8. Vogel C, Marcotte EM. Insights into the regulation of protein abundance from proteomic and transcriptomic analyses. Nat Rev Genet 2012;13(4):227–32.

9. Chen G, Gharib TG, Huang CC, et al. Discordant protein and mRNA expression in lung adenocarcinomas. Mol Cell Proteomics 2002;1(4):304–13.

10. Bair E. Identification of significant features in DNA microarray data. Wiley Interdiscip Rev Comput Stat 2013;5(4). http://dx.doi.org/10.1002/wics.1260.

11. Tusher VG, Tibshirani R, Chu G. Significance analysis of microarrays applied to the ionizing radiation response. Proc Natl Acad Sci U S A 2001;98(9): 5116–21.

12. Mootha VK, Lindgren CM, Eriksson KF, et al. PGC-1alpha-responsive genes involved in oxidative phosphorylation are coordinately downregulated in human diabetes. Nat Genet 2003;34(3):267–73.

13. Werner T. Bioinformatics applications for pathway analysis of microarray data. Curr Opin Biotechnol 2008;19(1):50–4.

14. Zhang W, Wang H, Song SW, et al. Insulin-like growth factor binding protein 2: gene expression microarrays and the hypothesis-generation paradigm. Brain Pathol 2002;12(1):87–94.

15. Eisen MB, Spellman PT, Brown PO, et al. Cluster analysis and display of genome-wide expression patterns. Proc Natl Acad Sci U S A 1998;95(25): 14863–8.

16. Cancer Genome Atlas Research Network. Comprehensive genomic characterization defines human glioblastoma genes and core pathways. Nature 2008;455(7216):1061–8.

17. Clark K, Vendt B, Smith K, et al. The Cancer Imaging Archive (TCIA): maintaining and operating a public information repository. J Digit Imaging 2013;26(6): 1045–57.

18. Mazurowski MA, Desjardins A, Malof JM. Imaging descriptors improve the predictive power of survival models for glioblastoma patients. Neuro Oncol 2013;15(10):1389–94.

19. Pope WB, Sayre J, Perlina A, et al. MR imaging correlates of survival in patients with high-grade gliomas. AJNR Am J Neuroradiol 2005;26(10): 2466–74.

20. Verhaak RG, Hoadley KA, Purdom E, et al. Integrated genomic analysis identifies clinically relevant subtypes of glioblastoma characterized by abnormalities in PDGFRA, IDH1, EGFR, and NF1. Cancer Cell 2010;17(1):98–110.

21. Phillips HS, Kharbanda S, Chen R, et al. Molecular subclasses of high-grade glioma predict prognosis, delineate a pattern of disease progression, and resemble stages in neurogenesis. Cancer Cell 2006;9(3):157–73.

22. Olar A, Aldape KD. Using the molecular classification of glioblastoma to inform personalized treatment. J Pathol 2014;232(2):165–77.

23. Stupp R, Mason WP, van den Bent MJ, et al. Radiotherapy plus concomitant and adjuvant temozolomide for glioblastoma. N Engl J Med 2005;352(10): 987–96.

24. Hegi ME, Diserens AC, Gorlia T, et al. MGMT gene silencing and benefit from temozolomide in glioblastoma. N Engl J Med 2005;352(10):997–1003.

25. Parsons DW, Jones S, Zhang X, et al. An integrated genomic analysis of human glioblastoma multiforme. Science 2008;321(5897):1807–12.

26. McCarthy N. Therapeutics: targeting an oncometabolite. Nat Rev Cancer 2013;13(6):383.

27. Cohen AL, Holmen SL, Colman H. IDH1 and IDH2 mutations in gliomas. Curr Neurol Neurosci Rep 2013;13(5):345.

28. Nicholas MK, Lukas RV, Chmura S, et al. Molecular heterogeneity in glioblastoma: therapeutic opportunities and challenges. Semin Oncol 2011;38(2): 243–53.

29. Patel AP, Tirosh I, Trombetta JJ, et al. Single-cell RNA-seq highlights intratumoral heterogeneity in primary glioblastoma. Science 2014;344(6190):1396–401.

30. Hobbs SK, Shi G, Homer R, et al. Magnetic resonance image-guided proteomics of human glioblastoma multiforme. J Magn Reson Imaging 2003; 18(5):530–6.

31. Raza SM, Fuller GN, Rhee CH, et al. Identification of necrosis-associated genes in glioblastoma by cDNA microarray analysis. Clin Cancer Res 2004;10(1 Pt 1):212–21.

32. Hammoud MA, Sawaya R, Shi W, et al. Prognostic significance of preoperative MRI scans in glioblastoma multiforme. J Neurooncol 1996;27(1):65–73.

33. Hardee ME, Zagzag D. Mechanisms of glioma-associated neovascularization. Am J Pathol 2012; 181(4):1126–41.

34. Lopci E, Grassi I, Chiti A, et al. PET radiopharmaceuticals for imaging of tumor hypoxia: a review of the

evidence. Am J Nucl Med Mol Imaging 2014;4(4): 365–84.

35. Mariani L, Beaudry C, McDonough WS, et al. Death-associated protein 3 (Dap-3) is overexpressed in invasive glioblastoma cells in vivo and in glioma cell lines with induced motility phenotype in vitro. Clin Cancer Res 2001;7(8):2480–9.

36. Hoelzinger DB, Mariani L, Weis J, et al. Gene expression profile of glioblastoma multiforme invasive phenotype points to new therapeutic targets. Neoplasia 2005;7(1):7–16.

37. Van Meter T, Dumur C, Hafez N, et al. Microarray analysis of MRI-defined tissue samples in glioblastoma reveals differences in regional expression of therapeutic targets. Diagn Mol Pathol 2006;15(4):195–205.

38. Barajas RF Jr, Hodgson JG, Chang JS, et al. Glioblastoma multiforme regional genetic and cellular expression patterns: influence on anatomic and physiologic MR imaging. Radiology 2010;254(2):564–76.

39. Carlson MR, Pope WB, Horvath S, et al. Relationship between survival and edema in malignant gliomas: role of vascular endothelial growth factor and neuronal pentraxin 2. Clin Cancer Res 2007;13(9): 2592–8.

40. Goel HL, Mercurio AM. VEGF targets the tumour cell. Nat Rev Cancer 2013;13(12):871–82.

41. Martinez de la Torre Y, Fabbri M, Jaillon S, et al. Evolution of the pentraxin family: the new entry PTX4. J Immunol 2010;184(9):5055–64.

42. Manley GT, Fujimura M, Ma T, et al. Aquaporin-4 deletion in mice reduces brain edema after acute water intoxication and ischemic stroke. Nat Med 2000;6(2):159–63.

43. Moriyama T, Kataoka H, Koono M, et al. Expression of hepatocyte growth factor/scatter factor and its receptor c-Met in brain tumors: evidence for a role in progression of astrocytic tumors (Review). Int J Mol Med 1999;3(5):531–6.

44. Chen J, Li Y, Yu TS, et al. A restricted cell population propagates glioblastoma growth after chemotherapy. Nature 2012;488(7412):522–6.

45. Pope WB, Chen JH, Dong J, et al. Relationship between gene expression and enhancement in glioblastoma multiforme: exploratory DNA microarray analysis. Radiology 2008;249(1):268–77.

46. Ligon KL, Huillard E, Mehta S, et al. Olig2-regulated lineage-restricted pathway controls replication competence in neural stem cells and malignant glioma. Neuron 2007;53(4):503–17.

47. Tso CL, Freije WA, Day A, et al. Distinct transcription profiles of primary and secondary glioblastoma subgroups. Cancer Res 2006;66(1):159–67.

48. Carrillo JA, Lai A, Nghiemphu PL, et al. Relationship between tumor enhancement, edema, IDH1 mutational status, MGMT promoter methylation, and survival in glioblastoma. AJNR Am J Neuroradiol 2012;33(7):1349–55.

49. Turcan S, Rohle D, Goenka A, et al. IDH1 mutation is sufficient to establish the glioma hypermethylator phenotype. Nature 2012;483(7390):479–83.

50. Diehn M, Nardini C, Wang DS, et al. Identification of noninvasive imaging surrogates for brain tumor gene-expression modules. Proc Natl Acad Sci U S A 2008;105(13):5213–8.

51. Kappadakunnel M, Eskin A, Dong J, et al. Stem cell associated gene expression in glioblastoma multiforme: relationship to survival and the subventricular zone. J Neurooncol 2010;96(3):359–67.

52. Ellingson BM, Lai A, Harris RJ, et al. Probabilistic radiographic atlas of glioblastoma phenotypes. AJNR Am J Neuroradiol 2013;34(3):533–40.

53. Palumbo S, Miracco C, Pirtoli L, et al. Emerging roles of microRNA in modulating cell-death processes in malignant glioma. J Cell Physiol 2014;229(3):277–86.

54. Zinn PO, Mahajan B, Sathyan P, et al. Radiogenomic mapping of edema/cellular invasion MRI-phenotypes in glioblastoma multiforme. PLoS One 2011;6(10): e25451.

55. Zhang R, Luo H, Wang S, et al. MicroRNA-377 inhibited proliferation and invasion of human glioblastoma cells by directly targeting specificity protein 1. Neuro Oncol 2014. [Epub ahead of print].

56. Lang MF, Yang S, Zhao C, et al. Genome-wide profiling identified a set of miRNAs that are differentially expressed in glioblastoma stem cells and normal neural stem cells. PLoS One 2012;7(4):e36248.

57. Othman N, Nagoor NH. The role of microRNAs in the regulation of apoptosis in lung cancer and its application in cancer treatment. Biomed Res Int 2014; 2014:318030.

58. Xie Q, Yan Y, Huang Z, et al. MicroRNA-221 targeting PI3-K/Akt signaling axis induces cell proliferation and BCNU resistance in human glioblastoma. Neuropathology 2014;34(5):455–64.

59. Vehlow A, Cordes N. Invasion as target for therapy of glioblastoma multiforme. Biochim Biophys Acta 2013;1836(2):236–44.

60. Pope WB, Mirsadraei L, Lai A, et al. Differential gene expression in glioblastoma defined by ADC histogram analysis: relationship to extracellular matrix molecules and survival. AJNR Am J Neuroradiol 2012;33(6):1059–64.

61. Grahovac J, Wells A. Matrikine and matricellular regulators of EGF receptor signaling on cancer cell migration and invasion. Lab Invest 2014;94(1): 31–40.

62. Zinn PO, Sathyan P, Mahajan B, et al. A novel volume-age-KPS (VAK) glioblastoma classification identifies a prognostic cognate microRNA-gene signature. PLoS One 2012;7(8):e41522.

63. Jain R, Poisson L, Narang J, et al. Genomic mapping and survival prediction in glioblastoma: molecular subclassification strengthened by hemodynamic imaging biomarkers. Radiology 2013;267(1):212–20.

64. Jain R, Poisson L, Narang J, et al. Correlation of perfusion parameters with genes related to angiogenesis regulation in glioblastoma: a feasibility study. AJNR Am J Neuroradiol 2012;33(7):1343–8.

65. Batchelor TT, Sorensen AG, di Tomaso E, et al. AZD2171, a pan-VEGF receptor tyrosine kinase inhibitor, normalizes tumor vasculature and alleviates edema in glioblastoma patients. Cancer Cell 2007; 11(1):83–95.

66. Gutman DA, Cooper LA, Hwang SN, et al. MR imaging predictors of molecular profile and survival: multi-institutional study of the TCGA glioblastoma data set. Radiology 2013;267(2):560–9.

67. Naeini KM, Pope WB, Cloughesy TF, et al. Identifying the mesenchymal molecular subtype of glioblastoma using quantitative volumetric analysis of anatomic magnetic resonance images. Neuro Oncol 2013;15(5):626–34.

68. Colen RR, Vangel M, Wang J, et al. Imaging genomic mapping of an invasive MRI phenotype predicts patient outcome and metabolic dysfunction: a TCGA glioma phenotype research group project. BMC Med Genomics 2014;7(1):30.

69. Jamshidi N, Diehn M, Bredel M, et al. Illuminating radiogenomic characteristics of glioblastoma multiforme through integration of MR imaging, messenger RNA expression, and DNA copy number variation. Radiology 2014;270(1):1–2.

70. Gevaert O, Mitchell LA, Achrol AS, et al. Glioblastoma multiforme: exploratory radiogenomic analysis by using quantitative image features. Radiology 2014;273:168–74.

71. Rafii A, Touboul C, Al Thani H, et al. Where cancer genomics should go next: a clinician's perspective. Hum Mol Genet 2014;23:R69–75.

72. Daemen A, Gevaert O, De Bie T, et al. Integrating microarray and proteomics data to predict the response on cetuximab in patients with rectal cancer. Pac Symp Biocomput 2008;166–77.

73. Porz N, Bauer S, Pica A, et al. Multi-modal glioblastoma segmentation: man versus machine. PLoS One 2014;9(5):e96873.

74. Pope WB, Young JR, Ellingson BM. Advances in MRI assessment of gliomas and response to anti-VEGF therapy. Curr Neurol Neurosci Rep 2011; 11(3):336–44.

75. Soh D, Dong D, Guo Y, et al. Consistency, comprehensiveness, and compatibility of pathway databases. BMC Bioinformatics 2010;11:449.

Neuroimaging and Genetic Influence in Treating Brain Neoplasms

L. Celso Hygino da Cruz Jr, MD[a],[*], Margareth Kimura, MD[b]

KEYWORDS

- High-grade gliomas • Glioblastoma • Gene expression • Radiogenomic • Treatment response
- Prognosis • Outcome • Pseudoprogression

KEY POINTS

- The inability of the traditional histopathologic brain neoplasm classification to define prognosis and treatment response determined the development of the genomic classification of brain neoplasms and radiogenomics.
- The major clinical importance of this molecular classification is that the same histopathologic type of brain tumor, glioblastoma multiforme, has different treatment response based on the molecular subtype classification.
- The same histopathologic tumor may differ in the molecular component and demonstrate different clinical behavior and outcome.
- Gene characteristics might be a better predictor of key outcomes than histopathologic classification.
- MR imaging findings may be correlated with molecular mutations of brain neoplasms and glioblastoma molecular subtypes.
- Radiogenomics is the combination of imaging and gene expression characteristics of brain neoplasms that has the potential to give insight into tumor biology.
- The major clinical importance of molecular classification of brain tumor, especially glioblastoma, is the capacity to evaluate treatment response, patient outcome, and prognosis.

INTRODUCTION

Glioblastoma multiforme (GBM) is the most common and aggressive primary brain tumor in adults. They account for 50% to 60% of all astrocytic gliomas, with an incidence of around 5 cases per 100,000 patients per year. Despite significant advances in treatment with aggressive multimodal therapy, GBM remains a deadly disease with a dismal prognosis, with a 2-year overall survival less than 10% and a median overall survival duration of 16 to 17 months.[1,2] The current standard of care is based on targeted surgical resection followed by concomitant radiation therapy and temozolomide (TMZ) treatment.[1,2] In recurrent cases, this treatment regimen is commonly followed by antiangiogenic therapy.[3] Nevertheless, after this new therapy approach, only a slight increase in overall survival has been observed, improved from 10 months to 16 to 17 months.

The identification of molecular genetic biomarkers has considerably increased the current understanding of glioma genesis, prognosis,

The authors have nothing to disclose.
[a] MRI Department of Clínica de Diagnostico por Imagem (CDPI) and IRM Ressonância Magnética, Av. das Américas, 4666 Sl 325, Centro Médico Barrashopping, Rio de Janeiro, RJ, Brazil; [b] MRI Department of Clínica de Diagnostico por Imagem (CDPI), Av. das Américas, 4666 Sl 325, Centro Médico Barrashopping, Rio de Janeiro, RJ, Brazil
* Corresponding author.
E-mail address: celsohygino@hotmail.com

evaluation, and treatment planning. Recent publications have pointed out that gene characteristics might be better predictors of key outcomes than histopathologic classification. Genetic and cellular features of high-grade glioma aggressiveness influence MR imaging. The heterogeneous aspect depicted by MR imaging can be secondary to underlying differences in intratumoral tissues and genetic expression patterns.[4] Improvement in treatment strategies has largely been based on the substantial progress in the identification of genetic alterations or profile in GBMs, which may enable the development of more individualized and specifically targeted therapy.

RADIOGENOMICS

An intriguing characteristic of glial brain tumors is their phenotypic variety. No isolated genetic event accounts for gliomagenesis, but rather the cumulative effects of several alterations that operate in a concerted manner and are responsible for the phenotypic and genotypic heterogeneity of these tumors. Radiogenomics can be referred to as a combination of imaging and gene expression and has the potential to give insight into tumor biology, which is harder to obtain from other techniques alone.

Glioblastoma was the first human cancer sequenced by The Cancer Genome Atlas (TGCA) network effort, resulting in a comprehensive characterization of the mutational spectrum of this neoplasm.[2,5,6] TCGA is a project supervised by the National Cancer Institute and the National Human Genome Research Institute to catalog genetic mutations responsible for cancer, using genome sequencing. It is a comprehensive and coordinated effort to accelerate the understanding of the molecular basis of cancer through the application of genome analysis technologies. The overarching goal is to improve the ability to diagnose, treat, and prevent cancer (https://wiki.nci.nih.gov/display/TCGA/The+Cancer+Genome+Atlas). The TCGA project has been established to generate a comprehensive catalog of genomic abnormalities driving tumorigenesis.[7]

Microarray is a tool used to characterize genomewide gene expression based on messenger RNA levels. This technique has been used to assess the correlation between gene-expression levels, MR imaging features, and outcome in GBM patients. Radiogenomics has been defined as the combination of imaging features and gene expression and has the potential to give insight regarding tumor biology, which may in turn be important to predict management and outcome.[8,9]

GENETIC EVALUATION OF BRAIN TUMORS

Great strides have been made in the characterization of regional GBM genetic expression patterns. Because of integrated genomic analysis, molecular classifications have been proposed with the intent of providing more uniform neoplasm subclasses from a biological standpoint. Imaging correlates of gene expression may provide important insight into brain tumor biology. Continued genomic sequencing may contribute to patient selection for trials and to developing more specific targeted therapies.

O^6-Methylguanine-DNA Methyltransferase

Epigenetic silence of the DNA repair O^6-methylguanine-DNA methyltransferase (MGMT) by promoter methylation is associated with a loss of its expression and has been related to longer overall survival in patients with high-grade gliomas.[10] Those patients treated with concomitant radiation therapy and alkylating agents, such as TMZ, have higher median survival (21.7 months) and 2-year survival (46%) rates when compared with those with unmethylated tumors.[11] Alkylating agents are highly reactive drugs that cause cell death by binding to DNA. MGMT inhibits the killing of tumor cells by alkylating agents by encoding a DNA repair protein to reverse alkylation at the DNA O^6 position of guanine, thereby averting the formation of lethal crosslinks.[12] A promoter controls MGMT activity, and methylation silences the gene in the neoplasm and thus diminishes DNA-repair activity. Through this mechanism, MGMT causes resistance to alkylating drugs (Fig. 1).

Methylation of the MGMT promoter in gliomas can be a useful predictor of tumor responsiveness to alkylating agents.[12] MGMT promoter methylation is an independent favorable prognostic factor that has been associated with longer survival in patients with newly diagnosed high-grade glioma after TMZ chemotherapy. Patients whose tumor contained a methylated MGMT promoter benefited from TMZ, whereas those with unmethylated tumors showed less benefit. Thus, MGMT methylation status may allow the selection of patients most likely to benefit from alkylating therapy. For those patients with unmethylated MGMT, alternative treatments using drugs with different mechanisms of action or methods of inhibiting MGMT should be used.[10]

The level of MGMT varies widely among different tumor types as well as among various samples of the same type of neoplasm. Approximately 30% of gliomas lack MGMT,[12] which may increase tumor sensitivity to alkylating treatment. High levels of MGMT in cancer cells may create

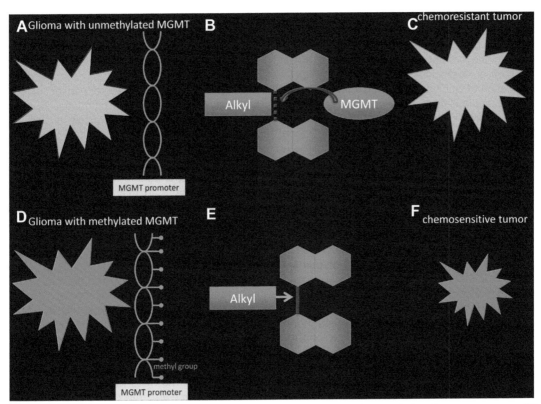

Fig. 1. Mechanism of inactivation of DNA repair-gene MGMT. Glioma with a methylated MGMT promoter (*A*). MGMT protein removes the alkylant agent from the DNA base guanine (*B*), cuts the DNA crosslinks, and results in resistance to chemotherapy (*C*). When the MGMT promoter is methylated (*D*), there is no active MGMT to repair the DNA crosslinks (*E*), leading to tumor cell death (*F*).

a resistant phenotype to alkylating agent treatment, which may become an important determinant of treatment failure.[10] The degree of intratumoral methylation varies among patients. The extent of methylation within the tumor has an association with survival. The degree of methylation impacts prognostic stratification directly, whereby the greatest methylation degree has the longest survival.[11] In a prior study, authors suggest that a cutoff level of 9% could be used to discriminate outcome between methylated and unmethylated tumors. Moreover, a methylation degree greater than 30% could benefit more tumors.

MGMT promoter methylation plays a key role in mechanisms conferring resistance to treatment with alkylating agents. Determination of the methylation status of the MGMT promoter may become an important molecular tool for identifying patients most likely to respond to the treatment and that might allow individually tailored therapy.[13] The methylation status of the MGMT promoter is determined by a polymerase-chain-reaction–specific analysis of tumor samples.[10] Furthermore,

new treatment regimens can be proposed using drugs capable of reactivating hypermethylated tumor suppressor genes or deactivating tumor promoting genes.

Isocitrate Dehydrogenase 1

Mutations in the isocitrate dehydrogenase 1 (IDH1) gene have been associated with improved outcome in patients with high-grade gliomas.[14] A better prognosis and reduced aggressiveness have been generally reported in glioma patients carrying IDH mutation.[15] Glioma patients with IDH1 mutations have a greater 5-year survival rate than patients with wild-type IDH1 gliomas (93% vs 51%).[16] Prior articles have reported treatment benefits for patients with IDH1 gene mutations. Early radiation therapy appears to be beneficial only in low-grade astrocytoma with IDH mutations.[14,17] IDH mutations have also been correlated with a higher rate of objective response to TMZ.[14,18]

Somatic mutations in isocitrate dehydrogenase 1 and 2 genes (IDH1 and IDH2) have been identified in primary brain cancers. These mutations result in the substitution of the arginine 132 codons by histidine in IDH1, which causes alterations in the normal enzymatic activities. IDH1 mutations are associated with alterations in DNA methylation of isocitrate, resulting in overproduction and accumulation of the putative oncometabolite 2-hydroxyglutarate (2-HG).[16] IDH1 appears to function as a tumor suppressor that, when mutationally inactivated, contributes to tumorigenesis partially through induction of the angiogenesis pathway (Fig. 2).[14]

Among low-grade gliomas, the incidence of mutation of arginine 132 (R132) in the IDH1 enzyme is much more evident and has been reported in more than 85% of grade II and III gliomas.[19] In a recent genome-wide analysis, mutations at codon 132 of IDH1 were found in less than 10% of primary GBMs, whereas this frequency is higher among secondary GBMs, accounting for more than 70%.[15] This gene has been associated with a distinct gene expression profile, especially in the proneural subset of glioblastoma, and is considered an independent prognostic indicator in these patients.[20]

The histopathologic difference between primary and secondary GBMs is hard to establish. However, secondary GBMs have subsets of genetic abnormalities different from primary GBMs. Hence, the in vivo detection of 2-HG could be a potential tool used to differentiate primary from secondary GBMs.[16] Noninvasive detection of 2-HG in glioma patients with IDH1 mutations may be of benefit in clinical management, because disease recurrence may be detected and may help in monitoring the treatment response (Fig. 3).[20] IDH1 mutations seem to occur early and are a key event in the pathogenesis of gliomas, with prognostic implications. It also may represent attractive targets for future pharmacologic inhibition.

Some authors have described that MR spectroscopy (MRS) is able to noninvasively measure 2-HG in gliomas and may serve as a potential biomarker for identifying patients with IDH1-mutant brain tumors.[15,20] Detection of 2-HG by MRS may provide insights into tumor progression and help monitor treatment effects (Fig. 4).[20] Prior reports have stated that this metabolite could be detected in almost all low-grade gliomas as well as in recurrent GBMs.[20] This finding has implications for diagnosis and monitoring treatment targeting IDH mutations. However, this in vivo MRS analysis is a technical challenge because of the complex spin-coupling features, which may lead to false-positive 2-HG detection.[15] Thus, to be performed, the MRS needs special postprocessing software and may clinically not be convenient for application.

More recently, diffusion-tensor MR imaging has been used to noninvasively detect genetic characteristics of gliomas, especially the IDH1 R132H

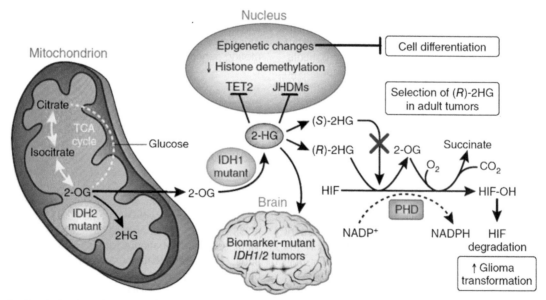

Fig. 2. Mechanism of IDH mutation. Tumors bearing mutations in IDH1/2 accumulate high amounts of the metabolite 2-HG. High levels of cellular 2-HG are hypothesized to drive the hydroxylation of HIF-α, leading to decreased HIF expression and increased glioma transformation. (*From* Young RM, Simon MC. Untuning the tumor metabolic machine: HIF-α: pro- and antitumorigenic? Nat Med 2012;18:1024; with permission.)

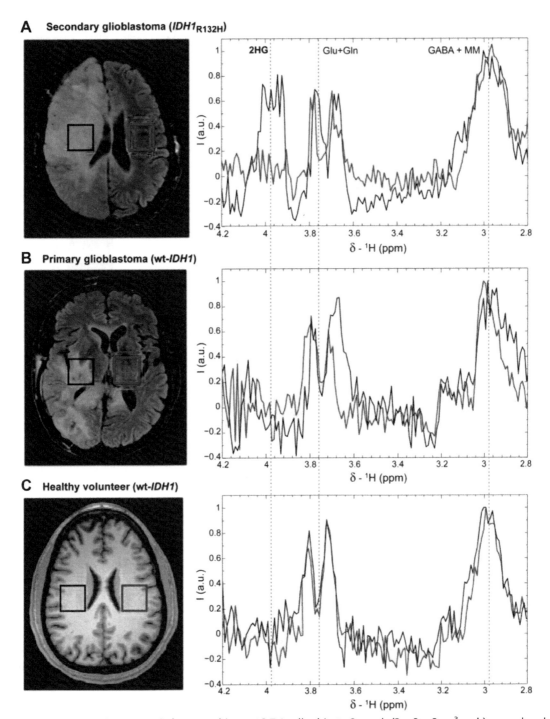

Fig. 3. 1D MEGA-LASER spectra in human subjects at 3 T. In all subjects, 2 voxels (3 × 3 × 3 cm³ each) were placed in both brain hemispheres, symmetrically from the middle line. (*A*) A secondary glioblastoma patient with *IDH1*R132H mutation. (*B, C*) The spectra from subjects with wt*IDH1*—primary glioblastoma (*B*) and a healthy volunteer (*C*). 2-HG is present only in the tumor voxel of the *IDH1*R132H patient. MM, denotes contamination of GABA signal with macromolecule signal. (*From* Andronesi OC, Kim GS, Gerstner E, et al. Detection of 2-hydroxyglutarate in IDH-mutated glioma patients by in vivo spectral-editing and 2D correlation magnetic resonance spectroscopy. Sci Transl Med 2012;4(116):116ra4; with permission)

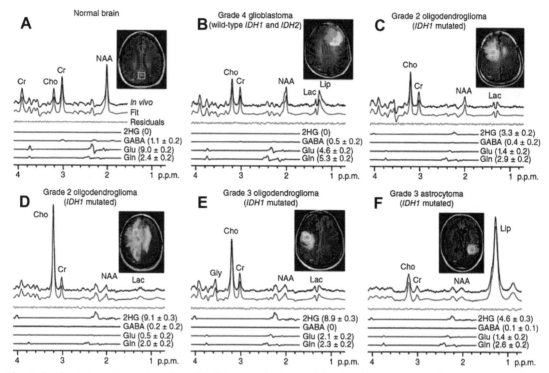

Fig. 4. In vivo 1H spectra and analysis. (A–F) In vivo single-voxel–localized PRESS spectra from normal brain (A) and tumors (B–F), at 3 T, are shown together with spectral fits (LCModel) and the components of 2-HG, GABA, glutamate, and glutamine as well as voxel positioning (2 × 2 × 2 cm³). Spectra are scaled with respect to the water signal from the voxel. Vertical lines are drawn at 2.25 ppm to indicate the H4 multiplet of 2-HG. Shown in parentheses is the estimated metabolite concentration (mM) ± SD. Cho, choline; Cr, creatine; Gln, glutamine; Glu, glutamate; Gly, glycine; Lac, lactate; Lip, lipids; NAA, N-acetylaspartate. Scale bars, 1 cm. (From Choi C, Ganji SK, DeBerardinis RJ, et al. 2-Hydroxyglutarate detection by magnetic resonance spectroscopy in IDH-mutated glioma patients. Nat Med 2012;18:627; with permission.)

mutation.[14] High fractional anisotropic (FA) values and low apparent diffusion coefficient (ADC) values were shown in a wild-type IDH1 group when compared with a mutation group in grade II and III gliomas. The authors found that, although FA and ADC values can detect IDH1 mutation, the ratio of minimal ADC is the best measurement for this proposal.[14]

Epidermal Growth Factor Receptor

Epidermal growth factor receptor (EGFR) amplification is a common molecular event in high-grade gliomas. Activation of the EGFR pathway in glioblastoma, and its overexpression and amplification, is a very frequent molecular event found in up to 50% of patients. It is associated with invasion and proliferation of neoplasm cells as well as apoptosis and angiogenesis. EGFR-amplified glioblastomas are relatively radiation-resistant and recur more frequently after therapy.[21]

EGFR amplification is more commonly observed in primary than secondary GBMs, especially the

classical glioblastoma subtype, found in up to 97% of patients in that subclass.[7] Thus, EGFR inhibitors could be used in the classical subtype of glioblastoma with better efficacy. Some morphologic MR imaging metrics have been correlated with amplification of EGFR. Higher ratios of the volume of T2-hyperintense lesion to the T1-enhancing volume and a decreased T2 border sharpness coefficient (fuzzier borders) have also been associated with EGFR overexpression prediction.[21] Other authors have suggested that this overexpression could be predicted by the ratio of contrast-enhancing tumor to necrotic tumor.[22] More recently, restricted diffusion has also been correlated with EGFR amplification, which could be a simpler analysis to be used in clinical practice, without the need for postprocessing.[2] Restricted diffusion in brain neoplasms can be secondary to increased neoplasm cellularity or ischemia. Moreover, EGFR status information can be used to predict the classical subtype of glioblastoma, which may in turn be useful to tailor therapy in selected patients.

1p19q

Oligodendrogliomas with 1p19q-deleted lesions have a favorable prognosis. In these genotype lesions, a better response to chemotherapy, duration of response to chemotherapy, progression-free survival after radiation therapy, and overall survival have been seen. Combined loss of 1p and 19q appears to define a treatment-sensitive malignant glioma, one which may often be curable with current therapies.[23]

These genotype neoplasms have a predilection for the frontal lobe location; the insular location is more common in lesions, which rarely or never delete 1p19q.[24] The allelic loss of chromosomal arms 1p19q has been associated with indistinct tumor borders in T1-weighted images, which may indicate invasiveness, and mixed signal intensity on T1-weighted and T2-weighted images (Fig. 5).[21,25] Calcification and hemorrhage might contribute to signal heterogeneity and susceptibility effect. Calcification is common among low-grade oligodendrogliomas and in anaplastic astrocytomas evolved from low-grade neoplasm, associated with 1p19q loss.[25,26]

YKL-40

Some prognostic factors must be taken into account for management of glioma patients. YKL-40, also denominated human cartilage glycoprotein-39 or CHI3L1, is a gene located on chromosome 1q32 that is considered one of the potential prognostic factors. Its expression has been used as an adjuvant tool to differentiate GBM from anaplastic oligodendroglioma.[27,28] YKL-40 has the ability to influence the processes of migration, invasion, and angiogenesis that underlie its capacity to stimulate proliferation.[28,29] In an earlier report, higher YKL-40 expression proved to be a negative prognostic marker associated with a lower response to radiation therapy and shorter overall survival.[27,28] Thus, the expression of YKL-40 predicts poor outcomes in glioblastoma. When combined with MGMT promoter methylation analysis, the prognostic value of these markers is closely related to the efficacy of adjuvant radiation therapy with chemotherapy, and this may influence patient selection for aggressive treatment regimens.[28]

Molecular Subclasses of High-Grade Glioma

The histopathologic characterization based on the World Health Organization classification still plays an important role in patient management and in defining the corresponding therapeutic approaches in gliomas. However, this classification fails to identify neoplasm subclasses with different aggressiveness within the same tumor grade. The genetic expression profile of brain neoplasms, especially the astrocytic tumors, varies among different degrees of malignancy and even among those of the same grade.[28]

There is an inability to define different patient outcomes because of histopathologic features. Because of integrated genomic analysis, a molecular classification with 4 different subtypes has been proposed with the intent of providing a more uniform molecular subclass classification of GBM. Verhaak and colleagues[7] proposed a gene expression–based molecular classification of glioblastoma of 4 subtypes: proneural, neural, classical, and mesenchymal, and integrated multidimensional genomic data to establish patterns of somatic mutations and DNA copy number.

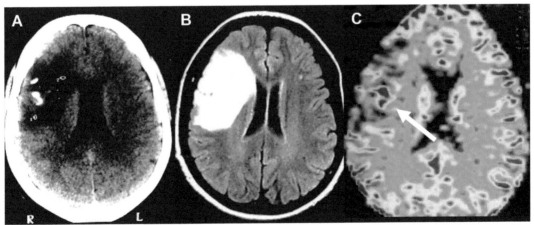

Fig. 5. Right frontal oligodendroglioma with 1p19q loss in a 54-year-old woman. An expansive and calcified lesion demonstrated on axial CT (A) and FLAIR (B) images, with areas of hyperperfusion on rCBV map (arrow, C).

The classical, mesenchymal, and proneural subtypes are defined, respectively, by aberrations and gene expression of EGFR, NF1, and PDGFRA/IDH1. High-level EGFR amplification is seen in the classical subtype and infrequently in other subtypes. Deletion of a region containing the NF1 gene predominantly occurs in the mesenchymal subtype. Two major features of the proneural class are alterations of PDGFRA and mutations in IDH1, in which younger patients are the majority and tend toward longer survival. Overexpression of neuron markers is seen in the neural subtype. The major clinical importance of this molecular classification is that the same histopathologic type of brain tumor, GBM, has a different treatment response based on the molecular subtype classification. Aggressive therapy performed with radiation therapy followed by TMZ showed the greatest benefit in classical GBM patients, whereas this treatment did not alter survival in the proneural subtype.[30] Most known secondary glioblastomas were classified as proneural.[7] Thus, the importance of detecting these subtypes relies on the tailored therapeutic approach that different subtypes may require (**Tables 1 and 2**).

IMAGING FEATURES

Noninvasive detection of gene expression before treatment can be an important way to predict outcome and to provide personalized therapy. Imaging correlates to gene expression may provide important insight into brain neoplasm, because MR imaging findings may be correlated with molecular mutations of a tumor. Moreover, some molecular signatures may be reflected in imaging features derived from standard MR imaging. Some tumor properties are associated with outcome, such as necrosis, contrast enhancement, and extent of edema. Although several reports have attempted to correlate imaging findings with molecular markers, no consistent associations have emerged and many imaging features lack any correlation with neoplasm molecular biology. Nevertheless, these preliminary findings are able to provide new insight for the clinical approach and management of brain neoplasm patients.

Although histopathology and immunohistochemistry guide the diagnosis and treatment of high-grade gliomas, tumor biology and genomic heterogeneity typify these lesions. Histopathologically similar tumors may differ in the molecular component and demonstrate different clinical behaviors and outcomes. Methods that evaluate molecular differences between glioblastomas hold promise for improving outcome and have the potential for individualizing patient management.

Undergrading of gliomas is a major problem in clinical practice accounting for about 30% of the cases, which can directly influence the management and outcome of those patients. Because of the heterogeneity of these lesions, unguided biopsy may be prone to sample errors. Although contrast enhancement is the MR imaging feature commonly used to assess glioblastoma, this imaging sequence has limited specificity in tumor grading. Advanced MR imaging techniques, like diffusion-weighted imaging, dynamic susceptibility-weighted contrast-enhanced imaging, and dynamic contrast-enhanced perfusion MR imaging, hold promise in quantitative evaluation of aggressiveness. Recent studies have suggested that genetic and cellular features of high-grade gliomas aggressiveness influence MR imaging, especially those advanced sequences, demonstrating low ADC values and increased relative cerebral blood volume (rCBV) in areas of angiogenesis and high cellularity (**Fig. 6**).[31]

The nonenhancing portion of the lesion is of upmost importance in clinical management, because it is commonly the site of recurrence after treatment. Therefore, these regions present with different genetic expressions when compared with the contrast-enhancing lesion. Prior investigators have found an up-regulation of genes associated with cell proliferation and infiltration, hypoxia, and angiogenesis in the contrast-enhanced portion of the lesion.[31] These findings

Table 1
Molecular subtype classification for glioblastoma multiforme based on gene expression

Gene Expression	Classical	Mesenchymal	Proneural	Neural
EGFR amplification	High level	Infrequent	Infrequent	Infrequent
NF1 deletion	No predominance	Predominance	No predominance	No predominance
PDGFRA/IDH1 alteration	Minor	Minor	Major	Minor
Neural markers expression	Expression	Expression	Expression	Overexpression

Table 2
Relationship between gene expression and treatment response, overall survival, and prognosis

Gene Expression	Tumor Biology	Radiation Therapy	Chemotherapy	Overall Survival	Prognostic Marker
MGMT methylation	GBM	Respond	Respond	Increases	Favorable
IDH1	Classical/mesenchymal/ proneural GBM/gliomas grade II, III	Respond	Respond	Increases	Favorable
EGFR	Primary GBM/classical GBM/high-grade gliomas	Resistant	Respond	Decreases	Unfavorable
1p19q	Oligodendroglioma	Respond	Respond	Increases	Favorable
YKL-40	GBM	Lower response	Respond	Decreases	Unfavorable

suggest that the genetic and biologic behaviors of gliomas significantly influence imaging features and thus have severe clinical implications. The techniques may add information to the contrast-enhanced MR image to better select the most appropriate location to biopsy the lesion, searching for the highest aggressive region (Fig. 7). Moreover, these imaging biomarkers may be used to noninvasively identify, prognosticate, and monitor clinically important features of glioma aggressiveness.[31] Some investigators have shown that

tumors classified as proneural demonstrated significantly less contrast enhancement than other subtypes. Similarly, the mesenchymal subtype also demonstrated less contrast enhancement.[32]

Perfusion parameters are considered a surrogate marker for angiogenesis. Recently, researchers have correlated hemodynamic and physiologic imaging biomarkers with the expression of genes regulating angiogenesis in glioblastoma. They concluded that angiogenic genes demonstrate a positive correlation with perfusion

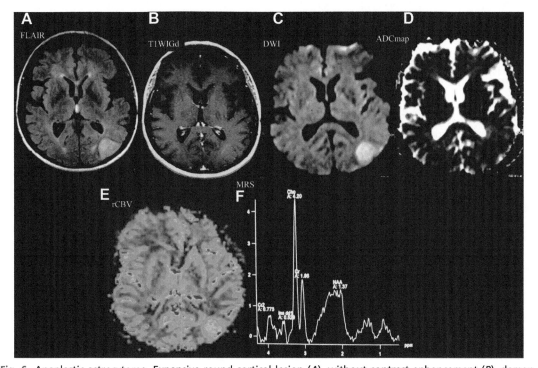

Fig. 6. Anaplastic astrocytoma. Expansive round cortical lesion (A), without contrast enhancement (B), demonstrating restricted diffusion (C) with low ADC values (D) and increased perfusion (E). MRS reveals a very high peak of choline and a reduction in NAA levels (F).

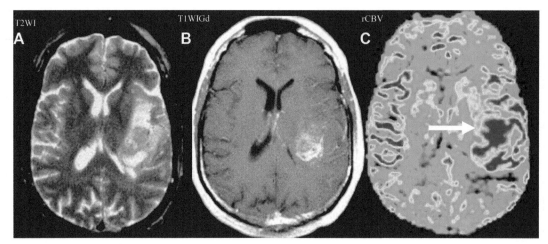

Fig. 7. GBM. Hyperperfusion is seen in parts of the tumor (*arrow, C*) that does not enhance after intravenous contrast administration (*B*), corresponding to angiogenesis and a higher aggressive component of heterogeneous lesion in left parieto-insular lobes (*A*).

parameters, whereas antiangiogenic genes showed an inverse correlation (**Fig. 8**).[33] The identification of key targets involved in the regulation and promotion of angiogenesis, like the vascular endothelial growth factor (VEGF) pathways, is crucial for the development of therapeutic antiangiogenic drugs.

Different from angiogenic gene expression associated with edema, necrosis, and a worse prognosis, IDH1 mutation and MGMT promoter methylation status are related to a favorable prognosis, associated with longer survival. Ring enhancement has been associated with unmethylation and primary glioblastoma, whereas irregular

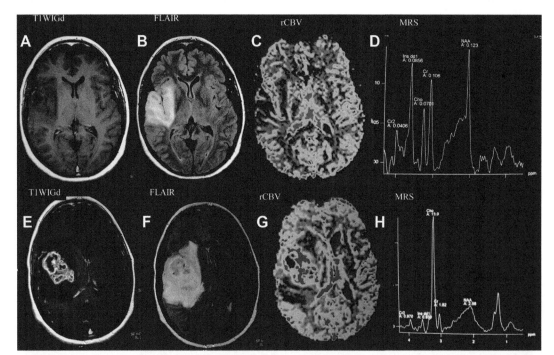

Fig. 8. A 55-year-old woman with a low-grade glioma in the right insular region (*A, B*). There is no hyperperfusion (*C*) and MRS reveals an elevation of myoinositol/creatine ratio (*D*). The follow-up MR examination, performed after clinical deterioration, demonstrates an enlargement of the lesion that has an irregular contrast enhancement (*E*), associated with vasogenic edema and infiltration (*F*). The lesion demonstrates hyperperfusion areas, related to neoangiogenesis (*G*). MRS shows a large peak of choline and peak of lipids/lactate (*H*).

and nodular enhancement has been related to methylated and secondary tumors (Fig. 9).[34]

Some earlier reports suggest that imaging features might be useful biomarkers able to predict IDH1 status. Neoplasms with IDH1 mutation have not demonstrated contrast enhancement and most of them have been located in the frontal lobe.[34] This molecular genotype has low vascular EGFR levels, as large regions of the lesion do not demonstrate contrast enhancement (Fig. 10). When there is a varying amount of oligodendroglioma component in association with 1p19q deletions, there is frontal lobe predilection as well as a better prognosis.[34] Tumor location seems to be a significant prognostic factor in glioblastoma, which may reflect the genetic profile of tumor precursor cells. Recently, authors suggested that the periventricular white matter tumor location was associated with short overall survival (Fig. 11). Moreover, this location also hosts most of the mesenchymal glioblastoma subtype, in which

there was lack of MGMT-promoter methylation and no amplification of IDH1 mutation, contributing to a poor prognosis.[35]

EGFR amplification tumors have a significantly higher contrast enhancement and hyperintense tumor volume when compared with nonamplification lesions.[35] A prior study identifies potential imaging biomarkers for different classes of anti-GBM therapeutic agents, including antiangiogenic and EGFR-based therapies.[22] Past reports have supported the idea that EGFR amplification has a negative prognosis.[35,36]

Diffusion-weighted images have been widely used to assess brain tumors. ADC histogram analysis can predict anti-VEGF treatment response to recurrent glioblastoma,[37] and ADC values have been reported as a prognostic factor of glioma outcome.[38] Patients with high-ADC tumors have had significantly poorer outcomes and have overexpressed genes for collagen and collagen-binding proteins.[37]

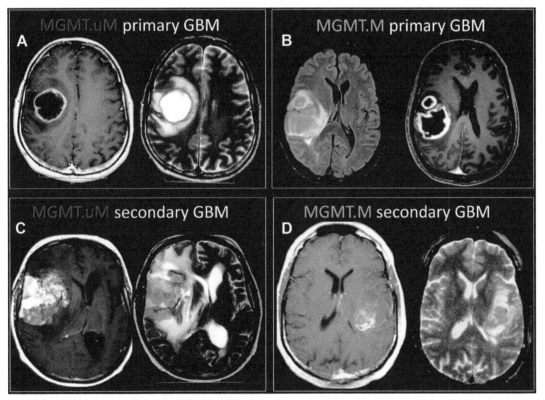

Fig. 9. Unmethylated primary GBM (A), an expanding, round necrotic cystic lesion, surrounded by a heterogenous hyperintense area on T2-weighted imaging. Methylated primary GBM (B), a more homogenous lesion in T2-weighted imaging, with an irregular rim of contrast enhancement, surrounded by vasogenic edema. Unmethylated secondary GBM (C). The hyperintense area is more homogenous and there is a nodular irregular contrast enhancement. Methylated secondary GBM (D). The hyperintense area in T2-weighted imaging is slightly inhomogeneous; the lesion also demonstrates an irregular contrast enhancement, with areas that do not enhance.

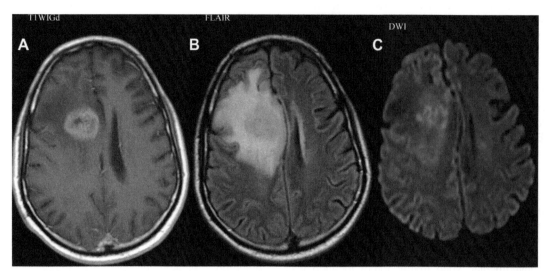

Fig. 10. GBM with IDH1 mutation. A round and expansive right frontal neoplasm, with a slight contrast enhancement (A), associated with vasogenic edema and peritumoral infiltrative region (B). Some areas of restricted diffusion are observed within the lesion (C).

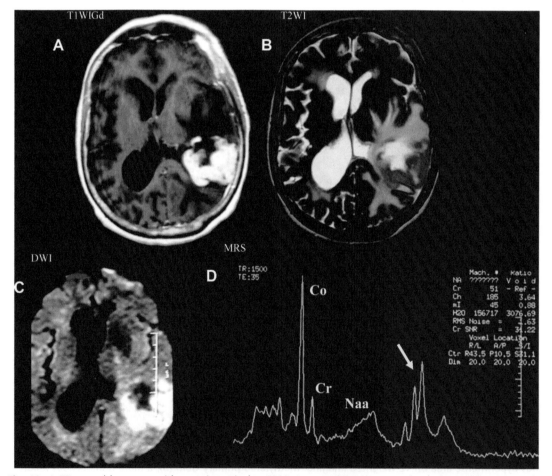

Fig. 11. A 75-year-old woman with a periventricular GBM. A necrotic/cystic expansive lesion, with an irregular contrast enhancement (A), surrounded by hyperintense area in T2-weighted imaging (B). The lesion has hypointensity on T2-weighted imaging and restricted diffusion (C) correlated with high cellularity. MRS shows a high choline peak, low NAA/creatine ratio, and a double peak of lipids and lactate (D).

PROGNOSTIC FEATURES

There are several prognostic factors related to glioblastoma prognosis that can help in the assessment of patients. The prognosis of GBM patients and their therapy responses are highly influenced by clinical and molecular genetic factors that are increasingly used for prognostic profiling and individualized risk-adapted treatment considerations.

Several imaging features have been shown to have potential prognostic value. The use of MR imaging parameters to noninvasively characterize the molecular status of the tumor is improving, mostly because new information provided by clinical research and modern imaging technologies has been added to daily clinical practice. Molecular tumor characterization may directly influence patient management and has the potential to improve the outcome. Imaging parameters can provide insights regarding molecular behavior, hypoxia, and angiogenesis related to different molecular tumor subclasses.[2] A significant correlation between overall survival, the degree of contrast enhancement, and the length of the tumor's major axis has been described.[32] Thus, MR imaging parameters have a potential value for patients in whom tumor sample analysis is not available.

Tissue samples are typically obtained from the contrast-enhanced portion of the lesion. However, there are some histopathologic features and quantitative MR imaging parameter differences between this enhanced portion and the nonenhanced component of the neoplasm.

Patients presenting with methylation of the MGMT promoter have a better prognosis than those with an unmethylated status. In a retrospective analysis, authors described a significantly improved clinical outcome in patients with newly diagnosed glioblastoma who had a methylated MGMT promoter and were treated with radiation therapy and TMZ. The 18-month survival rate reported was more than 60% among patients with a methylated status compared with less than 10% in the absence of promoter methylation.[39] The median survival rate among patients whose tumors had a methylated MGMT promoter status and were treated with radiation therapy and TMZ was greater than when treated only with radiotherapy (21.7 months compared with 15.3 months).[39]

TREATMENT
Current Treatment

Some progress has been made in the treatment of glioblastoma. Currently, standard of care for newly diagnosed glioblastoma is radiation therapy with concomitant and subsequent adjuvant TMZ for 5 days during each 28-day cycle for 12 cycles maximum.[1] This new regimen has improved 2-year survival from 11% to 27.3%, and 5-year survival from 1.9% to 9.8%. Moreover, progression-free survival also improved from 6.2 months to 10.6 months. However, no substantial improvement was observed in overall survival.[40]

Surgery

The extent of removal of brain neoplasm is one of the milestones of the treatment and is considered the first step. The presence of an infiltrative lesion makes it difficult to define tumor margins, because regions with malignant features are intermingled within functioning brain tissue that cannot be removed without severe detriment to the patient. Frequently, the major portion of the contrast-enhanced component of the lesion can be resected. However, it is quite impossible to achieve total resection of the nonenhancing component, which may explain the fact that a curative resection generally cannot be achieved. Therefore, there is a substantial residual nonenhancing tumor component, which may eventually become the site of focal recurrence. Thus, it is important to better define the burden of the lesion, especially the nonenhancing component.

Chemotherapy

Although the current standard therapy using an alkylating agent has considerably improved patients' outcome, recurrence can be frequent. Treatment options for these patients are limited and have a poor prognosis. For these patients, some strategies may be proposed, like repeated surgical resection, stereotactic radiosurgery, and chemotherapy using dose-intensified TMZ and antiangiogenic drugs, with mechanism of action based on the presence of an antibody to VEGF or an antibody to VEGF receptors.

A promising strategy for overcoming resistance mediated by MGMT seems to be depletion of MGMT by prolonged exposure to low doses of alkylating agents.[39]

Alkylating agents may cause blood toxicity, characterized by lymphopenia, which may lead to opportunistic infections, and thrombocytopenia. Therefore, it seems that regular lymphocyte counts and prophylaxis against opportunistic infections may be required when using this regimen.

Personalized Treatment

Individually tailored therapies for patients with high-grade gliomas are an important issue in current patient management. Efforts are geared toward finding factors identifying patients likely to benefit from the treatment chosen. The first step in this direction should be to determine clinically relevant molecular changes, which may contribute toward calculating its prognostic and predictive value.

MGMT methylation status can be a predictive factor for response to alkylating agent therapy. The addition of concomitant and adjuvant TMZ to radiation therapy improves the 2-year survival rate from 10% to more than 25% in a tumor with MGMT promoter methylation.[11] The tumor resistance mechanism to alkylating therapy has to be identified to propose additional treatment to those patients with unmethylated neoplasms. These patients may profit from other therapies based on different mechanisms of action and may be spared from the toxicity of alkylating agents. However, to date, no alternative treatment has yet been proposed and validated. Although differences in MGMT promoter methylation may determine the clinical course in patients with glioblastoma treated with TMZ, it is currently not recommended to use MGMT promoter methylation to determine who should or should not receive chemotherapy.[1,39]

Treatment Response

Noninvasive methods for monitoring growth or response to therapy would advance the practice of neuro-oncology.[32] Several imaging features have been shown to have potential prognostic value.

The Macdonald criteria are based on bidimensional measurements of enhancing lesions in conjunction with clinical evaluation and corticosteroid use and have been used to assess the post-therapeutic response of high-grade gliomas.[41] These criteria define tumor progression as an increase in the size of the contrast-enhancing lesion or the appearance of new enhancing lesions. However, there are significant recognized limitations to these criteria, like the difficulty in measuring irregularly shaped tumors and multifocal lesions, and lack of assessment of the nonenhancing portion of the neoplasm. Thus, tumor changes observed on FLAIR imaging characterized by the nonenhancing portion of the lesion are not assessed. Contrast enhancement in posttreatment brain neoplasms is a nonspecific finding and may not be considered a true surrogate marker for tumor response, because some treatment-related changes may be observed as a new area of contrast enhancement.

With the advent of novel treatment regimens, the limitations of Macdonald criteria have become acutely apparent. Pseudoprogression is defined as a transient increase in the nontumoral enhancing area related to treatment. It has been described in about 10% to 30% of high-grade gliomas treated with the current standard of care: surgical resection and radiation therapy plus concomitant chemotherapy, followed by cycles of adjuvant chemotherapy. Conversely, pseudoresponse is observed within 1 to 2 days after initiation of antiangiogenic therapies and is defined as a decrease in the enhancing tumor area. Some patients receiving antiangiogenic therapy may show evidence of recurrence with progressive increases in the nonenhancing component of the lesion on FLAIR imaging. Thus, these findings show that enhancement alone is not a measure of tumor activity but rather reflects a disturbed blood-brain barrier. The nonenhancing portion of the lesion should be analyzed to assess tumor response.[42]

The Response Assessment in Neuro-Oncology Criteria (RANO) more recently published updated guidelines for assessing response to therapy in gliomas.[43] Based on prior observation after brain tumor therapy, these response criteria suggest that the nonenhancing component of the tumor should also be taken into account when making assessments about progression or response. Hence, the major modification proposed by the RANO guidelines is the assessment of the nonenhancing area and the signal intensity changes on FLAIR imaging as evidence of tumor progression. The inclusion of a nonenhancing tumor in the determination of overall tumor burden improves the accuracy of determining tumor progression in the setting of antiangiogenic therapy.

Pseudoprogression
Pseudoprogression is defined as an increase in a contrast-enhancing lesion size just after completion of radiation therapy plus concomitant chemotherapy with TMZ in patients with high-grade tumors, followed by subsequent improvement or stabilization without any further treatment (Fig. 12).[44,45] This regimen is thought to be a subacute treatment-related reaction, mostly without clinical deterioration, instead of tumor progression. Although no report on a larger series of patients has yet been published, according to earlier reports, enlarged enhancing lesions may represent pseudoprogression in up to 45% to 65% of cases.[46] The RANO criteria proposed that within the first 12 weeks of completion of radiation therapy, when pseudoprogression is most prevalent, tumor progression can only be determined if most of the new enhancement is outside the radiation field or if there is pathologic confirmation.[43]

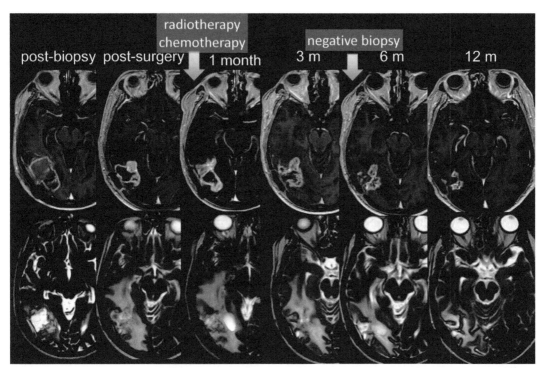

Fig. 12. Pseudoprogression. A 59-year-old man with GBM. An MR image obtained 1 month after radiotherapy-TMZ demonstrates an expansion of the right temporal lesion. Reductions in both the enhancing portion and the surrounding abnormal hyperintense area in the T2-weighted imaging were seen in the follow-up MR imaging examinations. (*Data from* Hygino da Cruz LC Jr, Rodriguez I, Domingues RC, et al. Pseudoprogression and pseudoresponse: imaging challenges in the assessment of posttreatment glioma. AJNR Am J Neuroradiol 2011;32(11):1981.)

The methylation status of the MGMT promoter has been shown to be a potent prognostic factor in high-grade gliomas patients. Patients benefit more from treatment if they have low MGMT expression, due to methylation of the promoter. A high association between pseudoprogression and MGMT promoter status has been described. Pseudoprogression has been demonstrated in more than 90% of high-grade gliomas with MGMT promoter methylation, while only 40% of unmethylated MGMT patients have developed it. Therefore, the MGMT methylation status is related to a high incidence of pseudoprogression as a consequence of higher sensitivity to treatment.[42] Hence, methylation of the MGMT promoter has been associated with a favorable prognosis and prolonged survival in adult patients with GBM treated with TMZ.[47]

Pseudoprogression is most prevalent within the first 12 weeks after completion of radiation therapy. Despite radiological evidence of lesion progression, patients often remain asymptomatic or only mildly symptomatic clinically.[10] This increase in contrast enhancement and peritumoral edema diminishes over time without any further treatment changes. Pseudoprogression is widely thought to be more frequent following concomitant radiotherapy with TMZ. However, it can occur following radiotherapy alone and, in some cases, it can also be associated with other chemotherapy regimens (**Fig. 13**).[42] Pathologically, pseudoprogression is characterized as reactive radiation-induced changes, vascular endothelium changes, increased blood-brain barrier permeability, necrosis, edema, and gliosis.[42]

Transient increases in contrast enhancement just after completion of chemoradiotherapy complicate the ability of the physician to determine whether to continue with standard adjuvant chemotherapy or to switch to a second-line treatment for recurrence. Pseudoprogression may represent an exaggerated response to effective therapy, and thus, it may not be misinterpreted as treatment failure leading to premature discontinuation of effective therapy. There are no currently definitive criteria to differentiate between true progression and pseudoprogression. The only way to diagnose pseudoprogression is based on combining clinical manifestations, follow-up MR imaging examinations, and pathologic findings.

No single imaging technique has been validated to recognize and adequately establish a diagnosis of pseudoprogression.[48] In the absence of definitive radiologic criteria diagnosis, an enlarging

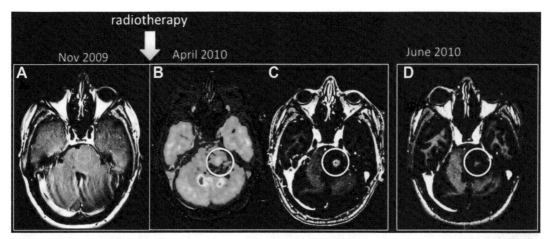

Fig. 13. Pseudoprogression. A 25-year-old man with a low-grade glioma in the left aspect of the pons (*A*) was treated with only radiotherapy (*arrow*). PET-MR imaging (*B*) showed hypermetabolism in the enhancing portion of the lesion (*C*). An MR imaging examination performed 1 month later (*D*) shows a reduction in the enhancing portion of the lesion. (*Data from* Hygino da Cruz LC Jr, Rodriguez I, Domingues RC, et al. Pseudoprogression and pseudoresponse: imaging challenges in the assessment of posttreatment glioma. AJNR Am J Neuroradiol 2011;32(11):1982.)

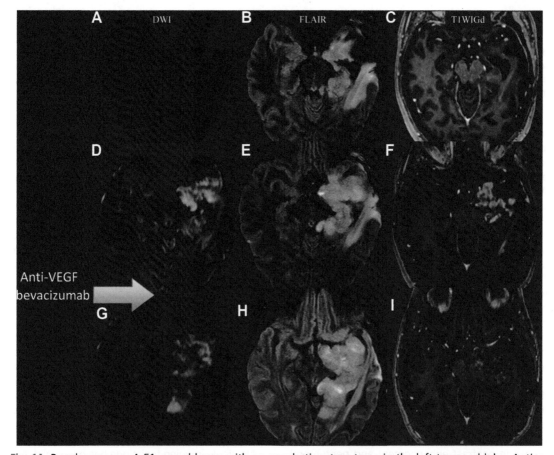

Fig. 14. Pseudoresponse. A 51-year-old man with an anaplastic astrocytoma in the left temporal lobe. Antiangiogenic therapy (*arrow*) was initiated after failure of initial treatment and tumoral recurrence (*A–F*). The contrast-enhancing portion of the lesion diminished dramatically (*G*), whereas there was an enlargement of the nonenhancing component seen on FLAIR (*H*) that has restricted diffusion (*I*).

lesion within the radiation field on the first post-chemoradiotherapy MR imaging represents a diagnostic dilemma to the oncologist. The presence of neurologic deterioration is more likely to be associated with true disease progression. Physicians may be tempted to include clinical data such as neurologic deterioration to help differentiate pseudoprogression from true neoplasm progression. Some authors recommend that 3 cycles of adjuvant TMZ be given before a decision is made about whether the initial imaging changes represent true disease progression or pseudoprogression.[49] More recent publications have suggested that rCBV obtained from a dynamic susceptibility contrast perfusion sequence may better predict a distinction between pseudoprogression and true tumor progression.[46,50–52]

Pseudoresponse

Antiangiogenic agents are used as second-line therapy for unresponsive or recurrent high-grade gliomas. These agents produce a rapid decrease in contrast enhancement, within hours, secondary to an antipermeability effect, with a pseudonormalization of the blood-brain barrier, rather than tumor reduction.[42] Thus, tumors appear to respond to treatment and tumor progression is more difficult to detect. This phenomenon is denominated pseudoresponse.[53] The pseudonormalization of the blood-brain barrier leads to a reduction in the vasogenic edema, which may improve the clinical symptoms and brain function. Although some patients display clinical improvement with a high response rate and progression-free survival, only modest effects on overall survival were noted. Patients may present with an enlargement of the nonenhancing portion of the lesion on T2-weighted and FLAIR sequences in follow-up MR imaging examinations, corresponding to tumor progression (**Fig. 14**).[54]

During antiangiogenic treatment, areas with restricted diffusion may be seen within the lesion and even outside the confines of an enhancing tumor. Diffusion restriction during treatment has been postulated to be a surrogate marker and a predictor of tumor progression, as development of a new focus of restricted diffusion may precede the development of a new enhancing tumor (**Fig. 15**).[55] In a more recent publication, restricted-diffusion lesions were generally stable

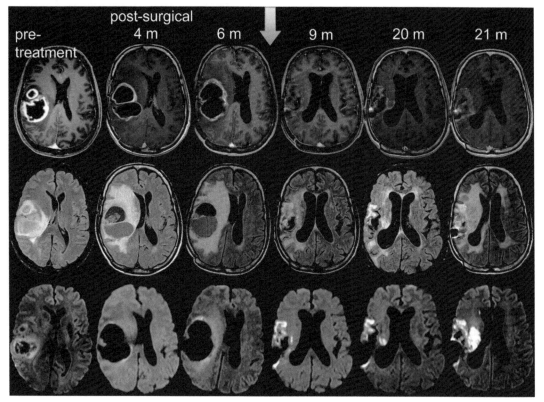

Fig. 15. A 58-year-old man with GBM. After failure of the previous treatment (surgery resection followed by concomitant radiochemotherapy), antiangiogenic therapy was initiated (*arrow*). In the follow-up MR imaging examination, new areas of restricted diffusion are observed that do not contrast-enhance. On imaging performed subsequently, the lesion continued to progress.

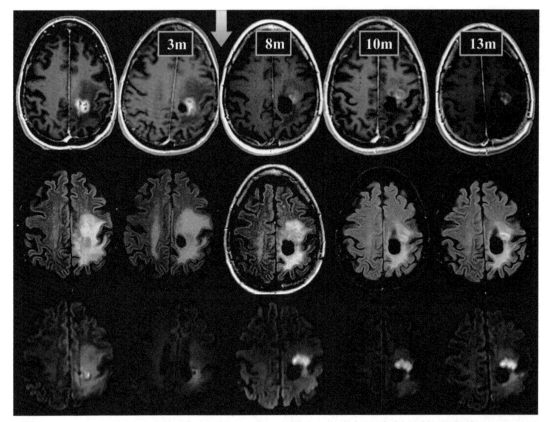

Fig. 16. Anaplastic astrocytoma in a patient who underwent surgical resection followed by radiotherapy. Antiangiogenic therapy was initiated (*arrow*). A new area of restricted diffusion is noted at the anterior margin of the surgical cavity that remains stable in size in the follow-up examinations.

and associated with improved outcomes, suggesting that they were not consistent with aggressive tumors (**Fig. 16**).[56] Although some investigations suggest that these lesions reflect hypercellular and aggressive tumor,[55] other studies suggest that these lesions represent chronic hypoxia and atypical gelatinous necrotic tissue.[56] These findings have implications for the management of patients with recurrent malignant gliomas.

SUMMARY

Significant advances have been made to understand the molecular mechanisms underlying the radiogenomics of gliomas better, with the ultimate goal of improving outcomes. Continued genomic sequencing efforts are expected to have expanding roles in the selection of patients for tailored treatment. In the future, patients may undergo molecular profiling for the identification of the individually altered key pathways that indicate the most beneficial therapeutic modality for the respective patient.

Much of the information encoded within neuroimaging studies remains unaccounted for and incompletely characterized at the molecular level. Phenotypic diversity of glioblastomas assessed by neuroimaging reflects underlying tumor gene expression differences, and the relationship could be uncovered by combining genome scale gene expression and MR imaging.

Efforts have been targeted toward discovering imaging biomarkers that could draw a parallel to underlying gene expression signatures. The identification of these imaging phenotype signatures will help advance individualized management.

REFERENCES

1. Stupp R, Mason WP, van den Bent MJ, et al. Radiotherapy plus concomitant and adjuvant temozolomide for glioblastoma. N Engl J Med 2005;352:987–96.
2. Young RJ, Gupta A, Shah AD, et al. Potential role of preoperative conventional MRI including diffusion measurements in assessing epidermal growth factor

receptor gene amplification status in patients with glioblastoma. AJNR Am J Neuroradiol 2013;34: 2271–7.

3. Cohen MH, Shen YL, Keegan P, et al. FDA drug approval summary: bevacizumab (Avastin) as treatment of recurrent glioblastoma multiforme. Oncologist 2009;14(11):1131–8.

4. Barajas RF, Phillips JJ, Parvataneni R, et al. Regional variation in histopathologic features of tumor specimens from treatment-naïve glioblastoma correlates with anatomic and physiologic MR imaging. Neuro Oncol 2012;14(7):942–54.

5. Mischel PS, Cloughesy TF, Nelson SF. DNA-microarray analysis of brain cancer: molecular classification for therapy. Nat Rev Neurosci 2004;5(10):782–92.

6. Hu LS, Eschbacher JM, Heiserman JE, et al. Reevaluation the imaging definition of tumor progression: perfusion MRI quantifies recurrent glioblastoma tumor fraction, pseudoprogression, and radiation necrosis to predict survival. Neuro Oncol 2012;14: 919–30.

7. Verhaak RG, Hoadley KA, Purdom E, et al. Integrated genomic analysis identifies clinically relevant subtypes of glioblastoma characterized by abnormalities in PDGFRA, IDH1, EGFR, and NF1. Cancer Cell 2010;17:98–110.

8. Pope WB, Mirsadraei L, Lai A, et al. Differential gene expression in glioblastoma defined by ADC histogram analysis: relationship to extracellular matrix molecules and survival. AJNR Am J Neuroradiol 2012;33:1059–64.

9. Pope WB, Prins RM, Thomas MA, et al. Non-invasive detection of 2-hydroxyglutarate and other metabolites in IDH1 mutant glioma patients using magnetic resonance spectroscopy. J Neurooncol 2012;107(1): 197–205.

10. Hegi ME, Diserens AC, Gorlia T, et al. MGMT gene silencing and benefit from temozolomide in glioblastoma. N Engl J Med 2005;352(10):997–1003.

11. Dunn J, Barborie A, Alam F, et al. Extent of MGMT promoter methylation correlates with outcome in glioblastomas given temozolomide and radiotherapy. Br J Cancer 2009;101(1):124–31.

12. Esteller M, Garcia-Foncillas J, Andion E, et al. Inactivation of the DNA-repair gene MGMT and the clinical response of gliomas to alkylating agents. N Engl J Med 2000;343(19):1350–4.

13. Hau P, Stupp R, Hegi ME. MGMT methylation status: the advent of stratified therapy in glioblastoma? Dis Markers 2007;23(1–2):97–104.

14. Tan WL, Huang WY, Yin J, et al. Can diffusion tensor imaging noninvasively detect IDH1 gene mutations in astrogliomas? A retrospective study of 112 cases. AJNR Am J Neuroradiol 2014;35:920–7.

15. Esmaeili M, Vettukattil R, Bathen TF. 2-Hydroxyglutarate as a magnetic resonance biomarker for glioma subtyping. Transl Oncol 2013;6(2):92–8.

16. Yan H, Parsons DW, Jin G, et al. IDH1 and IDH2 mutations in gliomas. N Engl J Med 2009;360(8): 765–73.

17. Juratli TA, Kirsch M, Robel K, et al. IDH mutations as an early and consistent marker in low-grade astrocytomas WHO grade II and their consecutive secondary high-grade gliomas. J Neurooncol 2012;108: 403–10.

18. SongTao Q, Lei Y, Si G, et al. IDH mutations predict longer survival and response to temozolomide in secondary glioblastoma. Cancer Sci 2012;103:269–73.

19. Andronesi OC, Kim GS, Gerstner E, et al. Detection of 2-hydroxyglutarate in IDH-mutated glioma patients by in vivo spectral-editing and 2D correlation magnetic resonance spectroscopy. Sci Transl Med 2012;4(116):116ra4.

20. Lazovic J, Soto H, Piccioni D, et al. Detection of 2-hydroxyglutaric acid in vivo by proton magnetic resonance spectroscopy in U87 glioma cells overexpressing isocitrate dehydrogenase-1 mutation. Neuro Oncol 2012;14(12):1465–72.

21. Aghi M, Gaviani P, Henson JW, et al. Magnetic resonance imaging characteristics predict epidermal growth factor receptor amplification status in glioblastoma. Clin Cancer Res 2005;11(24):8600–5.

22. Diehn M, Nardini C, Wanf DS, et al. Identification of noninvasive imaging surrogates for brain tumor gene-expression modules. Proc Natl Acad Sci U S A 2008;105(13):5213–8.

23. Ino Y, Betensky RA, Zlatescu MC, et al. Molecular subtypes of anaplastic oligodendroglioma: implications for patient management at diagnosis. Clin Cancer Res 2001;7:839–45.

24. Goze C, Rigau V, Gilbert L, et al. Lack of complete 1p19q deletion in a consecutive series of 12 WHO grade II glioma involving the insula: a marker of worse prognosis? J Neurooncol 2009;99:57–64.

25. Megyesi JF, Kachur E, Lee Dh, et al. Imaging correlation of molecular signatures in oligodendrogliomas. Clin Cancer Res 2004;10:4303–6.

26. van den Bent MJ, Looijenga LH, Langenberg K, et al. Chromosomal anomalies in oligodendroglial tumors are correlated to clinical features. Cancer 2003;97:1276–84.

27. Pelloski CE, Lin E, Zhang L, et al. Prognostic associations of activated mitogen-activated protein kinase and Akt pathways in glioblastoma. Clin Cancer Res 2006;12(13):3935–41.

28. Salvati M, Pichierri A, Piccirilli M, et al. Extent of tumoral removal and molecular markers in cerebral glioblastoma: a combined prognostic factors study in a surgical series of 105 patients. J Neurosurg 2012;117:204–11.

29. Nutt CL, Betensky RA, Brower MA, et al. YKL-40 is a differential diagnostic marker for histologic subtypes of high-grade gliomas. Clin Cancer Res 2005;11(6): 2258–64.

30. Philips HS, Kharbanda S, Chen R, et al. Molecular subclasses of high-grade glioma predict prognosis, delineate a pattern of disease progression, and resemble stages in neurogenesis. Cancer Cell 2006;9:157–73.

31. Barajas RF, Hodgson JG, Chang JS, et al. Glioblastoma multiforme regional genetic and cellular expression patterns: influence on anatomic and physiologic MR imaging. Radiology 2010;254(2):564–76.

32. Gutman DA, Cooper LA, Hwang SN, et al. MR imaging predictors of molecular profile and survival: multi-institutional study of the TCGA glioblastoma data set. Radiology 2013;267(2):560–9.

33. Jain R, Poisson L, Narang J, et al. Correlation of perfusion parameters with genes related to angiogenesis regulation in glioblastoma: a feasibility study. AJNR Am J Neuroradiol 2012;33:1343–8.

34. Carrillo JA, Lai A, Nghiemphu PL, et al. Relationship between tumor enhancement, edema, IDH1 mutation status, MGMT promoter methylation, and survival in glioblastoma. AJNR Am J Neuroradiol 2012;33:1349–55.

35. Elligson BM, Lai A, Haaris RJ, et al. Probabilistic radiographic atlas of glioblastoma phenotypes. AJNR Am J Neuroradiol 2013;34:533–40.

36. Etienne MC, Formento JL, Lebrun-Frenay C, et al. Epidermal growth factor receptor and labeling index are independent prognostic factor in glial tumor outcome. Clin Cancer Res 1998;4:2383–90.

37. Pope WB, Kim HJ, Huo J, et al. Recurrent glioblastoma multiforme: ADC histogram analysis predicts response to bevacizumab treatment. Radiology 2009;252(1):182–9.

38. Higano S, Yun X, Kumabe T, et al. Malignant astrocytic tumors: clinical importance of apparent diffusion coefficient in prediction of grade and prognosis. Radiology 2006;241:839–46.

39. Hegi ME, Liu L, Herman JG, et al. Correlation of O^6-methylguanine methyltransferase (MGMT) promoter methylation with clinical outcomes in glioblastoma and clinical strategies to modulate MGMT activity. J Clin Oncol 2008;26(25):4189–99.

40. Thon N, Kreth S, Kreth F. Personalized treatment strategies in glioblastoma: MGMT promoter methylation status. Onco Targets Ther 2013;6:1363–72.

41. Macdonald DR, Cascino T, Schold SJ, et al. Response criteria for phase II studies of supratentorial malignant glioma. J Clin Oncol 1990;8:1277–80.

42. Hygino da Cruz LC Jr, Rodriguez I, Domingues RC, et al. Pseudoprogression and pseudoresponse: imaging challenges in the assessment of posttreatment glioma. AJNR Am J Neuroradiol 2011;32(11): 1978–85.

43. Wen PY, Macdonald DR, Reardon DA, et al. Updated response assessment criteria for high-grade gliomas: response assessment in neuro-oncology working group. J Clin Oncol 2010;28:1963–72.

44. Brandsma D, Stalpers L, Taal W, et al. Clinical features, mechanisms, and management of pseudoprogression in malignant glioma. Lancet Oncol 2008;9:453–61.

45. de Wit MC, de Bruin HG, Eijkenboom W, et al. Immediate post-radiotherapy changes in malignant glioma can mimic tumor progression. Neurology 2004;63:535–7.

46. Cha J, Kim ST, Kim HJ, et al. Differentiation of tumor progression from pseudoprogression in patients with posttreatment glioblastoma using multiparametric histogram analysis. AJNR Am J Neuroradiol 2004;35(7):1309–17.

47. Essig M, Anzalone N, Combs SE, et al. MR Imaging of neoplastic central nervous system lesions: review and recommendations for current practice. AJNR Am J Neuroradiol 2012;33:803–17.

48. Singh AD, Easaw JC. Does neurologic deterioration help to differentiate between pseudoprogression and true disease progression in newly diagnosed glioblastoma multiforme? Curr Oncol 2012;19:295–8.

49. Chang DT, Ng RY, Siu DY, et al. Pseudoprogression of malignant glioma in chinese patients receiving concomitant chemoradiotherapy. Hong Kong Med J 2012;18:221–5.

50. Chaski C, Neyns B, Michotte A, et al. Pseudoprogression after radiotherapy with concurrent temozolomide for high-grade glioma: clinical observations and working recommendations. Surg Neurol 2009; 72:423–8.

51. Kong DS, Kim ST, Kim EH, et al. Diagnostic dilemma of pseudoprogression in the treatment of newly diagnosed glioblastomas: the role of assessing relative cerebral blood flow volume and oxygen-6-methylguanine-DNA methyltransferase promoter methylation status. AJNR Am J Neuroradiol 2011; 32:382–7.

52. Tsien C, Galbán CJ, Chenevert TL, et al. Parametric response map as an imaging biomarker to distinguish progression from pseudoprogression in high-grade glioma. J Clin Oncol 2010;28(13):2293–9.

53. Batchelor TT, Sorensen AG, di Tomaso E, et al. AZD2171, a pan-VEGF receptor tyrosine kinase inhibitor, normalizes tumor vasculature and alleviates edema in glioblastoma patients. Cancer Cell 2007;11:83–95.

54. Norden AD, Young GS, Setayesh K, et al. Bevacizumab for recurrent malignant gliomas: efficacy, toxicity, and patterns of recurrence. Neurology 2008;70:779–87.

55. Gupta A, Young RJ, Karimi S. Isolated diffusion restriction precedes the development of enhancing tumor in a subset of patients with glioblastoma. AJNR Am J Neuroradiol 2011;32:1301–6.

56. Mong S, Ellingson BM, Nghiemphu PL, et al. Persistent diffusion-restricted lesions in bevacizumab-treated malignant gliomas are associated with improved survival compared with matched controls. AJNR Am J Neuroradiol 2012;33:1763–70.

Imaging Genomics of Glioblastoma
State of the Art Bridge Between Genomics and Neuroradiology

Mohamed G. ElBanan, MD[a], Ahmed M. Amer, MD[a],
Pascal O. Zinn, MD, PhD[b], Rivka R. Colen, MD[a],*

KEYWORDS

- Glioblastoma • Imaging genomics • Genetic biomarkers • Radiogenomics • MGMT • IDH1
- EGFR • 1p/19q

KEY POINTS

- Glioblastoma constitutes a major challenge being the most aggressive and therapy-resistant malignant brain tumor.
- Personalized targeted treatment protocols are the focus of research as underlying genomic and molecular pathways are continuously being identified.
- Imaging genomics represents a new branch in science that links currently used imaging modalities to predict and correlate genomic profiles in glioblastoma tumors noninvasively.

GLIOBLASTOMA, OVERCOMING THE CHALLENGE

Glioblastoma (GBM; World Health Organization [WHO] grade IV astrocytoma) is the most common malignant primary brain tumor accounting for 45.2% of malignant primary brain tumors and for about 15.6% of all primary brain tumors.[1,2] The best current standard of care for GBM includes surgical resection followed by adjuvant local radiotherapy and systemic chemotherapy with temozolomide (TMZ).[3] Despite this aggressive multimodal treatment, the relative survival estimates for GBM are low; less than 5% of patients survived 5 years postdiagnosis.[2] The median overall survival duration for patients ranges from 12.2 to 15.9 months.[3,4] This is thought to be attributed to the highly infiltrative nature and the heterogeneity that GBM exhibits on molecular and genomic

levels, which lead to differences in individual treatment response and prognosis.[5] Approximately 90% of GBM tumors recur at the site of surgical resection because of invasive tumor cells that were left behind after resection and managed to avert the radiation therapy.[6,7]

Although considered one histologic group, high-grade gliomas exhibit genetic and molecular heterogeneity to the extent that the "one-size-fits all" model for treatment of GBM is no longer valid; thus, research is now being directed toward a more personalized approach in treatment of patients with GBM.[8,9] Establishment of this personalized treatment approach requires thorough understanding of the disease processes and underlying genomic and molecular pathways in the development of GBM along with identification of molecular features of the tumor that can predict response so that selection of patients who are

The authors have nothing to disclose.
[a] Department of Diagnostic Radiology, MD Anderson Cancer Center, University of Texas, 1400 Pressler Street, Houston, TX 77030, USA; [b] Department of Neurosurgery, Baylor College of Medicine, One Baylor Plaza, Houston, TX 77030, USA
* Corresponding author. Department of Radiology, MD Anderson Cancer Center, 1400 Pressler Street, Unit 1482, Room # FCT 16.5037, Houston, TX 77030.
E-mail address: rcolen@mdanderson.org

most likely to benefit from a particular treatment can be done.[6,10]

THE CANCER GENOME ATLAS AND GENETIC BIOMARKER IDENTIFICATION

Atkinson and colleagues[11] defined a biomarker as "a characteristic that is objectively measured and evaluated as an indicator of normal biological processes, pathogenic processes, or pharmacologic responses to a therapeutic intervention." Predictive biomarker compares the effect of a certain intervention for marker-positive versus marker-negative patients and predicts the differential effect of this intervention on the outcome (ie, indicate whether the patient is likely or unlikely to benefit from a specific drug or regimen). Prognostic biomarker provides information about the patient's probable long-term outcome (overall survival), either untreated or with a standard treatment.[12,13]

With the change in perception of cancer as a disease of genetic alterations, it has been concluded that the time interval between initial development of malignancy and the initial diagnosis and intervention allows multiple genetic alterations to accumulate.[14] Accordingly, most cancers now are associated with change in the expression of multiple genes and not just a single gene.[14,15] This diversity in genetic alterations renders identification of certain predictive and prognostic genetic biomarkers for GBM a great challenge. During the last decade, the use of microarray-based high-output sequencing methods that allowed simultaneous measurement of many genes and their products, and further quantitative analysis of the entire gene networks has deepened the insight of the processes underlying the development of GBM.[15]

Thorough analysis of the Cancer Genome Atlas (TCGA) data concluded that GBM harbors more than 60 genetic alterations including genetic mutations and chromosomal aberrations.[16–18] TCGA, which began in 2006, is a publicly available large-scale multi-institutional collaborative effort funded by the National Cancer Institute and the National Human Genome Research Institute to establish a better understanding of the molecular alterations of cancer associated with pathologic and radiologic features and response to therapy. GBM was the first cancer examined by TCGA. By identification of specific genetic mutations and microRNA expressions in nearly 500 tumor samples, TCGA-driven studies increased awareness of the significance of the genetic and molecular pathways in the pathogenesis of GBM and the identification of potential novel molecular

therapeutic targets.[6,16] Typical identified alterations included mutations affecting epidermal growth factor receptor (EGFR), tumor protein 53 (TP53), cyclin-dependent kinase inhibitor 2a, cyclin-dependent kinase 4, retinoblastoma 1, and phosphatase and tensin homolog (PTEN) genes and deletions on several chromosomal arms including 1p, 9p, 10p, 10q, 13q, 17p, 19q, and 22.[19] Some of the most significant GBM genetic biomarkers that have been identified include EGFR, O^6-methylguanine–DNA methyltransferase (MGMT)-promoter methylation, isocitrate dehydrogenase-1 (IDH1) mutation, 1p/19q co-deletion, and TP53 mutation.

MOLECULAR CLASSIFICATION OF GLIOBLASTOMA

This breakthrough in genetic identification paved the path for explaining the difference in survival and response to treatment among patients of GBM through replacing the classical classification of GBM with another molecularly based classification.[5,20] Classically, GBM was classified into primary GBM (which presents at the time of diagnosis as advanced cancers with no previous evidence of lower-grade lesion) and secondary GBM (those who have clinical, radiologic, or histopathologic evidence of malignant progression from a pre-existing lower-grade tumor).[21] Based on the differences in genetic aberrations and gene-expression, further classification of GBM identified four molecular subtypes: classical, mesenchymal, proneural, and neural, which are different in gene expression of EGFR, neurofibromin 1 (NF1), alpha-type platelet-derived growth factor receptor (PDGFRA/IDH1), and ERBB2, respectively.[5,6,22,23] Patients of the classical and mesenchymal subtypes of GBM showed significantly reduced mortality and improved survival with the use of aggressive concurrent chemoradiotherapy.[5] However, survival was not altered in the proneural subtype.[5] Molecular analysis of low-grade gliomas is currently underway, and it is anticipated that the data will provide similar molecular subclassification of low-grade gliomas.

PRINCIPAL GENETIC BIOMARKERS IN GLIOBLASTOMA

It is important that radiologists understand common genetic alterations. Certain imaging features of GBMs may correlate with certain gene expressions.[17] Imaging can provide a noninvasive technique to assess spatial and temporal changes in gene expression.[17] Understanding the molecular changes that occur in GBMs is helpful in explaining imaging findings in patients undergoing molecular targeted therapies.[17]

TMZ, an alkylating therapeutic agent used in treatment of GBM, acts through methylation of the O^6 position of guanine, thus triggering cytotoxicity and apoptosis of cancer cells.[24] Although O^6-alkylguanine is not the main lesion induced by alkylating agents, it seems to be the most cytotoxic one.[25] Cellular protection against the effect of such alkylating agents is mediated through the MGMT gene, located on chromosome 10q26, which encodes for a DNA repair protein (MGMT) that is responsible for removing the alkyl groups from the O^6 position of guanine.[24,26] Epigenetic slicing of MGMT gene by promoter methylation suppresses the gene expression, leading to reduction of the amount of MGMT protein and subsequently reduces the DNA repair capacity of the cell. This renders the cell more prone to the action of alkylating therapeutic agents because of the accumulation of O^6-alkylguanine, which subsequent to incorrect pairing with thymidine triggers mismatch repair, thereby inducing DNA damage and, eventually, cell death.[24,25] Cancer cells harboring higher levels of MGMT gene expression, which blunts the effect of alkylating therapeutic agents, are considered to be a treatment-resistant group and patients belonging to this group are less likely to benefit from treatment with alkylating agents.[24] Accordingly, MGMT-promoter methylation status is considered to be the strongest prognostic factor for outcome in patients with newly diagnosed GBM, and is a powerful predictor of response to alkylating chemotherapy.[24,25,27–29]

IDH enzyme plays an important role in the cellular protection against oxidative damage. IDH exists in three isoforms: IDH1, which is strictly cytosolic, and IDH2 and IDH3, which are located inside the mitochondria. These enzymes are responsible for conversion of isocitrate to α-ketoglutarate, a process that is accompanied by reduction of $NADP^+$ into NADPH (NAD^+ into NAD in case of IDH3).[30] Only mutations of IDH1 and IDH2 were found in high proportions in gliomas, with IDH1 mutations being much more common than IDH2.[18,31] In fact, gliomas are considered to be the most likely cancer type to show IDH gene mutation. Altered IDH1 enzyme found in tumor cells consists of dimer between the wild and the mutated enzymes.[32] Mutated IDH1 enzyme contributes to the pathogenesis of gliomas through different mechanisms, most prominent of which is reduction of α-ketoglutarate into 2-hydroxyglutarate resulting in inhibition of the activity of a variety of dioxygenases (eg, prolyl hydroxylase), with subsequent activation of hypoxia-inducible factor (HIF)-1α transcription factor and promotion of vascular endothelial growth factor (VEGF)–mediated angiogenesis, eventually leading to greater tumor growth.[32–35] IDH1 mutations have shown to be an independent prognostic biomarker in patients with glioma.[31,36] Patients with mutated IDH1 have shown a better prognosis (5-year survival rate, 93%) than those without the mutation (5-year survival rate, 51%) in terms of overall and progression-free survival.[37] Recent studies have showed that IDH1 mutation also can have a potential predictive role. In secondary patients with GBM, IDH1 mutations and MGMT-promoter methylation status were strongly correlated with increased overall survival.[38] Patients with both IDH1 mutation and MGMT-promoter methylation had the best response rate to TMZ (median progression-free survival, 13.4 months) followed by patients with IDH1 mutation alone (10.2 months), and finally patients with none of these genetic alterations had the worst response rate to TMZ (6.1 months).[38] Because of its value as a biomarker, IDH1 mutation status is likely to result in revisions to the current WHO classification scheme for GBM.[39]

VEGF is one of the most critical proangiogenic factors that play an integral role in brain angiogenesis.[40] The VEGF gene contains a hypoxia-responsive element within its promoter that binds HIF-1α, thereby activating transcription. VEGF is responsible for directing nearby angiogenesis. It was proved that inhibition of this HIF/VEGF pathway suppresses tumor growth experimentally. Once expressed and secreted, extracellular VEGF binds to its high-affinity receptors, VEGFR-1 and VEGFR-2, which are upregulated on endothelial cells of high-grade gliomas, but not present in normal brain. Receptor activation then leads to angiogenesis in regions adjacent to tumor cells leading to the high vascularity noted in GBM tumors.[40]

EGFR is a transmembrane tyrosine kinase receptor.[41] EGFR gene overexpression is found in more than 50% of patients with GBM, and EGFR amplification and mutation are strongly associated with GBM transformation.[41] EGFR normally exists as a monomer that transforms into homodimers on binding to EGF with consequent kinase activation and autophosphorylation.[42] This leads to activation and phosphorylation of EGFR variant III (EGFRvIII).[41–43] EGFRvIII is found in a subgroup of patients (20%–40%) who undergo EGFR gene rearrangements and it lacks the extracellular domain.[44] Activated EGFR stimulates EGFRvIII resulting in activation of downstream signaling pathways, such as receptor tyrosine kinase, phosphoinositide 3-kinase, and PTEN eventually leading to augmentation of tumor angiogenesis, cell proliferation, and cell survival.[41,43] Heimberger and colleagues[45] found that EGFRvIII has a negative prognostic value in patients surviving more than 1 year. Therapies have been developed that are directed at the overexpressed *EGFR* in GBM.[46] Multiple studies demonstrate how *EGFR* status affects GBM response to treatment.[47,48] Mellinghoff and colleagues[48] demonstrated that GBMs characterized by coexpression of *EGFRvIII* and *PTEN* yield the best response to therapy using *EGFR* inhibitors. Accordingly, it might become important to determine the *EGFR* status of patients with GBM before therapy to stratify patients into clinical trials and also to predict which group of patients would benefit most of the treatment.

1p/19q loss of heterozygosity (LOH) is the genetic hallmark of oligodendrogliomas and anaplastic oligodendrogliomas (WHO grades II and III, respectively). It is found in 40% to 90% of the patients with oligodendrogliomas and it is linked to longer survival. It also predicts a favorable response to chemotherapy and radiotherapy.[49–51] However, in GBM, the prognostic value of these alterations is still debatable.[51] In GBM, 1p/19q codeletion is primarily associated with GBM with oligodendroglial component (GB-O). The percentage of GB-O cases in GBM population ranges from 4.2% to 27.2%.[52–54] The presence of 1p/19q codeletion was observed in 22% to 28% of GB-O patients,[55] whereas LOH 1p was observed in 24% of patients with GBM and LOH 19q was detected in 5% to 33% of patients with GBM.[51,55] However, the impact of LOH 1p on survival is unclear and the results of previous studies are inconsistent. Homma and colleagues[56] studied 209 patients with GBM. A total of 21% of these patients were LOH 1p and/or 19q positive. LOH 1p patients showed longer survival than patients without LOH 1p (13.2 ± 10.8 vs 9.6 ± 7.4 months; $P = .0536$). After age and gender adjustment, multivariate analysis showed longer survival in patients with LOH 1p (hazard ratio, 0.7; 95% confidence interval, 0.5–1.0).

BASICS OF IMAGING OF GLIOBLASTOMA
Histopathologic Imaging

Despite the diversity of appearances, the single most important pathologic characteristic of GBM that discriminates it from lower-grade astrocytomas is the presence of central necrosis (**Fig. 1**).[57] GBM is also characterized by the presence of significant necrosis, microvascular proliferation, and invasion in addition to other feature of anaplastic astrocytomas including cellularity, nuclear atypia, and mitotic activity.[6] GBM is also

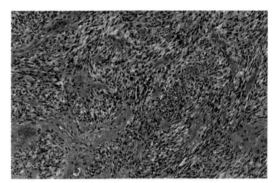

Fig. 1. Histopathologic image of cerebral glioblastoma. (*From* Berkeley Morphometric Visualization and Quantification from H&E sections, sponsored by the Lawrence Berkeley National Laboratory. Available at: http://tcga.lbl.gov/biosig/tcgadownload.do. Accessed March 1, 2014.)

characterized by "pseudopalisading," in which areas of viable neoplastic cells form an irregular border surrounding areas of necrotic debris.[57] This characteristic pathology reflects the basis of the imaging findings of GBM. Out of all available imaging modalities, MR imaging stands as the imaging modality of choice for diagnosis, pretreatment surgical planning, and posttreatment monitoring of GBM.[58]

MR Imaging

MR imaging techniques of GBM are shown in **Table 1**. Classically, GBM is described on MR imaging as a thick irregular ring of heterogeneous enhancement surrounding a central nonenhancing core of necrosis and surrounded by an area of peritumoral hyperintensity, the latter more evident on FLAIR and T2-weighted sequences, representing the region of tumor infiltration and vasogenic edema (**Fig. 2**).[58,59] In fact, neoplastic cells extend beyond the detected imaging changes and in areas of normal-appearing white matter.[59]

Advanced imaging techniques including magnetic resonance (MR) diffusion, perfusion, and spectroscopy enhance the anatomic data

Table 1 MR imaging techniques for glioblastoma	
Conventional Techniques	**Advanced Techniques**
T1-weighted imaging	MR perfusion imaging
T2-weighted imaging	MR spectroscopy imaging
FLAIR imaging sequence	MR diffusion-weighted imaging

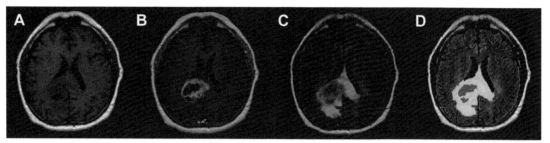

Fig. 2. MR imaging features of adult GBM. (*A*) Precontrast T1 sequence. (*B*) Postcontrast T1 sequence. (*C*) FLAIR sequence. (*D*) Segmented image of a typical GBM tumor as shown by three-dimensional Slicer software (www. slicer.org), where *red* represents central necrosis, *yellow* represents the contrast-enhancing portion of the tumor, and *blue* represents the surrounding abnormal signal intensity corresponding to edema and invasion.

supplied by conventional MR imaging and provide physiologic information, such as cellularity, microperfusion, and metabolism, respectively.[58,60] Diffusion-weighted imaging measures the diffusion of water molecules in a voxel. In GBM, diffusion is restricted in areas with a high density of cell packing/tumor cells and high nuclear-to-cytoplasm ratios (**Fig. 3**).[61] Findings on diffusion-weighted echoplanar MR images can be used to distinguish nonenhancing tumor from peritumoral edema when these abnormalities are located in white matter and to differentiate various components of tumor (enhancing, nonenhancing, cystic, or necrotic).[62] MR perfusion imaging assesses angiogenesis and blood-brain barrier permeability, which can be predictive of the tumor grade and higher malignant histology (**Fig. 4**).[63,64] Moreover, as novel therapeutic agents targeting angiogenesis in brain tumors are being developed, the role of perfusion imaging as an important tool for diagnosis and follow-up becomes more evident.[65] Lastly, MR spectroscopy measures the changes in metabolites in the region of interest based on chemical information obtained from the MR signal.[66]

These characteristic imaging findings correspond to the unique pathologic features that GBM exhibits.[57] Interestingly, regional genetic and cellular expression patterns of GBM were found to influence the anatomic and physiologic MR imaging.[67] This significant relationship plays an important role in the potential value of the use of MR imaging as a noninvasive surrogate for identification of these genetic alterations.

IMAGING GENOMICS: A NEW DIMENSION FOR DIAGNOSTIC IMAGING

Genetic profiling of GBM as the basis of the personalized treatment approach necessitates obtaining tissue specimens from the tumor with subsequent histologic and immunohistochemical analysis. Accordingly, obtained results depend on the surgical procurement of the specimen, the part of the tumor from which this specimen biopsy was obtained, and the analysis methods used for genetic identification.[15] Because of the heterogeneity of genetic expression that GBM exhibits in between the different tumor components, the results obtained from the tumor sample only reflect

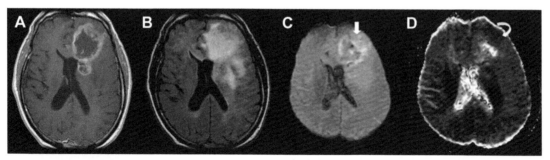

Fig. 3. Diffusion-weighted imaging MR image of a patient with GBM. (*A*) Postcontrast T1-weighted image shows well-defined ring-enhancing lesion in the deep left temporoparietal region with subependymal extension. (*B*) FLAIR sequence shows peritumoral edema and invasion. The mass demonstrates restricted diffusion evident by hyperintensity (*straight arrow*) on (*C*) diffusion-weighted MR image with drop of signal on the (*D*) ADC map (*curved arrow*).

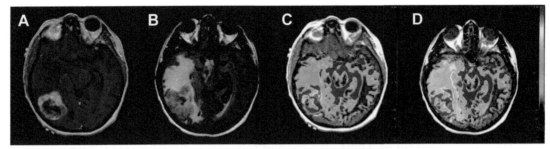

Fig. 4. MR image DSC perfusion of GBM. Thick, irregularly enhancing GBM on postcontrast T1-weighted image (*A*) with perilesional edema and cell infiltration on (*B*) T2/FLAIR images. (*C, D*) Perfusion maps superimposed on the T1 postgadolinium and FLAIR sequences, respectively, demonstrating increased relative cerebral blood volume values corresponding to the ring-enhancing area. Note the intermediate relative cerebral blood volume value over the edema and cell infiltration region.

the genetic alterations in this part of the tumor and not the tumor as a whole, leading to inaccurate results.[5,15] Moreover, this technique, being invasive, carries a lot of risks and drawbacks. It involves the risk of pain, infection, hemorrhage, and the complications associated with any surgical procedure. Also it is not always possible to obtain a sample of the tumor especially if it is located in a risky or inaccessible location of the brain tissue. It became clear that this technique for genetic profiling is unsuitable for routine use for every patient with GBM.[15] Consequently, the need for a safer, noninvasive, accurate, and comprehensive alternate for genetic identification has drawn attention to other techniques that can be routinely used with minimal risks and complications. MR imaging of the brain has been demonstrated to have a strong potential as a surrogate for GBM genetic profiling.[58] This interconnection between radiologic imaging and genomics is described by the term "imaging genomics."

Imaging genomics is a new field in science that bidirectionally links specific imaging traits, better called radiophenotypes, to genomic profiles thus providing a novel bridge between two entities, namely imaging and genomics, that until recently had not been well-elucidated.[15,58] In imaging genomics imaging traits obtained from routine imaging studies are being associated with certain gene expression patterns so these traits can be used as a noninvasive surrogate for providing molecular information about the tumor's genetic profiles.[15] This may further strengthen the integration of multiple data (Fig. 5).

Great interest has been shown in the use of MR imaging for noninvasive genetic profiling of patients with GBM.[68–73] Aside from being noninvasive, the routine use of MR imaging in the diagnosis, pretreatment planning, and posttreatment follow-up empowers the value of MR imaging as an important tool for genetic profiling.

Moreover, it was demonstrated that the intratumoral imaging heterogeneity could also reflect the associated intratumoral genetic heterogeneity in GBM and so MR imaging can give a comprehensive picture of genetic expression of the tumor as a whole.[15,22] Using GBM samples obtained by image-guided stereotactic biopsies, Van Meter and colleagues[74] revealed differences in the expression of 623 genes between samples obtained from the enhancing core and those obtained from the periphery of tumors. Furthermore, with the introduction of advanced MR imaging sequences, MR imaging captures multidimensional, in vivo portraits of GBMs because of its ability to extract structural, compositional, physiologic, and functional information.[68]

VISUALLY ACCESSIBLE REMBRANDT IMAGES

For these imaging traits to be an effective applicable predictor of the underlying genetic profile,

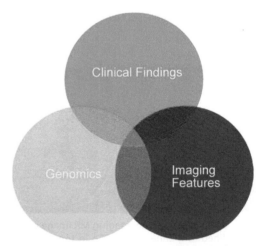

Fig. 5. Schematic drawing depicts the basic domains of imaging genomics. Integration of multidimensional data.

they should be assessed in a standardized reproducible fashion that is independent of the interpreting radiologist and can be validated by multiple observers. A barrier against this was the absence of controlled terminologies that describe the pathologic findings. This lack of consistency meant that results of individual studies might remain isolated because results are often not directly comparable with one another. Collaborative effort for defining a rich set of qualitative and quantitative imaging biomarkers led to the emergence of the Visually Accessible Rembrandt Images (VASARI) GBM feature set.[75,76] The goal of VASARI is to develop reproducible methods to classify MR imaging of glioma tumors and provide linkages between those images, histology, and genetic data obtained from brain cancer specimens. This comprehensive feature set consists of 26 observations (grouped under four categories) familiar to neuroradiologists to describe the morphology of brain tumors on routine contrast-enhanced MR imaging. Features included tumor location, side of lesion center, eloquent brain, enhancing proportion, necrosis proportion, multifocality, and multicentricity and others.[75] Other quantitative features, which were not included in the VASARI feature set, including necrosis volume, enhancing tumor volume, and surrounding edema volume, are also being investigated.[77] Using a controlled set of imaging features has been shown statistically to improve prediction of survival in patients with GBM over clinical features alone.[78]

QUALITATIVE MR IMAGING GENOMICS OF GLIOBLASTOMA

The first MR imaging–based neuroimaging genetics study was reported by Bookheimer and colleagues[79] in 2000 as a test of the effect of variation within the apolipoprotein E gene, associated with risk for Alzheimer disease, on brain activity during memory tasks measured by functional MR imaging in healthy older adults with intact cognition.[80] During the following years, because of the successful identification of predictive and prognostic molecular biomarkers of GBM and their incorporation into the daily clinical practice, the concept of imaging genomics was adopted by neuroradiologists and researchers and accordingly multiple neuroimaging genomics studies were conducted to extract neuroimaging signatures that can be used as a noninvasive predictor of the molecular biomarkers status in patients with GBM.

Tumor enhancement characteristics and their correlation with certain genetic expressions in GBM has been the focus of many researchers. A study by Barajas and colleagues[67] discovered that 359 genes were significantly overexpressed at least two-fold on average in contrast-enhancing samples relative to peritumoral nonenhancing samples and conversely, 684 probe sets were significantly overexpressed at least two-fold on average in peritumoral nonenhancing samples relative to enhancing samples. Those 359 genes that were overexpressed in contrast-enhancing samples tended to be associated with regulation of mitosis, angiogenesis, and apoptosis.[67] Diehn and colleagues[68] described the correlation between contrast-enhanced radiophenotype and the genetic expression of genes involved in tumor hypoxia and angiogenesis (eg, VEGF [$P = .012$]) and found that EGFR overexpression was associated with a high ratio of contrast enhancement to necrosis within the same tumor ($P = .019$). Pope and colleagues[69] showed that interleukin-8 and VEGF were overexpressed in completely enhancing tumors when compared with incompletely enhancing ones. Moreover, tumors associated with low TP53 gene expression (<50% as shown by immunohistochemical staining) demonstrated heterogeneous enhancement and ill-defined borders on postcontrast T1-weighted images, whereas those with higher TP53 gene expression demonstrated well-defined borders and typical ring enhancement pattern on postcontrast T1-weighted images.[81] IDH1 mutation proved to be associated with non–contrast-enhancing tumors in a study by Carrillo and colleagues[82] in which they showed that imaging features including larger tumor size and non–contrast-enhancing tumors could be used to determine IDH1 mutational status with 97.5% accuracy but can poorly predict the MGMT promoter methylation status. However, Drabycz and colleagues[83] found that ring enhancement was associated with unmethylated MGMT-promoter status ($P = .006$). A multi-institutional study of the TCGA GBM data set by Gutman and colleagues[76] stated that the proneural subtype was associated significantly with low levels of contrast enhancement (contrast enhancement <5%) than other tumor types ($P<.01$) and that the mesenchymal subtype was noted to show consistently fewer nonenhancements than the other tumor subtypes ($P<.01$).

Other imaging features in patients with GBM were also investigated for possible correlation with underlying genetic expressions. Diehn and colleagues[68] in their previously mentioned study identified correlation between the mass effect radiophenotype and the proliferation gene-expression signature ($P = .0017$). Regarding tumor location, Carrillo and colleagues[82] in their study stated that *IDH1* mutation is most commonly seen in GBM tumors located in the frontal lobe. Ellingson and colleagues[84] described that *MGMT* methylated tumors with the *IDH1* mutation tended to occur in the left frontal lobe, whereas *EGFR* amplified and *EGFR* variant 3–expressing tumors occurred most frequently in the left temporal lobe, a region that was associated with favorable response to radiochemotherapy and increased survival. In another study, Ellingson and colleagues[85] found that GBM tumors with unmethylated *MGMT*-promoter tend to localize in the right cerebral hemisphere. Eoli and colleagues[86] found that patterns of enhancement and tumor location could allow a preoperative differentiation between primary and secondary GBM where primary GBM, which are large lesions with ring enhancement and large necrotic cysts, are most frequently located in the temporal lobe, and secondary GBM, which are more homogeneously enhancing lesions, are mainly located in the frontal lobes.

QUANTITATIVE MR IMAGING GENOMICS OF GLIOBLASTOMA

Although most of the studies discussed examined qualitative MR imaging features of GBM, others stressed the significance of the quantitative imaging features. In 2011, Zinn and colleagues[77] published the first comprehensive radiogenomic analysis using quantitative MR imaging volumetrics and large-scale gene and microRNA expression profiling in GBM. This study examined gene-expression analysis in high versus low FLAIR groups and revealed top genes and microRNAs. The top upregulated gene identified in the high FLAIR was *PERIOSTIN*, a gene that was proved to be involved in invasion and mesenchymal transition in vitro (Fig. 6).[77,87] Zinn and colleagues[73] also proposed the volume-age-Karnofsky classification system in which tumors were categorized based on the total volume of tumor on preoperative MR imaging, the patient's age, and the patient's Karnofsky performance score. GBM *MGMT*-promoter methylation status and *TP53* expression were correlation with patients' survival differences in this study.[73]

Naeini and colleagues[70] found that the volume of contrast enhancement, volume of central necrosis, combined volume of contrast enhancement and central necrosis, and the ratio of T2/FLAIR to contrast enhancement and necrosis were significantly different in mesenchymal molecular subtype compared with other molecular subtypes of GBM ($P<.05$). They stated that the volume ratio of T2 hyperintensity to contrast enhancement and central necrosis was significantly lower in mesenchymal versus nonmesenchymal GBM and was actually a significant predictor of the mesenchymal subtype ($P<.0001$).[70] Ellingson and colleagues[85] described a volumetric difference between GBM tumors harboring *MGMT*-promoter methylation and those who lack it. They observed a significant difference in T2/FLAIR hyperintense volume between *MGMT*

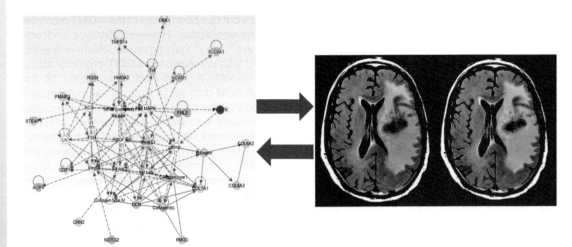

Fig. 6. Ingenuity pathway analysis in the high edema and invasion radiophenotype patient group. The gene network showing the top upregulated mRNAs in the high versus low FLAIR volume groups. (*From* Zinn PO, Mahajan B, Sathyan P, et al. Radiogenomic mapping of edema/cellular invasion MR imaging-phenotypes in glioblastoma multiforme. PLoS One 2011;6(10):e25451.)

methylated and unmethylated tumors where *MGMT*-promoter methylated tumors have less edema compared with *MGMT* unmethylated tumors (*P* = .0092).

ADVANCED MR IMAGING GENOMICS OF GLIOBLASTOMA

With the incorporation of the advanced MR imaging techniques into the routine clinical practice, researchers started investigating the correlation between the parameters obtained from these advanced techniques and underlying differences in genetic expression patterns. Maia and colleagues[72] confirmed the correlation of relative cerebral blood volume (rCBV) measurements, *VEGF* expression, and histopathologic grade in nonenhancing gliomas. Barajas and colleagues[67] found correlation between rCBV and the histopathologic features of gliomas aggressiveness. They found that contrast-enhancing regions had rCBV values that were significantly elevated compared with those in peritumoral nonenhancing regions and those contrast-enhancing regions had significant upregulation of genes associated with infiltrative processes, hypoxia, and angiogenesis (*P*<.01).[67] Jain and colleagues[71] stated that rCBV measurements in GBM tumors showed statistically significant correlation with overall survival independent of the molecular subclassification systems.[5] Hirai and colleagues[88] also showed that high-grade gliomas with higher rCBV (>2.3) had significantly lower 2-year overall survival compared with those with lower rCBV. Colen and colleagues[89] uncovered genes and the corresponding molecules

that were significantly associated with invasion and angiogenesis in patients with high CBV (**Fig. 7**).

Pope and colleagues[90] discussed the use of MR imaging to detect metabolites associated with specific genetic mutation in GBM. Using MR spectroscopy they were able to detect multiple metabolites, in particular 2-hydroxyglutarate, which were produced in GBM tumors harboring *IDH1* mutation.[90] Other researchers were also able to detect 2-hydroxyglutarate in *IDH1* mutant GBM using MR spectroscopy, which empowers the potential for further research on using these advance MR techniques as noninvasive predictors of genetic expression profiles.[91,92]

Regarding diffusion MR imaging, Moon and colleagues[93] found that in preoperative imaging apparent diffusion coefficient ratio was significantly higher, and the fractional anisotropy and fractional anisotropy ratios were significantly lower in the methylated group than in the unmethylated group. Pope and colleagues[94] concluded in their study that GBM tumors with high apparent diffusion coefficient showed greater extracellular matrix protein gene expression compared with low apparent diffusion coefficient GBM, although the underlying link between them is still unclear and the relationship between this molecule and the proinvasive phenotype is still to be further investigated. Colen and colleagues studied the correlations between apparent diffusion coefficient values and genomic data. They identified the top upregulated gene networks associated with proliferation and increased tumor aggressiveness (**Fig. 8**).[95]

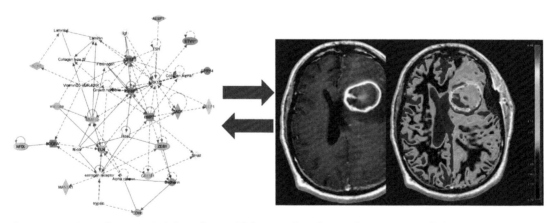

Fig. 7. Ingenuity pathway analysis in patients with increased perfusion. The gene network demonstrating the top upregulated mRNAs in patients with high versus low relative cerebral blood volume values. (*From* Colen R, TCGA Phenotype Group, Zinn P. Perfusion imaging genomic mapping uncovers potential genomic targets involved in angiogenesis and invasion. Poster presented at Society for Neuro-Oncology. San Francisco, November 21–24, 2013.)

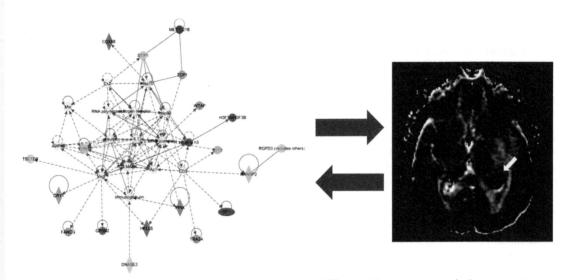

Fig. 8. Ingenuity pathway analysis in patients with restricted diffusion. The gene network demonstrating top upregulated mRNAs in patients with low versus high ADC values. *Arrow* pointing to a region of the tumor showing restricted diffusion on ADC map. (*From* Thomas G, Wang J, Mahmood Z, et al. Diffusion imaging genomic mapping identifies genomic targets involved in invasion and poor prognosis. Poster presented at American Society of Neuroradiology. Montreal, Canada, May 17–22, 2014.)

SUMMARY

Imaging genomics is a relatively new branch in clinical science and is expected to play an important role as an integral part of the diagnosis, preoperative planning, and postoperative follow-up of patients with GBM. Being bidirectional, imaging genomics has the potential to reveal novel genetic and molecular targets for new therapies that might improve the well-being and overall survival of patients with GBM. Further research is needed and the introduction of new neuroimaging techniques into the routine patient care further extends the possibilities for imaging genomics. Further research should be directed toward incorporation of multiple quantitative and qualitative imaging parameters to create unique imaging signatures that can predict specific genetic profiles with high degree of accuracy and reliability, which will accordingly pave the way for noninvasive genomic identification of GBM tumors.

REFERENCES

1. Louis DN, Ohgaki H, Wiestler OD, et al. The 2007 WHO classification of tumours of the central nervous system. Acta Neuropathol 2007;114(2):97–109.
2. Ostrom QT, Gittleman H, Farah P, et al. CBTRUS statistical report: primary brain and central nervous system tumors diagnosed in the United States in 2006-2010. Neuro Oncol 2013;15(Suppl 2):ii1–56.
3. Stupp R, Mason WP, van den Bent MJ, et al. Radiotherapy plus concomitant and adjuvant temozolomide for glioblastoma. N Engl J Med 2005;352(10):987–96.
4. Stupp R, Hegi ME, Mason WP, et al. Effects of radiotherapy with concomitant and adjuvant temozolomide versus radiotherapy alone on survival in glioblastoma in a randomised phase III study: 5-year analysis of the EORTC-NCIC trial. Lancet Oncol 2009;10(5):459–66.
5. Verhaak RG, Hoadley KA, Purdom E, et al. Integrated genomic analysis identifies clinically relevant subtypes of glioblastoma characterized by abnormalities in PDGFRA, IDH1, EGFR, and NF1. Cancer Cell 2010;17(1):98–110.
6. Agnihotri S, Burrell KE, Wolf A, et al. Glioblastoma, a brief review of history, molecular genetics, animal models and novel therapeutic strategies. Arch Immunol Ther Exp (Warsz) 2013;61(1):25–41.
7. Berens ME, Giese A. "…those left behind." Biology and oncology of invasive glioma cells. Neoplasia 1999;1(3):208–19.
8. Corwin D, Holdsworth C, Rockne RC, et al. Toward patient-specific, biologically optimized radiation therapy plans for the treatment of glioblastoma. PLoS One 2013;8(11):e79115.
9. Mischel PS, Shai R, Shi T, et al. Identification of molecular subtypes of glioblastoma by gene expression profiling. Oncogene 2003;22(15):2361–73.
10. Weller M, Stupp R, Hegi M, et al. Individualized targeted therapy for glioblastoma: fact or fiction? Cancer J 2012;18(1):40–4.
11. Biomarkers Definitions Working Group. Biomarkers and surrogate endpoints: preferred definitions and conceptual framework. Clin Pharmacol Ther 2001; 69(3):89–95.

12. Težak Ž, Kondratovich MV, Mansfield E. US FDA and personalized medicine: in vitro diagnostic regulatory perspective. Per Med 2010;7(5):517–30.

13. Simon R. Clinical trial designs for evaluating the medical utility of prognostic and predictive biomarkers in oncology. Per Med 2010;7(1):33–47.

14. Alizadeh AA, Staudt LM. Genomic-scale gene expression profiling of normal and malignant immune cells. Curr Opin Immunol 2000;12(2):219–25.

15. Rutman AM, Kuo MD. Radiogenomics: creating a link between molecular diagnostics and diagnostic imaging. Eur J Radiol 2009;70(2):232–41.

16. Cancer Genome Atlas Research Network. Comprehensive genomic characterization defines human glioblastoma genes and core pathways. Nature 2008;455(7216):1061–8.

17. Belden CJ, Valdes PA, Ran C, et al. Genetics of glioblastoma: a window into its imaging and histopathologic variability. Radiographics 2011;31(6):1717–40.

18. Parsons DW, Jones S, Zhang X, et al. An integrated genomic analysis of human glioblastoma multiforme. Science 2008;321(5897):1807–12.

19. Schmidt MC, Antweiler S, Urban N, et al. Impact of genotype and morphology on the prognosis of glioblastoma. J Neuropathol Exp Neurol 2002;61(4):321–8.

20. Phillips HS, Kharbanda S, Chen R, et al. Molecular subclasses of high-grade glioma predict prognosis, delineate a pattern of disease progression, and resemble stages in neurogenesis. Cancer Cell 2006;9(3):157–73.

21. Ohgaki H, Kleihues P. The definition of primary and secondary glioblastoma. Clin Cancer Res 2013;19(4):764–72.

22. Liang Y, Diehn M, Watson N, et al. Gene expression profiling reveals molecularly and clinically distinct subtypes of glioblastoma multiforme. Proc Natl Acad Sci U S A 2005;102(16):5814–9.

23. Colman H, Aldape K. Molecular predictors in glioblastoma: toward personalized therapy. Arch Neurol 2008;65(7):877–83.

24. Hegi ME, Diserens AC, Gorlia T, et al. MGMT gene silencing and benefit from temozolomide in glioblastoma. N Engl J Med 2005;352(10):997–1003.

25. Weller M, Stupp R, Reifenberger G, et al. MGMT promoter methylation in malignant gliomas: ready for personalized medicine? Nat Rev Neurol 2010;6(1):39–51.

26. Pegg AE. Repair of O(6)-alkylguanine by alkyltransferases. Mutat Res 2000;462(2–3):83–100.

27. Esteller M, Garcia-Foncillas J, Andion E, et al. Inactivation of the DNA-repair gene MGMT and the clinical response of gliomas to alkylating agents. N Engl J Med 2000;343(19):1350–4.

28. Hegi ME, Diserens AC, Godard S, et al. Clinical trial substantiates the predictive value of O-6-methylguanine-DNA methyltransferase promoter methylation in glioblastoma patients treated with temozolomide. Clin Cancer Res 2004;10(6):1871–4.

29. Weller M, Felsberg J, Hartmann C, et al. Molecular predictors of progression-free and overall survival in patients with newly diagnosed glioblastoma: a prospective translational study of the German Glioma Network. J Clin Oncol 2009;27(34):5743–50.

30. Frezza C, Tennant DA, Gottlieb E. IDH1 mutations in gliomas: when an enzyme loses its grip. Cancer Cell 2010;17(1):7–9.

31. Yan H, Parsons DW, Jin G, et al. IDH1 and IDH2 mutations in gliomas. N Engl J Med 2009;360(8):765–73.

32. Hodges TR, Choi BD, Bigner DD, et al. Isocitrate dehydrogenase 1: what it means to the neurosurgeon: a review. J Neurosurg 2013;118(6):1176–80.

33. Dang L, White DW, Gross S, et al. Cancer-associated IDH1 mutations produce 2-hydroxyglutarate. Nature 2009;462(7274):739–U752.

34. Zhao S, Lin Y, Xu W, et al. Glioma-derived mutations in IDH1 dominantly inhibit IDH1 catalytic activity and induce HIF-1alpha. Science 2009;324(5924):261–5.

35. King A, Selak MA, Gottlieb E. Succinate dehydrogenase and fumarate hydratase: linking mitochondrial dysfunction and cancer. Oncogene 2006;25(34):4675–82.

36. Sanson M, Marie Y, Paris S, et al. Isocitrate dehydrogenase 1 codon 132 mutation is an important prognostic biomarker in gliomas. J Clin Oncol 2009;27(25):4150–4.

37. van den Bent MJ, Dubbink HJ, Marie Y, et al. IDH1 and IDH2 mutations are prognostic but not predictive for outcome in anaplastic oligodendroglial tumors: a report of the European Organization for Research and Treatment of Cancer Brain Tumor Group. Clin Cancer Res 2010;16(5):1597–604.

38. SongTao Q, Lei Y, Si G, et al. IDH mutations predict longer survival and response to temozolomide in secondary glioblastoma. Cancer Sci 2012;103(2):269–73.

39. von Deimling A, Korshunov A, Hartmann C. The next generation of glioma biomarkers: MGMT methylation, BRAF fusions and IDH1 mutations. Brain Pathol 2011;21(1):74–87.

40. Plate KH. Mechanisms of angiogenesis in the brain. J Neuropathol Exp Neurol 1999;58(4):313–20.

41. Fan QW, Cheng CK, Gustafson WC, et al. EGFR phosphorylates tumor-derived EGFRvIII driving STAT3/5 and progression in glioblastoma. Cancer Cell 2013;24(4):438–49.

42. Jura N, Endres NF, Engel K, et al. Mechanism for activation of the EGF receptor catalytic domain by the juxtamembrane segment. Cell 2009;137(7):1293–307.

43. Zadeh G, Bhat KP, Aldape K. EGFR and EGFRvIII in glioblastoma: partners in crime. Cancer Cell 2013; 24(4):403–4.

44. Emlet DR, Gupta P, Holgado-Madruga M, et al. Targeting a glioblastoma cancer stem cell population defined by EGF receptor variant III. Cancer Res 2014;74:1238–49.

45. Heimberger AB, Hlatky R, Suki D, et al. Prognostic effect of epidermal growth factor receptor and EGFRvIII in glioblastoma multiforme patients. Clin Cancer Res 2005;11(4):1462–6.

46. Yang RY, Yang KS, Pike LJ, et al. Targeting the dimerization of epidermal growth factor receptors with small-molecule inhibitors. Chem Biol Drug Des 2010;76(1):1–9.

47. Wachsberger PR, Lawrence RY, Liu Y, et al. Epidermal growth factor receptor (EGFR) mutation status and Rad51 determine the response of glioblastoma (GBM) to multimodality therapy with cetuximab, temozolomide and radiation. Front Oncol 2013;3:13.

48. Mellinghoff IK, Wang MY, Vivanco I, et al. Molecular determinants of the response of glioblastomas to EGFR kinase inhibitors. N Engl J Med 2005; 353(19):2012–24.

49. Gladson CL, Prayson RA, Liu WM. The pathobiology of glioma tumors. Annu Rev Pathol 2010;5:33–50.

50. Nutt CL. Molecular genetics of oligodendrogliomas: a model for improved clinical management in the field of neurooncology. Neurosurg Focus 2005; 19(5):E2.

51. Kaneshiro D, Kobayashi T, Chao ST, et al. Chromosome 1p and 19q deletions in glioblastoma multiforme. Appl Immunohistochem Mol Morphol 2009; 17(6):512–6.

52. Pinto LW, Araújo MB, Vettore AL, et al. Glioblastomas: correlation between oligodendroglial components, genetic abnormalities, and prognosis. Virchows Arch 2008;452(5):481–90.

53. Salvati M, Formichella AI, D'Elia A, et al. Cerebral glioblastoma with oligodendrogliomal component: analysis of 36 cases. J Neurooncol 2009;94(1): 129–34.

54. Vordermark D, Ruprecht K, Rieckmann P, et al. Glioblastoma multiforme with oligodendroglial component (GBMO): favorable outcome after postoperative radiotherapy and chemotherapy with nimustine (ACNU) and teniposide (VM26). BMC Cancer 2006;6:247.

55. Jesionek-Kupnicka D, Szybka M, Potemski P, et al. Association of loss of heterozygosity with shorter survival in primary glioblastoma patients. Pol J Pathol 2013;64(4):268–75.

56. Homma T, Fukushima T, Vaccarella S, et al. Correlation among pathology, genotype, and patient outcomes in glioblastoma. J Neuropathol Exp Neurol 2006;65(9):846–54.

57. Rees JH, Smirniotopoulos JG, Jones RV, et al. Glioblastoma multiforme: radiologic-pathologic correlation. Radiographics 1996;16(6):1413–38.

58. Zinn PO, Colen RR. Imaging genomic mapping in glioblastoma. Neurosurgery 2013;60(Suppl 1):126–30.

59. Osborn AG, Salzman KL, Barkovich AJ. Diagnostic imaging: brain. Amirsys; 2010.

60. Al-Okaili RN, Krejza J, Wang S, et al. Advanced MR imaging techniques in the diagnosis of intraaxial brain tumors in adults. Radiographics 2006; 26(Suppl 1):S173–89.

61. Le Bihan D, Turner R, Douek P, et al. Diffusion MR imaging: clinical applications. AJR Am J Roentgenol 1992;159(3):591–9.

62. Tien RD, Felsberg GJ, Friedman H, et al. MR imaging of high-grade cerebral gliomas: value of diffusion-weighted echoplanar pulse sequences. AJR Am J Roentgenol 1994;162(3):671–7.

63. Le Bihan D. Theoretical principles of perfusion imaging. Application to magnetic resonance imaging. Invest Radiol 1992;27(Suppl 2):S6–11.

64. Law M, Yang S, Babb JS, et al. Comparison of cerebral blood volume and vascular permeability from dynamic susceptibility contrast-enhanced perfusion MR imaging with glioma grade. AJNR Am J Neuroradiol 2004;25(5):746–55.

65. Covarrubias DJ, Rosen BR, Lev MH. Dynamic magnetic resonance perfusion imaging of brain tumors. Oncologist 2004;9(5):528–37.

66. Cho YD, Choi GH, Lee SP, et al. (1)H-MRS metabolic patterns for distinguishing between meningiomas and other brain tumors. Magn Reson Imaging 2003;21(6):663–72.

67. Barajas RF Jr, Hodgson JG, Chang JS, et al. Glioblastoma multiforme regional genetic and cellular expression patterns: influence on anatomic and physiologic MR imaging. Radiology 2010;254(2): 564–76.

68. Diehn M, Nardini C, Wang DS, et al. Identification of noninvasive imaging surrogates for brain tumor gene-expression modules. Proc Natl Acad Sci U S A 2008;105(13):5213–8.

69. Pope WB, Chen JH, Dong J, et al. Relationship between gene expression and enhancement in glioblastoma multiforme: exploratory DNA microarray analysis. Radiology 2008;249(1):268–77.

70. Naeini KM, Pope WB, Cloughesy TF, et al. Identifying the mesenchymal molecular subtype of glioblastoma using quantitative volumetric analysis of anatomic magnetic resonance images. Neuro Oncol 2013;15(5):626–34.

71. Jain R, Poisson L, Narang J, et al. Genomic mapping and survival prediction in glioblastoma: molecular subclassification strengthened by hemodynamic imaging biomarkers. Radiology 2013;267(1):212–20.

72. Maia AC Jr, Malheiros SM, da Rocha AJ, et al. MR cerebral blood volume maps correlated with

vascular endothelial growth factor expression and tumor grade in nonenhancing gliomas. AJNR Am J Neuroradiol 2005;26(4):777–83.

73. Zinn PO, Sathyan P, Mahajan B, et al. A novel volume-age-KPS (VAK) glioblastoma classification identifies a prognostic cognate microRNA-gene signature. PLoS One 2012;7(8):e41522.

74. Van Meter T, Dumur C, Hafez N, et al. Microarray analysis of MRI-defined tissue samples in glioblastoma reveals differences in regional expression of therapeutic targets. Diagn Mol Pathol 2006;15(4): 195–205.

75. The Cancer Imaging Archive. VASARI Research Project. 2013. Available at: https://wiki.cancerima gingarchive.net/display/Public/VASARI+Research+ Project. Accessed March 1, 2014.

76. Gutman DA, Cooper LA, Hwang SN, et al. MR imaging predictors of molecular profile and survival: multi-institutional study of the TCGA glioblastoma data set. Radiology 2013;267(2):560–9.

77. Zinn PO, Mahajan B, Sathyan P, et al. Radiogenomic mapping of edema/cellular invasion MRI-phenotypes in glioblastoma multiforme. PLoS One 2011; 6(10):e25451.

78. Mazurowski MA, Desjardins A, Malof JM. Imaging descriptors improve the predictive power of survival models for glioblastoma patients. Neuro Oncol 2013;15(10):1389–94.

79. Bookheimer SY, Strojwas MH, Cohen MS, et al. Patterns of brain activation in people at risk for Alzheimer's disease. N Engl J Med 2000;343(7):450–6.

80. Bigos KL, Weinberger DR. Imaging genetics: days of future past. Neuroimage 2010;53(3):804–9.

81. Mut M, Turba UC, Botella AC, et al. Neuroimaging characteristics in subgroup of GBMs with p53 over-expression. J Neuroimaging 2007;17(2):168–74.

82. Carrillo JA, Lai A, Nghiemphu PL, et al. Relationship between tumor enhancement, edema, IDH1 mutational status, MGMT promoter methylation, and survival in glioblastoma. AJNR Am J Neuroradiol 2012;33(7):1349–55.

83. Drabycz S, Roldan G, de Robles P, et al. An analysis of image texture, tumor location, and MGMT promoter methylation in glioblastoma using magnetic resonance imaging. Neuroimage 2010;49(2):1398–405.

84. Ellingson BM, Lai A, Harris RJ, et al. Probabilistic radiographic atlas of glioblastoma phenotypes. AJNR Am J Neuroradiol 2013;34(3):533–40.

85. Ellingson BM, Cloughesy TF, Pope WB, et al. Anatomic localization of O6-methylguanine DNA methyltransferase (MGMT) promoter methylated

and unmethylated tumors: a radiographic study in 358 de novo human glioblastomas. Neuroimage 2012;59(2):908–16.

86. Eoli M, Menghi F, Bruzzone MG, et al. Methylation of O6-methylguanine DNA methyltransferase and loss of heterozygosity on 19q and/or 17p are overlapping features of secondary glioblastomas with prolonged survival. Clin Cancer Res 2007;13(9): 2606–13.

87. Mikheeva SA, Mikheev AM, Petit A, et al. TWIST1 promotes invasion through mesenchymal change in human glioblastoma. Mol Cancer 2010;9:194.

88. Hirai T, Murakami R, Nakamura H, et al. Prognostic value of perfusion MR imaging of high-grade astrocytomas: long-term follow-up study. AJNR Am J Neuroradiol 2008;29(8):1505–10.

89. Colen R, TCGA Phenotype Group, Zinn P. Perfusion imaging genomic mapping uncovers potential genomic targets involved in angiogenesis and invasion. Poster presented at: Society for Neuro-Oncology. San Francisco, November 21–24, 2013.

90. Pope WB, Prins RM, Albert Thomas M, et al. Noninvasive detection of 2-hydroxyglutarate and other metabolites in IDH1 mutant glioma patients using magnetic resonance spectroscopy. J Neurooncol 2012;107(1):197–205.

91. Choi C, Ganji SK, DeBerardinis RJ, et al. 2-hydroxy-glutarate detection by magnetic resonance spectroscopy in IDH-mutated patients with gliomas. Nat Med 2012;18(4):624–9.

92. Andronesi OC, Kim GS, Gerstner E, et al. Detection of 2-hydroxyglutarate in IDH-mutated glioma patients by in vivo spectral-editing and 2D correlation magnetic resonance spectroscopy. Sci Transl Med 2012;4(116):116ra114.

93. Moon WJ, Choi JW, Roh HG, et al. Imaging parameters of high grade gliomas in relation to the MGMT promoter methylation status: the CT, diffusion tensor imaging, and perfusion MR imaging. Neuroradiology 2012;54(6):555–63.

94. Pope WB, Mirsadraei L, Lai A, et al. Differential gene expression in glioblastoma defined by ADC histogram analysis: relationship to extracellular matrix molecules and survival. AJNR Am J Neuroradiol 2012;33(6):1059–64.

95. Thomas G, Wang J, Mahmood Z, et al. Diffusion imaging genomic mapping identifies genomic targets involved in invasion and poor prognosis. Poster presented at: American Society of Neuroradiology. Montreal, Canada, May 17–22, 2014.

Index

Note: Page numbers of article titles are in **boldface** type.

A

Alpers disease, 37
Alzheimer's disease, 17–22
    early onset, molecular imaging and, 18–20
    late-onset, apolipoprotein E e3/e4-associated
        genetic risk for, molecular imaging and, 20–21
        family history of, molecular imaging and, 21–22
        molecular imaging and, 20–22
Aneurysmal vasculopathy, 69
Aneurysm(s), 69–73
    giant partially thrombosed, 69, 71
    giant patent unruptured, 69, 70
    intracranial, 70–73
        rupture of, 73
    partially thrombosed, 69, 70
    saccular, 70–71
Apolipoprotein E, in multiple sclerosis, 88–89, 90
Arteriovenous malformations, in hemorrhagic
    hereditary telangiectasia, 73–74
Astrocytoma, 97–98
    anaplastic, 128, 129
        treatment of, pseudoresponse to, 136, 137–138

B

Brain imaging, and genetic risk, in pediatric
    population, **31–51, 53–67**
Brain neoplasms, treating of, neuroimaging and
    genetic influence in, **121–140**
Brain tumors, genetic evaluation of, 122–128
    imaging of, future directions in, 116
        genomics of, **105–119**
        radiogenomics of, 122–128

C

Cancer genome atlas, and genetic biomarker
    identification, 141–142
    history of, and visually accessible rembrandt
        images feature set, 108, 109
Capillary malformation-arteriovenous malformation,
    73–74
Central nervous system, congenital malformations of,
    31–32, 53–54
Cerebral autosomal dominant arteriopathy, with
    subcortical infarcts and leukoencephalopathy, 91
Cerebral cavernous malformation, 77–79
Cerebrovascular malformations, influence of genetic
    markers on, **69–82**

Children, brain imaging and genetic risk in, congenital
    malformations of central nervous system, **53–67**
        inherited metabolic diseases, **31–51**
Cobblestone malformation, 57
Corpus callosum, agenesis of, 54–55
Cortical development, malformations of, 55–59
Cortical dysgenesis, with abnormal cell proliferation
    but without neoplasia, 57
Cytogenetics, classic, 7, 8

D

Dandy-Walker malformation, 59
Devic disease, 91–92
DNA, chromosomal aberrations of, 5–6
    genome instability and loss of heterozygosity in,
        6–7
    methylation of, 3
    point mutations, insertions, deletions, and
        duplications in, 6
    role of cromatin structure in, 3
    sequence variation, 4–5
    single nucleotide polymorphism of, 4–5
    telomere maintenance mechanism of, 7
    to protein, 2–4
    transcription and translation, intracellular
        mechanism of, 4, 5
DNA methylation, epigenetics in, 6
DNA replication, molecular abnormalities in, 4–7
DNA sequencing, 9–10, 11
DNA transcription, control of gene expression in, 2–3
Duane syndrome, 62

E

Encephalomyopathy, mitochondrial, lactic acidosis
    and strokelike episodes in, 36–37
Encephalopathy, mitochondral neurogastrointestinal,
    40
Energy metabolism, disorders involving, MR
    phenotype-genotype correlation in, 33–40
    MR phenotype-genotype in disorders not related
        to, 38–39, 40–49
Epidermal growth factor receptor, 126
    in glioblastoma, 143–144
Epilepsy, myoclonus, with ragged red fibers, 40

F

Fragile X syndrome, 13

Neuroimag Clin N Am 25 (2015) 155–157
http://dx.doi.org/10.1016/S1052-5149(14)00117-8
1052-5149/15/$ – see front matter © 2015 Elsevier Inc. All rights reserved.

G

Gene expression, assessment of, using microarray
 analysis, 105, 106
 genomic information as measure of, 105
Genes, discovery of, 1
Genetic abnormalities, technologies to identify, 7–12
  array comparative genomic hybridization,
   11–12, 13
  classic cytogenetics, 7, 8
  fluorescence in situ hybridization, 8
  microarray tools, 11, 12
  polymerase chain reaction, 8–9
  sequencing, 9–10, 11
Genetic code, 7
Genetic markers, and their influence on
 cerebrovascular malformations, **69–82**
Genetics, in neuroimaging, understanding of, **1–16**
 molecular imaging in, **17–29**
Genetics/genome project, history of, 1–2
Genomic data, interpretation of, caveats in, 107, 108
Genomic hybridization, array comparative, 11–12, 13
Genotype-phenotype correlation, 32–33
Glioblastoma multiforme, 97, 98, 121–122
  current standard of care for, 141
  hyperperfusion in, 129, 130
  molecular characterization of, clinical applications
   and technological trends, 100–102
   genetic alterations, 98–99
   transcriptomes, 99–100
  molecular subtype classification of, 128
  periventricular, 131, 132
  pseudoprogression of, 134–137
  survival in, 141
  treatment of, personalized approach to,
   141–142
   pseudoresponse to, 137
  unmethylated primary, 130–131
  with IDH1 mutation, 131, 132
Glioblastoma(s), advanced MR imaging genomics of,
 149, 150
  association of imaging, clinical, molecular, and
   histopathologic features in, 112
  axial images of, 113, 114
  genetic biomarkers in, 142–144
  histopathologic imaging of, 144
  imaging genomics of, **141–153**
   new dimension in, 145–146
  imaging of, 144–145
  knowledge for referring physician, 102
  molecular classification of, 109–110, 142
  molecular genetics of, **97–103**
  molecular heterogeneity of, 110
  MR imaging of, 144–145, 146
  prognostic features of, 133
  qualitative MR imaging genomics of, 147–148
  quantitative MR imaging genomics of, 148–149

relationship between gene expression and
 treatment response, 128, 129
 rembrandt images in, visually accessible, 146–147
 sequencing of, 122
 treatment of, chemotherapy in, 133
  current, 133
  personalized, 133–134
  response to, 134–138
  surgical, 133
Glioma(s), 97
 clinical trials of, 101
 high-grade, molecular subclasses of, 127–128
 imaging features of, 128–133
 imaging-genomic analyses for, 110–116
 low-grade, 129–130
 pseudoprogression of, 135, 136
Glutamate, in multiple sclerosis, 89
Glycoprotein-39, denominated human cartilage
 (YKL-40), 127

H

Hemorrhagic hereditary telangiectasia, 73–74
Hindbrain, axon guidance disorders of, 60–63
Holoprosencephaly, 54
Hybridization, fluorescence in situ, 8, 9
Hydrocephalus, X-linked, 54–55

I

IDH enzyme, in glioblastoma, 143
Imaging-genomics, 105, 106
 advantages of, 107
Inborn errors of metabolism, intoxication symptoms
 in, 38–39, 40
 neuroimaging in, 33
 related to large molecule abnormalities, 40–49
Isocitrate dehydrogenase 1, 123–126
 mutations in, mechanism of, 124, 125

J

Joubert syndrome, 59–60, 61

K

Kallmann syndrome, 62–63
Kearns-Sayre syndrome, progressive external
 ophthalmoplegia and, 37–40

L

Leber hereditary optic neuropathy, 36, 92
Leigh syndrome, 36
Leucine-rich repeat kinase 2, 22–25
Leukodystrophies, with genetic inheritance,
 46–48, 49
Lymphatic malformations, 79–80
Lymphedema, 79

M

Magnetic resonance imaging, advanced, genomics
  of glioblastoma, 149, 150
    in multiple sclerosis, 90, 91
  of brain, multiple sclerosis susceptibility genes
    and, 85–88
  of glioblastoma, 144–145, 146
    qualitative, genomics of glioblastoma, 147–148
    quantitative, genomics of glioblastoma, 148–149
Maple syrup urine disease, 40, 41
Megalencephalic leukoencephalopathy with
  subcortical cysts, 49
Megaloencephaly, 56–57
Metabolic diseases, inherited, 31, 32
    neuroimaging in, 33
O6-Methylguanine-DNA methyltransferase, 122, 123
Microarray technology, 105, 122
  limitations of, 105–107
Microarray tools, of DNA chips, 11, 12
Microcephaly, 55–56
Midbrain, and hindbrain, malformations of, 59–63
Mitochondrial diseases, neuroimaging in, 33–34, 35
Mitochondrial respiratory chain defect disorders, 34, 35
Mitochondriopathy, 33–34, 35
Moebius syndrome, 62
Molecular imaging, in genetics, **17–29**
mRNA processing (splicing), 3
Multiple sclerosis, advanced MR imaging in, 90, 91
  apolipoprotein E in, 88–89, 90
  brain-derived neurotrophic factor in, 88, 89
  future perspectives in, 92–93
  genetics of, 84
  glutamate in, 89
  imaging of, 84–85, 86
  imaging phenotypes in, **83–96**
  neurodegeneration in, genetic associations with,
    88–89, 90
  primary progressive, 83
  relapsing-remitting, 83
  secondary progressive, 83
  spinal cord lesions in, genetics of, 89–90
  susceptibility genes, and brain MR imaging, 85–88
Multiple sclerosis-related diseases, and mimics,
  genetics of, 90
Myoclonus epilepsy, with ragged red fibers, 40

N

Neuroependymal abnormalities, malformations
  with, 57
Neurogenetics, 32–33
Neuroimaging, genetics in, understanding of, **1–16**
Neurologic disorders, genetics and epigenetics of,
  12–14
  genome abnormalities associated with, 13, 14
Neurotrophic factor, brain-derived, in multiple
  sclerosis, 88, 89

O

Oligodendroglioma, 97–98
  with 1p19q-deleted lesions, 127, 144
Ophthalmoplegia, progressive external, and
  Kearns-Sayre syndrome, 37–40
Osler-Rendu-Weber syndrome, 73–74

P

Parkinson disease, 22–27
  asymptomatic patients, radiotracers and changes
    in, 26–27
  dominantly inherited mutations in, 22–25
  genetic forms of, 24
  monogenic forms of, 22–25
    dopaminergic neurotransmission in, molecular
      imaging of, 25–27
  symptomatic patients, radiotracers and changes
    in, 25–26
Periventricular heterotopia, 57
Pial limiting membrane, abnormal terminal migration
  and defects in, malformations caused by, 57
Polymerase chain reaction, 8–9
Polymerase DNA directed y, 35–36
Polymicrogyria, 57–59
Protein, from DNA to, 2–4
Protein synthesis, 4
  translation and post-transcriptional mechanisms
    of control, 4

R

Radiogenomics, of brain tumors, 122–128
Rhombencephalosynapsis, 59, 60
RNA, noncoding, 3–4
RNA/microRNA, interfering, in protein synthesis, 4
RNA subtypes, noncoding RNA, 3–4

S

Single nucleotide polymorphism, 4–5
Spinal cord lesions, genetics of, in multiple sclerosis,
  89–90
Sturge-Weber syndrome, 75–77

T

Transmantle migration, generalized abnormal,
  malformations caused by, 57
Tuberous sclerosis, and vascular anomalies, 71, 72

V

Vascular endothelial growth factor, in glioblastoma,
  143
Venous malformations, 79
Ventral induction, malformations of, 54–55

Moving?

Make sure your subscription moves with you!

To notify us of your new address, find your **Clinics Account Number** (located on your mailing label above your name), and contact customer service at:

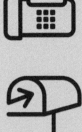

Email: journalscustomerservice-usa@elsevier.com

800-654-2452 (subscribers in the U.S. & Canada)
314-447-8871 (subscribers outside of the U.S. & Canada)

Fax number: 314-447-8029

Elsevier Health Sciences Division
Subscription Customer Service
3251 Riverport Lane
Maryland Heights, MO 63043

*To ensure uninterrupted delivery of your subscription,
please notify us at least 4 weeks in advance of move.

Printed and bound by CPI Group (UK) Ltd, Croydon, CR0 4YY

03/10/2024

01040379-0014